ENDOCRINE DISRUPTORS

Effects on Male and Female Reproductive Systems

ENDOCRINE DISRUPTORS

Effects on Male and Female Reproductive Systems

edited by

Rajesh K. Naz

CRC Press

Boca Raton   London   New York   Washington, D.C.

Acquiring Editor:	Barbara Norwitz
Project Editor:	Maggie Mogck
Marketing Manager:	Becky McEldowney
Cover design:	Jonathan Pennell

Library of Congress Cataloging-in-Publication Data

Endocrine disruptors : effects on male and female reproductive systems / edited by Rajesh K. Naz.

    p. cm.
    Includes bibliographical references and index.
    ISBN 0-8493-3164-1 (alk. paper)
    1. Reproductive toxicology.   2. Endocrine toxicology.   I. Naz, Rajesh K.
    [DNLM: 1. Infertility--chemically induced.   2. Estrogens--metabolism.
  3. Environmental pollutants--adverse effects.   WP570E556   1999]
    RA1224.2.E63   1999
    616.6'92—dc21
    DNLM/DLC
    for Library of Congress

          98-36723
          CIP

Preface

Recently there has been an alarming concern among the scientific community, policy makers, and general public regarding the reproductive and health hazards of the endocrine disrupting environmental chemicals. "Each man in this room is half the man his grandfather was." These were the words recently quoted during a Congressional hearing reporting the startling and controversial finding that a serious decline in the quality and quantity of human spermatozoa has occurred over the past 50 years. Another report from Scotland revealed that men born after 1970 had a sperm count 25% lower than those born before 1959 — an average annual decline of 2.1%. Similar concerns have been reported for women with an increased incidence of infertility and early menopause. These data have led scientists and environmentalists to believe that the human species is approaching a fertility crisis, while others think that the available data are insufficient to deduce worldwide conclusions. Nevertheless, the topic of gonadotoxicity remains a real challenge and concern to almost everyone, both men and women.

Gonadotoxicity has recently been the subject of a number of reviews, with a myriad environmental agents now being classified as reproductive toxicants. Reduced fertility, embryo/fetal loss, birth defects, and other postnatal structural and functional abnormalities are the potential outcomes of exposures to such toxicants. However, the database for establishing safe exposure levels and risk assessment for such outcomes remains limited.

The declining fertility and teratogenic effects are not the only indicators that the human population is at risk. A marked increase in the incidence of cancers associated with the reproductive systems in men (prostate/testicular) and women (breast/ovarian) is also an associated/causative factor of these exposures. The tissues/organs associated with the reproductive systems are the most sensitive to these toxicants' exposure, making breast cancer one of the most prevalent and leading causes of death in women, and prostate cancer as the leading cause of death in men. These deleterious effects have been attributed to environmental toxicants, many of which act as "estrogens". The "estrogen hypothesis" has inspired a number of debates and investigations. The list of potential estrogenic chemicals continues to grow, although it is not known what exact levels and combinations may be hazardous to the reproductive functions, including the development of carcinogenic potentials. Besides, several synthetic chemicals termed *endocrine disruptors/impostors* exert a variety of toxic effects on the gonads, sexual, and reproductive function and behavior, in addition to carcinogenic effects. Thus far, over 50 such hormone impostors referred to as persistent organic pollutants (OPOs) have been identified, the most common of which are organochlorines (DDT, PCBs) and dioxins.

The study of gonadotoxicity and carcinogenesis is an escalating concern not only to andrologists, urologists, and reproductive endocrinologists, biologists, gynecologists, and oncologists, but also to environmentalists, as well as the public at large. This book is timely and unique and covers these pertinent and controversial topics from epidemiology to etiology, concluding with future directions. The contributors are leading authorities in their fields, making the book an interesting treatise. At this time, there is no scientifically creditable and comprehensive book available on this topic, making it the first of its kind.

The book is divided into two main sections. The first section deals with the effects of various environmental toxicants including dietary toxicants on the female reproductive system with special emphasis on effects and mechanism(s) of their action on the sex differentiation during development, fertility, and breast cancer. This section is comprised of seven chapters written by eminent scientists who are experts in the field of female endocrinology and carcinogenesis. The first chapter elegantly discusses the effects and mechanism(s) of action of endocrine disruptors on the hypothalamus-pituitary-gonadal axis and provides an overview of how the disruption of this axis can lead to various reproductive dysfunction and health abnormalities (P. Thomas). The second chapter describes how the diethylstilbestrol (DES) and environmental estrogens influence the developing female reproductive system (R. Newbold). Endocrine disruption can be caused directly via interference of the hypothalamus-pituitary-gonadal axis and/or indirectly through extensive oocyte destruction resulting in premature ovarian failure (POF). The third chapter focuses on the toxicants that destroy ovarian follicles resulting in POF, an early menopause. POF can cause an increased risk of osteoporosis, cardiovascular disease, and ovarian cancer (P.B. Hower). The fourth chapter describes the estrogenic compounds called phytoestrogens that are present in plants and thus, can disrupt the endocrine milieu through dietary sources (H.B. Patisaul and P.L. Whitten). Discussed in the fifth chapter are the effects and mechanisms of estrogens and xenoestrogens on the development of breast cancer (A.M. Soto and C. Sonnenschein). The sixth chapter suggests that the potential molecular mechanism(s) for the toxicity of environmental estrogens involves differential regulation of gene expression through various cis- and transacting elements (S.M. Hyder, J.L. Kirkland, D.S. Loose-Mitchell, S. Makela, and G.M. Stancel). The last chapter in this section focuses on the effects and mechanism of action of 2,3,7,8-tetrachlorodibenzo-p-dioxin (TCDD) and related environmental antiestrogens on tumorigenesis and breast cancer (S.M. Safe).

The second section of this book deals with the effects of endocrine disruption by various environmental toxicants on the male reproductive system, focusing on male fertility and development of benign prostate hyperplasia (BPH) and prostate cancer. It includes five chapters. The first chapter describes the effects of endocrine disruptors on male fertility and discusses recent controversial issues regarding the global decline in fertility of men (S.C. Sikka and R.K. Naz). The second chapter elegantly describes the effects and mechanism(s) of action of antiandrogens on sex differentiation and testicular function including androgen biosynthesis. The third chapter in this section deals with the effects of endocrine disruptors (antiestrogens as well as anitandrogens) on erectile dysfunction in men (S.C. Sikka and R.K Naz). The fourth chapter describes the role of natural and manmade estrogens in prostate development (F.S. vom Saal and B.G. Timms). The last chapter in this section focuses on the effects of environmental metal ion contaminates on the development of BPH and prostate cancer (S.-M. Ho).

In conclusion, this book is a unique and comprehensive treatise, offering up-to-date information on a topic that is currently becoming a major concern among the scientific community and general public. The authors of this book are expert investigators who are pioneers in their fields and have presented the data in a dynamic manner that undoubtedly establishes this book as a model source of authentic, vital, and viable scientific information.

Editor

Rajesh K. Naz, Ph.D., is Professor of Obstetrics and Gynecology, and Physiology, as well as Director of the Division of Research at the Medical College of Ohio in Toledo.

Dr. Naz received his B.S. and M.S. degrees in biochemistry in 1973 and 1975, respectively. He received his Ph.D. in immunology in 1980 from the prestigious All India Institute of Medical Sciences in New Delhi, under the guidance of the renowned reproductive endocrinologist G. P. Talwar. In 1984, following postdoctoral work in reproductive immunology at the University of Michigan Medical School in Ann Arbor and then at the Oregon Regional Primate Research Center at Beaverton, he was appointed Assistant Professor and Director of the *In Vitro* Fertilization and Andrology Laboratories at George Washington University in Washington, D.C. He joined the Albert Einstein College of Medicine in 1987 and was promoted to Associate Professor and Director of Research in 1989. He moved to the Medical College of Ohio in 1996.

Dr. Naz is a member of the Society of Gynecologic Investigation, American Society of Biochemistry and Molecular Biology, American Society for the Immunology of Reproduction, International Society for the Immunology of Reproduction, American Fertility Society, American Society of Andrology, Society for the Study of Reproduction, American Association for the Advancement of Science, and the New York Academy of Sciences.

Dr. Naz has lectured on reproductive immunology at numerous national and international symposia and at various conferences. He has received many prestigious awards and honors, and is a scientific reviewer for various grant proposals and research manuscripts for journals. He also is the member of the editorial boards of seven journals including *Biology of Reproduction, Archives of Andrology*, and is the associate editor of *Frontiers in BioScience*.

He has served in several study sections of the National Institutes of Health, including chairman of the Special Emphasis Panel SBIR Study Section. He is a regular member of NIH's Reproductive Endocrinology Study Section.

Dr. Naz has published over 125 articles in scientific journals, as well as authoring and editing three books: *Immunology of Reproduction, Male Reproductive Medicine: From Spermatogenesis to Sperm Function and Modulation of Fertility*, and *Prostate: Basic and Clinical Aspects*. His current interests include the molecular mechanisms underlying endocrinologic control of fertility and infertility, and benign prostate hyperplasia (BPH) and prostate cancer in humans. He is especially interested in how the endocrine disrupters and environmental toxins can modify the male and female reproductive systems.

Contributors

L. Earl Gray, Jr.   U.S. Environmental Protection Agency, Research Triangle Park, North Carolina

Shuk-Mei Ho   Tufts University, Medford, Massachusetts

Patricia B. Hoyer   University of Arizona, Tuscon, Arizona

Salman M. Hyder   University of Texas Medical School, Houston, Texas

William R. Kelce   Monsanto Company, St. Louis, Missouri

John L Kirkland   Baylor College of Medicine, Houston, Texas

David S. Loose-Mitchell   University of Texas Medical School, Houston, Texas

Sari Mäkelä   Univseristy of Turku, Institute of Biomedicine, Kiinamyllynkatu, Finland

Rajesh K. Naz   Medical College of Ohio, Toledo, Ohio

Retha R. Newbold   National Institute of Environmental Health Sciences, Research Triangle Park, North Carolina

Heather B. Patisaul   Emory University, Atlanta, Georgia

Stephen A. Safe   Texas A&M University, College Station, Texas

Suresh C. Sikka   Tulane University School of Medicine, New Orleans, Louisiana

Carlos Sonnenschein   Tufts University School of Medicine, Boston, Massachusetts

Ana M. Soto   Tufts University School of Medicine, Boston, Massachusetts

George M. Stancel   University of Texas Medical School, Houston, Texas

Peter Thomas   Marine Science Institute, Port Aransas, Texas

Barry B. Timms   University of South Dakota, Vermillion, South Dakota

Frederick S. vom Saal   University of Missouri-Columbia, Columbia, Missouri

Patricia L. Whitten   Emory University, Atlanta, Georgia

Acknowledgments

The considerable support and encouragement from friends and colleagues who have contributed to this book is gratefully acknowledged. I am thankful to Linda Wagner for providing excellent secretarial help. Special thanks to Abhi and Manu Naz for love and understanding. I am grateful to Puchy for providing exciting and delightful impetus to compile this book.

I am also deeply indebted to the support from my department and medical school, and from the National Institutes of Health (HD24425) for making publication of this volume possible.

Contents

Dedication

This book is dedicated to our search for realization

of Absolute Truth and Knowledge

Section I

Effect on the Female Reproductive System

1

Nontraditional Sites of Endocrine Disruption by Chemicals on the Hypothalamus–Pituitary–Gonadal Axis: Interactions with Steroid Membrane Receptors, Monoaminergic Pathways, and Signal Transduction Systems

Peter Thomas

CONTENTS

0-8493-3164-1/99/$0.00+$.50
© 1999 by CRC Press LLC

1.1   Introduction

Recently, there has been a heightened awareness and concern among the scientific community, policy makers, and the general public over the reproductive hazards of endocrine-disrupting environmental chemicals, particularly xenobiotic estrogens, to fish, wildlife, and humans.[1,2] Feminization of male birds, alligators, and fish and the production of the estrogen-induced yolk precursor, vitellogenin, in male freshwater fish have been reported after environmental exposure to xenobiotic estrogens, such as o,p'-DDT and kepone, and to pulp kraft mill effluent and sewage containing nonylphenols.[1,3-5] In humans estrogenic effects of kepone were detected in male workers at a pesticide manufacturing plant.[1] Xenobiotic estrogens also have been implicated in the recent increase in breast cancer, one of the leading causes of death in women,[6] and in the purported decrease in average sperm counts in semen samples collected from men over the past 50 years.[7]

Extensive research over the past decade has identified a rapidly growing list of environmental contaminants that disrupt reproductive processes in vertebrates primarily by exerting estrogenic or antiestrogenic actions.[1,8,9] Most of these estrogenic xenobiotics, such as dichlorodiphenyl-trichloroethane (DDT) and its isomers, PCBs and their hydroxylated metabolites, kepone, methoxychlor metabolites, nonylphenol, and bisphenyl A, are considered to exert their estrogenic effects primarily by binding to nuclear estrogen receptors.[8,10-14] However the genomic actions of estrogens also can be influenced by other signaling mechanisms (receptor cross-talk) such as growth factors.[15,16] Dioxin (2,3,7,8-tetrachlorodibenzo-p-dioxin, TCDD) and related dibenzo-p-dioxins, dibenzofurans, and PCBs are thought to induce antiestrogenic effects indirectly by binding to the aryl hydrocarbon (Ah) receptor[17] and subsequently interfering with estrogen receptor binding to DNA response elements.[18] In addition, a variety of xenobiotic compounds are capable of binding to nuclear androgen and progesterone receptors.[19,13] For example, vinclozolin metabolites and the DDT analog, p,p'-DDE, are effective competitors of androgen binding to the androgen receptor and have antiandrogenic actions in mammals.[20,13]

Although interference with the genomic actions of steroid hormones is considered to be the principal mechanism of endocrine disruption by many xenobiotics, chemicals could potentially act via different mechanisms at other sites on the hypothalamus–pituitary–gonadal axis to disrupt reproductive function.[21,22] Monoaminergic and amino acid neurotransmitter pathways in the hypothalamus modulate the synthesis and secretion of gonadotropin-releasing hormone (GnRH), which in turn regulates the secretion of gonadotropins from the pituitary. Therefore, neuropharmacological and neurotoxic chemicals that alter hypothalamic neurotransmitter function[23-25,14] could influence GnRH secretion[26] and secondarily alter gonadotropin secretion, resulting in disruption of the reproductive cycle. Alternatively, chemicals could exert direct effects on GnRH neuronal activity.[27] In addition, direct actions of heavy metals have been demonstrated at the pituitary to alter gonadotropin secretion[28,29] and at the gonadal level to disrupt steroidogenesis.[30,14] Xenobiotics also potentially could interfere with nongenomic actions of steroids mediated by binding to steroid membrane receptors on oocytes and sperm plasma membranes[31,32] or could interfere with binding of catecholstrogens to catecholamine receptors in the brain.[33]

In this chapter, some nontraditional sites and mechanisms of chemical interference with hypothalamus–pituitary–gonadal function, identified in a well-characterized vertebrate model of reproductive endocrine toxicology, the Atlantic croaker (*Micropogonias undulatus*), are discussed. The characteristics of maturation-inducing steroid receptors on plasma membranes of oocytes and sperm and their physiological roles in final maturation of gametes are described. Evidence of binding of xenobiotic estrogens to the membrane receptors and disruption of final gamete maturation is presented, and the potential susceptibility of steroid membrane receptors to interference by lipophilic xenobiotic estrogens is discussed. In addition, some mechanisms of endocrine disruption by heavy metals are described. Evidence is presented that lead, which is neurotoxic, can disrupt neuroendocrine function and gonadotropin secretion in croaker by altering hypothalamic monoaminergic function. Finally, *in vitro* studies demonstrating direct stimulatory actions of cadmium at the pituitary and gonadal levels to increase hormone secretion are described. The results suggest cadmium stimulation of gonadotropin secretion and steroidogenesis is probably mediated by alterations in signal transduction pathways and calcium homeostasis.

1.2 Steroid Membrane Receptors

1.2.1 Nongenomic Actions of Steroids

The classic model of hormone action for all known classes of steroids and many xenobiotic estrogens involves diffusion or transport of the steroid or xenobiotic across the plasma membrane, its binding to intracellular receptors in target cells, activation of the receptor, and tight association of the hormone-receptor complex and associated proteins to specific nuclear binding sites, resulting in alteration of gene transcription.[34,8] However, recently many different laboratories using a wide variety of animal and cell models have obtained convincing evidence that some steroid effects are too rapid to be explained by a genomic action and that steroids can also exert nongenomic actions by binding to membranes and membrane-bound receptors.[35-37] For example, estrogen causes rapid prolactin release from pituitary cell lines,[38] rapid release of intracellular calcium in rat granulosa cells,[39] and short-term electrophysiological changes in various brain regions.[40] Progesterone also induces rapid effects, such as calcium influx into human sperm[41,42] and dopamine release from the corpus striatum,[43] whereas glucocorticoids have been shown to cause rapid electrophysiological effects on mammalian neurons,[44] behavioral effects,[45] and lysis of lymphoma cells.[46] Although there is still considerable debate over which of these steroid effects are mediated by specific steroid receptors and which are the results of membrane potential changes due to disruption of the lipid bilayer, steroid membrane receptors have been positively identified in many tissues where rapid nongenomic steroid effects have been observed. Specific plasma membrane receptors for estrogens have been identified in rat pituitary, liver, and uterine tissues,[47,48] for glucocorticoids in liver, brain and lymphoma cells,[49,46,45] and for progesterone in rat brain cell membranes.[50] In addition, a steroid recognition site which is functionally coupled to the $GABA_A$-benzodiazepene receptor has been identified, which suggests both specific membrane locations and functions for these receptors.[51]

1.2.2 Oocyte Maturation in Amphibians and Fish

1.2.2.1 Role of Oocyte Maturation-Inducing Steroid (MIS) Membrane Receptors

The nongenomic actions of progestogen maturational steroids in amphibians and fishes and the roles of receptors on the oocyte plasma membrane as intermediaries in progestogen action have been recognized widely for nearly two decades[52,53] and currently are the most thoroughly characterized models of membrane receptor-mediated steroid action. The discovery that steroids could induce meiotic maturation of amphibian and teleostean oocytes in simple *in vitro* incubation systems stimulated intensive research on the natural maturation-inducing steroids in these vertebrate groups and their mechanisms of action.[52,54] It was shown that the amphibian MIS, progesterone, was ineffective in inducing final oocyte maturation when microinjected in *Xenopus laevis* and *Rana pipiens* oocytes,[55,56] but it was effective when applied externally bound to beads or in a polymer form.[57,58] Identical results were obtained with the teleostean MIS, 17,20β-dihydroxy-4-pregnen-3-one (17,20β-P) in goldfish oocytes.[59] Moreover, inhibitors of transcription did not prevent 17,20β-P-induced final oocyte maturation in teleosts, which supports the concept that the action of the MIS is nongenomic.[54,60] The finding that increases in cyclic AMP levels by pharmacological agents block MIS stimulation of oocyte maturation *in vitro* also suggests that the action of the MIS is nongenomic and instead involves a second messenger signal transduction pathway.[60] A decrease in cyclic AMP is required for MIS induction of final oocyte maturation in rainbow trout, which appears to involve a guanine nucleotide-binding G-protein in the signal transduction pathway across the oocyte plasma membrane to the cytoplasm. A cytoplasmic factor, named maturation-promoting factor, composed of cdc 2 kinase and cyclin B, is formed and is the intracellular mediator of oocyte maturation.[60]

Direct evidence for the presence of a membrane receptor for the MIS and its involvement in final oocyte maturation was first obtained in amphibians, *Xenopus*[53,61,62] and *Rana*,[63] primarily using photoaffinity labeling with the synthetic progestin, R5020. The existence of a high affinity ($K_d = 10^{-9}$M) progesterone receptor in the plasma membrane of *Xenopus* oocytes has since been confirmed using a membrane filtration technique,[64] although it was found that the ligand used in earlier studies, R5020, recognizes a different binding site than the natural MIS.

1.2.2.2 Characteristics of Ovarian MIS Membrane Receptors in Fishes

The first convincing evidence for the existence of a high affinity ($K_d = 10^{-9}$M), low capacity (10^{-13}–10^{-12} mol/g ovary) membrane receptor for the teleost MIS was obtained in spotted seatrout (*Cynoscion nebulosus*) ovaries for 17,20β, 21-trihydroxy-4-pregnen-3-one (20β-S), the natural MIS in this species.[65,66] Subsequently, specific binding of the salmonid MIS, 17,20β-P, and R5020 to ovarian and oocyte membrane preparations has been reported in brook trout and rainbow trout[67,68] and for the perciform MIS, 20β-S in striped bass.[69] The membrane receptor for the MIS in spotted seatrout ovaries shows the greatest steroid specificity, and only structurally similar C21 steroids have similar binding affinities,[65,70] whereas most other MIS membrane receptors investigated to date also show significant binding to androgens and estrogens.[64,67,68]

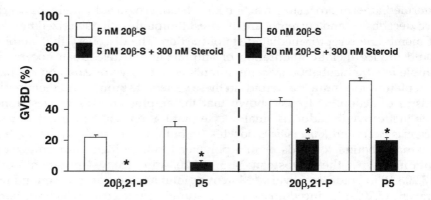

FIGURE 1.1
Effects of coincubating 20β,21-dihydroxy-4-pregnen-3-one (20β,21-P) and pregnenolone (P5) with 20β-S for 1 min on subsequent final maturation of spotted seatrout oocytes *in vitro*. % GVBD — percent oocytes that completed germinal vesicle breakdown. Asterisks denote treatments significantly different from corresponding 20β-S treatment alone (N = 6).

A close correlation has been demonstrated between the receptor-binding affinities of steroids for the MIS membrane receptor in spotted seatrout ovaries and their agonist and antagonist activities in *in vitro* final oocyte maturation (FOM) bioassays. The presence of hydroxyl groups at both the 17 and 20β positions on the progesterone nucleus appears to be essential for agonist activity in the seatrout final oocyte maturation bioassay, whereas hydroxyls at both the 20β and 21 positions are required for high binding affinity for the receptor.[70] The presence of hydroxyls at all three positions (17, 20β, and 21 positions, i.e., 20β-S) results in greatest affinity for the receptor and the most potent induction of oocyte maturation in the bioassay. The action of 20β-S is rapid; 1-min exposure to 20β-S is sufficient to induce FOM, which is consistent with its rapid rate of association with the receptor.

The effects of incubating follicle-enclosed seatrout oocytes with the MIS (20β-S) in the presence of two steroids with high relative binding affinities (rba's) for the receptor but lacking maturation-inducing activity, 20β, 21-dihydroxy-4-pregnen-3-one (20β, 21-P) and pregnenolone, are shown in Figure 1.1. Germinal vesicle breakdown (GVBD, i.e., disappearance of the nucleus) was used as the end point in the final oocyte maturation bioassay.[71] Induction of GVBD by 1-min exposure to 5 nM and 50 nM 20β-S was inhibited by coincubation with 300 nM 20β, 21-P, which has hydroxyls on the 20 and 21 positions of the progesterone nucleus (rba 50%), and 300 nM pregnenolone, which has a hydroxyl on the 3β position (rba 96%). Other steroids that displaced 50% or more of the bound, tritiated 20β-S from its receptor at a concentration of 300 nM also significantly inhibited 20β-S-induced GVBD.[70] Only one other steroid, 17,20β-P, caused significant induction of FOM after 1-min exposure; but its potency was much lower than that of 20β-S, which is consistent with its low rba (<1.0%). These studies demonstrate that the 1-min GVBD *in vitro* bioassay with seatrout oocytes is highly specific for the natural MIS, 20β-S. No other steroids are capable of inducing GVBD at physiological concentrations. The ability of the bioassay to detect antagonism of MIS action by other steroids also indicates its potential for examining the consequences of interference of 20β-S action on the oocyte membrane receptor by xenobiotic chemicals.

1.2.2.3 Xenobiotic Estrogen Binding to the Ovarian MIS Membrane Receptor in Fish

A broad range of xenobiotic organic compounds have been shown to disrupt early development as well as endocrine and reproductive functions in vertebrates by binding to nuclear steroid receptors, particularly estrogen receptors, and mimicking or antagonizing the actions of the endogenous hormones.[9,11,13,14] However, practically no information is currently available on whether these organic compounds can also bind to steroid membrane receptors and disrupt steroid action at the level of the plasma membrane. Xenobiotic interactions with steroid membrane receptors cannot be predicted from their affinities for nuclear receptors because their steroid ligand specificities differ, especially for synthetic antihormones.[36,72] For example, the steroid specificity of the nuclear progestogen receptor in seatrout ovarian tissue, which mediates 20β-S induction of ovulation, differs considerably from that of the seatrout ovarian 20β-S membrane receptor.[70,73,74]

The development of a reliable filter assay for the 20β-S membrane receptor and the availability of large amounts of starting material (seatrout ovaries weigh up to 1 kg) have permitted detailed investigations of the interactions of xenobiotics with steroid membrane receptors to be conducted. The displacement of 5 nM [³H]-20β-S by the organochlorines kepone, methoxychlor, o,p'-DDD, and o,p'-DDE over a broad range of concentrations (1 nM to 1 mM) was investigated in competition assays. The organochlorines were added to the assay buffer dissolved in ethanol (final concentration 1%), which did not affect receptor binding. The ovarian membrane preparations were incubated with the organochlorines and [³H]-20β-S for 30 min at 4°C before separation of bound from free by filtration through glass microfiber filters. All the organochlorines displaced the [³H]-20β-S in a concentration-dependent manner. Displacement curves for o,p'-DDD and kepone are shown in Figure 1.2. Significant displacement of 20β-S was observed with o,p'-DDD at a concentration of 100 μM. Kepone had a lower binding affinity in this assay, although in several other receptor assays binding affinity was tenfold higher. To determine if this decrease in [³H]-20β-S binding is due to disruption of the plasma membrane and loss of binding sites, membrane preparations were incubated with o,p'-DDD, kepone, or buffer alone for 30 min and subsequently washed thoroughly four times to remove any of the compounds prior to conducting the 20β-S receptor assay. It was found that

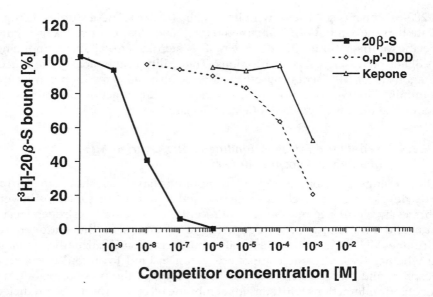

FIGURE 1.2
Competition by the xenoestrogens o,p'-DDD and kepone for [³H]-20β-S binding to the spotted seatrout ovarian MIS membrane receptor. Binding is expressed as a percentage of total binding (binding suppressed by 300 nM 20β-S).

prior exposure to these compounds did not alter the [³H]-20β-S binding capacity of membrane receptor preparations, thereby indicating that they did not destroy binding sites and that the inhibition of receptor binding is reversible.

To determine whether inhibition of binding by kepone was competitive, Scatchard plot analyses of [³H]-20β-S binding were performed in the presence of kepone.[75] Different concentrations of kepone (0.2, 1, and 10 μM) altered the K_D value of [³H]-20β-S binding to the receptor without changing the B_{max}, which suggests that the binding is competitive. However, Scatchard analysis with other organochlorines suggests that xenobiotic binding to the receptor is often noncompetitive. Recent studies indicate that a broad range of xenobiotic organic compounds, including many that are estrogenic, are capable of displacing [³H]-20β-S from the membrane receptor. Estrogenic hydroxylated PCB congeners such as 2',5'-PCB-3-OH cause 50% displacement of 20β-S from the receptor at a concentration of 10 μM, similar to their affinities for the seatrout hepatic nuclear estrogen receptor (unpublished observation). Nonylphenol and the mycotoxin estrogen, zearalenone, diethylstilbestrol, and several other synthetic estrogens and antiestrogens have tenfold higher relative binding affinities for the receptor, causing significant displacement in the high nanomolar concentration range. Estradiol has a similar binding affinity, displacing 13% of [³H]-20β-S at a concentration of 300 nM.[70] We conclude, therefore, that the seatrout progestin membrane receptor is susceptible to interference by a variety of estrogenic xenobiotic compounds.

1.2.2.4   Xenobiotic Estrogen Interference with MIS Induction
of Oocyte Maturation

Bioassays of final oocyte maturation were conducted with xenobiotics that bound to the seatrout receptor to determine whether they displayed agonist activities or antagonized the actions of 20β-S. Ovarian tissue from Atlantic croaker, a closely related species belonging to the same family as seatrout, was used for the *in vitro* bioassays. Approximately 50 follicle-enclosed oocytes were preincubated for 9 h in culture medium in the presence of gonadotropin to induce maturational competence, i.e., the ability of oocytes to undergo final maturation in response to the MIS.[71,76] One critical component of this process induced by the periovulatory surge in gonadotropin secretion is upregulation of the oocyte membrane MIS receptor.[77,78] The culture medium was removed at the end of the preincubation period, replaced with fresh medium containing either 20β-S alone or 20β-S in combination with various concentrations of kepone or o,p'-DDD (dissolved in ethanol, final concentration 0.1%), and the "primed" oocytes were incubated for an additional 12 h to allow them to complete final maturation. Dissolution of the nucleus or germinal vesicle GVBD was scored by visual examination under low power magnification at the end of the incubation.

Nearly all of the oocytes had completed GVBD after incubation in 290 nM 20β-S alone (Figure 1.3A); the lipid globules in the ooplasm had fused and the oocytes were fully hydrated. Final maturation of the majority of the oocytes in response to 20β-S was inhibited by exposure to 100 μM kepone or o,p'-DDD for 12 h (Figure 1.3A). Maturation was abnormal and arrested at early stages in most of the oocytes.[32] The oocytes in the xenobiotic-exposed groups that completed GVBD had an abnormal appearance; incomplete clearing of the ooplasm, hydration, and oil droplet formation were often observed.[32] The inhibition of GVBD by kepone and o,p'-DDD in response to 290 nM 20β-S was concentration-dependent, with significant inhibition occurring at concentrations of 1 and 10 nM (Figure 1.3A). Almost identical concentration-response relationships were observed when seatrout oocytes were incubated with these xenobiotics (results not shown). The two xenobiotics did not act as agonists on GVBD at any of the concentrations tested. A variety of other organochlorines, including methoxychlor, DDT derivatives, and hydroxylated PCBs, also inhibited GVBD of croaker and seatrout oocytes in a concentration-dependent manner (unpublished observation).

The finding that some of the oocytes underwent GVBD even at the highest kepone and o,p'-DDD concentrations tested (100 μM) suggests that the xenobiotics are not merely toxic to the oocytes but instead may antagonize the actions of 20β-S. Association of 20β-S with the membrane receptor is rapid with a $t_{1/2}$ of less than 2 min.[65] Consequently, incubation of maturationally competent croaker oocytes with 20β-S for 1–5 min is sufficient to induce GVBD.[70] Short-term incubations were therefore conducted with the xenobiotics to limit the possible contribution of nonspecific toxic actions to the effects observed. Co-incubation of the oocytes with 20β-S and o,p'-DDD or

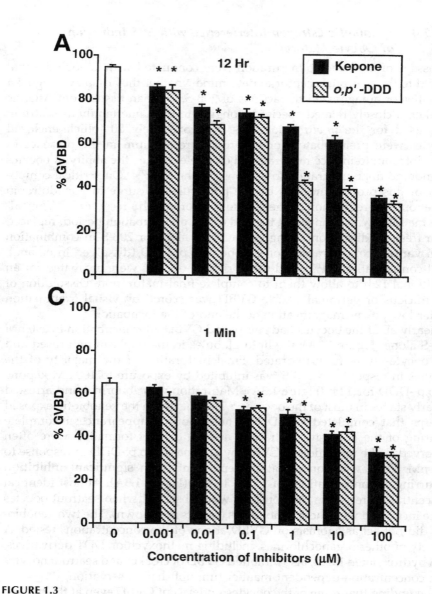

FIGURE 1.3
Concentration-dependent effects of kepone and o,p'-DDD on 20β-S-induced GVBD of primed Atlantic croaker oocytes *in vitro*. (A) 12-h and (C) 1-min exposure to both xenobiotics in the presence of 290 nM 20β-S or 20β-S alone (clear bar). (B) 5-min exposure to kepone, and (D) 5-min exposure to o,p'-DDD in the presence of 290, 29, and 2.9 nM 20β-S. Bars represent means ± S.E.M. of six observations. Asterisks denote means significantly different from controls ($p < 0.05$, Tukey's HSD test). (From Ghosh, S. and Thomas, P., *Mar. Environ. Res.*, 39, 159, 1995. With permission.)

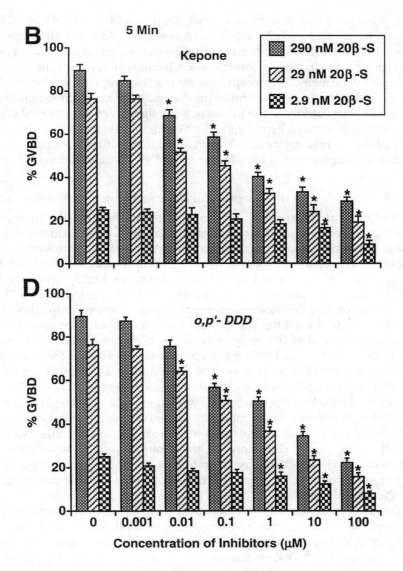

FIGURE 1.3 (continued)

kepone for 1 min followed by 5 min of repeated washing and an additional 12-h incubation in media alone resulted in a concentration-dependent inhibition of GVBD (Figure 1.3C). The functional integrity of the oocytes was not impaired after exposure to the xenobiotics because subsequent exposure to 20β-S completely restored the ability of the oocytes to undergo GVBD.

More pronounced inhibitory effects of kepone and o,p′-DDD on GVBD induced by 29 and 290 nM 20β-S were observed after a 5-min exposure (Figure 1.3B, D). Although the concentration-dependent inhibition of GVBD by the xenobiotics in these bioassays is consistent with an antagonistic action mediated by the membrane receptor, additional experiments will be required to confirm this mechanism of endocrine disruption. Recent refinements have increased the sensitivity of the bioassay, with significant induction of GVBD occurring after a 1 min exposure to 5 nM 20β-S, close to its K_d.[70] Thus it is now possible to investigate xenobiotic antagonism with steroid action at the membrane receptor over a broader range of 20β-S concentrations.

1.2.2.5   Significance of Receptor Location in Plasma Membrane

The finding that the majority of xenobiotics that bind to the membrane progestin receptor in seatrout ovaries display little or no affinity for the nuclear progestin receptor in this species[74] suggests that localization of the receptor in the plasma membrane may be important for xenobiotic binding activity. Many of the xenobiotic estrogens tested are highly lipophilic and readily interact with biological membranes, which are rich in lipids.[79,80] Techniques to solubilize the membrane receptor and measure competition with 20β-S binding to the solubilized protein were developed to investigate this possibility. Removal of the receptor from the plasma membrane by solubilization did not alter the binding affinities of natural and synthetic steroids, whereas it did result in a complete loss of binding to a variety of xenobiotic estrogenic compounds, such as DDT analogs, and hydroxylated PCBs. In a separate study, the binding of organic compounds lacking estrogenic activity with different degrees of lipophilicity (octanol/water coefficients) to the membrane receptor was investigated in competition assays. The two most lipophilic compounds, dibenzofuran and biphenyl, caused significant displacement of [^{3}H]-20β-S at a concentration of 100 nM, whereas none of the other organic compounds were effective competitors at this concentration (unpublished observation).

In conclusion, these studies demonstrate that the MIS membrane receptor is susceptible to interference by estrogenic xenobiotic compounds and also by highly lipophilic nonestrogenic organic compounds. These xenobiotics act as antagonists, blocking the induction of final oocyte maturation in response to 20β-S. The finding that localization of the receptor in the plasma membrane is a requirement for binding to xenobiotic antagonists but not for binding to steroids suggests that the binding sites for these two classes of ligands differ. However, information on the primary structure of steroid membrane receptors will be required to model likely binding sites for natural and xenobiotic ligands. Finally, these results suggest that steroid membrane receptors are potentially susceptible to interference by lipophilic organic compounds, particularly estrogenic xenobiotics, and may be additional targets for these xenobiotics.

1.2.3   Sperm Activation in Mammals and Fish

1.2.3.1   *Rapid Actions of Progesterone on Sperm Membranes in Mammals*

Studies over the past decade have demonstrated that progesterone exerts direct and rapid nongenomic actions on human sperm, resulting in hyperactive motility and induction of the acrosome reaction, increased binding to the zona pellucida, and fusion with the oocyte.[81,82] This activation of sperm by progesterone has been shown by several laboratories to be mediated by an influx of calcium.[83-85] Moreover, the increase in intracellular calcium concentrations is rapid, occurring within seconds, and is concentration dependent,[41,86,87] which suggests that progesterone exerts a nongenomic action by binding to a specific cell surface receptor on sperm.[83,85] The increase in calcium in sperm after exposure to progesterone activates phospholipase C,[41] resulting in rapid changes in swimming direction (hyperactivation) and the acrosome reaction. One of the possible functions of hyperactive motility in mammalian sperm is to provide increased thrust necessary for the penetration of the oocyte zona.[88] Although this receptor has not yet been characterized,[85,89] several other lines of evidence also suggest the existence of a specific progesterone membrane receptor on mammalian sperm. Progesterone is still able to increase sperm calcium concentrations and calcium influx when it is bound to bovine serum albumin (BSA) and unable to traverse the plasma membrane, suggesting a cell surface site of action.[42,90] Histological studies using fluorescein-isothiocynate labeling of the progesterone BSA complex have confirmed that the binding sites are on the plasma membrane of the sperm head.[91,92] Studies on the structure-activity relationships for calcium influx and the acrosome reaction have suggested that the steroid specificity of the putative progesterone membrane receptor differs considerably from that of the classical nuclear progesterone receptor.[83,93,94] However, the steroid binding of this putative receptor has not been fully characterized.

1.2.3.2   *Characteristics of Sperm MIS Membrane Receptor in Fish*

Recently MIS receptors were identified and fully characterized on plasma membranes of spotted seatrout and Atlantic croaker sperm[95,96] using a modification of the protocol developed for assaying the ovarian membrane MIS receptor in these species.[65,70] Saturation analysis showed the presence of saturable 20β-S binding in the membrane fractions of seatrout and croaker sperm and testes; complete saturation was achieved with approximately 20 nM 20β-S[95,96] (Table 1.1). Scatchard analyses indicated the presence of a single class of high affinity (K_d = 18–22 nM), low capacity (B_{max} = 0.09 to 0.003 nM ml^{-1}milt) binding sites in the membrane preparations (Figure 1.4). The [^{3}H]-20β-S binding was readily displaced with excess cold 20β-S. The rates of association and dissociation were extremely rapid; each had a $t_{1/2}$ of less

TABLE 1.1

Characteristics of Atlantic Croaker 20β-S Sperm Membrane Receptor

Receptor Criteria	Binding Characteristics
1. High affinity, single receptor site	K_d = 25.5 nM, single class binding sites (by Scatchard analysis)
2. Low capacity, saturable binding	B_{max} = 0.085 nM ml^{-1} milt; saturated with 20 nM [^{3}H]-20β-S
3. Displaceable binding	Association $T_{1/2}$ = 2 min
	Dissociation $T_{1/2}$ = 2.5 min
4. High steroid specificity	RBA[a]: 17,20β-P, Prog., S-<0.11; T-<0.11; T-<0.01; E$_2$, F no binding
5. Tissue specificity[b]	Sperm, testis, ovary, liver, not in gill
6. Biological validation	1.5-2.5× increase receptor conc. after incubation with GtH

[a] RBA — relative binding affinity, calculated from concentration of 20β-S causing 50% displacement.
[b] Data also from Patiño and Thomas (1990) in spotted seatrout tissue.

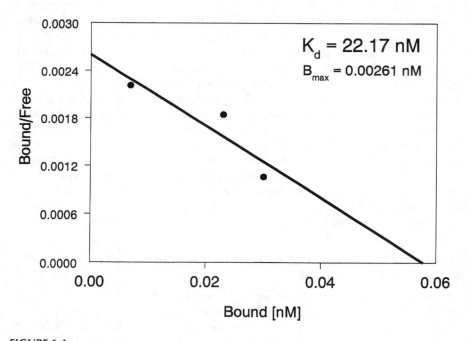

FIGURE 1.4
Representative Scatchard plot of the specific binding of [^{3}H]-20β-S to a spotted seatrout spermatozoa plasma membrane extract, K_d = 22.17 nM, B_{max} = 0.00261 nmol mL^{-1} milt. (From Thomas, P., Breckenridge-Miller, D., and Detweiler, C., *Fish, Physiol. Biochem.*, 17, 109, 1997. With permission.)

than 2.5 min. These rapid rates of association/dissociation are characteristic of plasma membrane receptors. The binding was highly specific for 20β-S (Figure 1.5); all the other C21 steroids tested had relative binding affinities of less than 15% for the seatrout receptor (Figure 1.5). The binding affinity

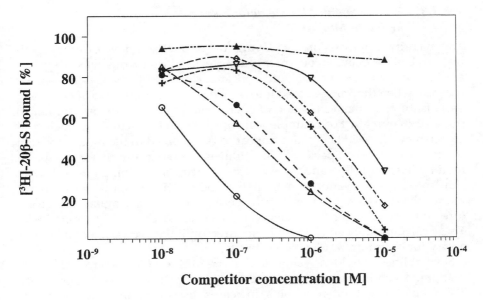

FIGURE 1.5

Steroid binding specificity of spotted seatrout testicular plasma membrane preparations. Membranes were incubated for 30 min with 20 nM [³H]-20β-S and 10 nM-10 μM competitor: ○ – ○ 20β-S, Δ – Δ 17,20β-P, • – •, progesterone, + – + 11- deoxycortisol, Δ – Δ cortisol, ∇ – ∇ estradiol, ◇ – ◇ testosterone. (From Thomas, B., Breckenridge-Miller, D., and Detweiler, C., *Fish. Physiol. Biochem.* 17, 109, 1997. With permission.)

of testosterone was two orders of magnitude lower, whereas estradiol and cortisol were ineffective at displacing 20β-S from the binding sites on croaker sperm.[96] Estradiol had a slightly higher affinity for the seatrout sperm and testes receptor (rba 0.4%, Figure 1.5), but the specificities of the receptors for the other steroids were practically identical.[95] This pattern of steroid binding affinity is similar to that of the ovarian MIS membrane receptor[65,70] but differs notably from that of the nuclear progestin receptor in seatrout testes, in which several C21 steroids display higher affinities.[73,74] Specific 20β-S binding was limited primarily to reproductive tissues, with small amounts also present in the liver (Table 1.1).

The final criteria that need to be satisfied for a binding moiety to be designated as a receptor are that changes in receptor abundance are consistent with its proposed physiological functions. In male fish the prespawning surge in plasma gonadotropin levels causes increases in MIS production and milt volume. It was found that hormonal stimulation of gonadotropin secretion by luteinizing hormane-releasing hormone (LHRH) injection caused a two- to three-fold increase in sperm 20β-S concentrations 2 d later, which was accompanied by an increase in milt volume. Similarly, incubation of minced croaker and seatrout testicular tissues with gonadotropin for 18 h increased sperm receptor levels several fold compared to controls.[95,96] Therefore, sperm membrane 20β-S binding in both species fulfill all the criteria for their designation as hormone receptors.

1.2.3.3   Role of Sperm MIS Membrane Receptor
in Sperm Motility

The majority of teleosts are egg laying (oviparous) and have external fertilization. Unlike mammalian sperm, the sperm of oviparous teleost species are immotile in the seminal fluid and are activated by changes in osmotic pressure when they are released into the external medium.[97] However, many basic features of the acquisition of sperm motility in teleosts are similar to those of mammals. For example, calcium influx via calcium channels and elevated cyclic AMP levels also appear to be involved in the final activation of sperm in teleost species.[98,99] Calcium is a potent stimulator of sperm motility in teleosts[100,101] and increases the velocity and turning rate of sperm, similar to hyperactivation of mammalian sperm. However, calcium does not induce the acrosome reaction in fish sperm, since fish sperm lack this structure and instead enter the oocyte via a specialized channel, the micropyle. These calcium-induced changes in sperm motility are considered to be necessary for optimum fertilization capacity.

Several lines of evidence suggest that the MIS receptor on croaker sperm is an important intermediary on sperm activation. Incubation of sperm with 20β-S, but not with other steroids, increases the percentage that are motile, as well as sperm velocity and their turning rate. This stimulatory effect of 20β-S is concentration-dependent and is enhanced if 20β-S receptor concentrations on croaker sperm are upregulated by prior *in vivo* treatment with LHRH (unpublished observation). Incubation with 20β-S also causes rapid increases in intrasperm free calcium concentrations. These studies suggest, therefore, that 20β-S activates croaker sperm by elevating intracellular free calcium levels and that the process is dependent upon sufficient numbers of MIS sperm membrane receptors and functional calcium channels. Thus, it is proposed that the basic mechanism of sperm activation by progestins in the male reproductive tract of a teleost species with external fertilization is similar to that induced by progesterone in the female tract of a vertebrate group with internal fertilization, the mammals.

1.2.3.4   Xenobiotic Estrogen Binding to Sperm MIS
Membrane Receptor

The ability of the xenobiotic estrogens, kepone, o,p'-DDE, and 2'4'6'-PCB-4-OH, and a mycotoxin estrogen, zearalenone, to displace [³H]-20β-S from the croaker sperm membrane MIS receptor was examined in competitive binding assays.[32,95] Sperm membrane preparations were incubated in the presence of [³H]-20β-S with or without various amounts of unlabeled 20β-S or the estrogenic compounds (concentration range: 10 nM to 1 mM) for 30–60 min at 4°C. Maximum specific binding was expressed as the binding suppressed by 100-fold excess unlabeled 20β-S.

All four estrogenic compounds were effective competitors for [³H]-20β-S binding to the sperm membrane MIS receptor (Figure 1.6). Zearalenone and kepone caused significant displacement at a concentration of 100 nM. None

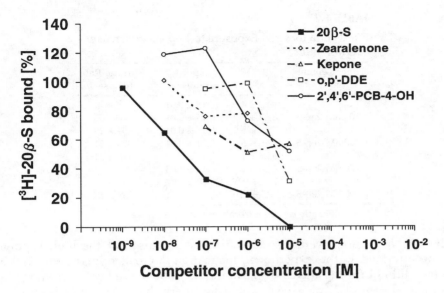

FIGURE 1.6

Competition by xenobiotic estrogens, kepone, o,p'-DDE, and 2',4',6'-PCB-4-OH, and a my-cotoxin estrogen, zearalenone, for [³H]-20β-S binding to the Atlantic croaker sperm MIS membrane receptor. Binding is expressed as a percentage of total binding (binding sup-pressed by 300 nM 20β-S). (From Thomas, P., Breckenridge-Miller, D., and Detweiler, C., *Mar. Environ. Res.*, in press. With permission.)

of the estrogenic compounds were capable of completely displacing 20β-S from the receptor and only one, o,p'-DDE, caused more than 50% displace-ment under these assay conditions. In addition, the slopes of their competition curves were not parallel to that of 20β-S, which suggests that the xenobiotic binding is of the noncompetitive type.

1.2.3.5 Effects of a Xenobiotic Estrogen, Kepone, on Sperm Motility

The effects of acute exposure to one of the estrogenic compounds, kepone, on the motility of croaker sperm was investigated in a preliminary study.[32] The sperm were diluted 50-fold in a physiological saline and incubated with various concentrations of kepone (0, 50, 100, 200, 1000 μM) in the presence or absence of 100 nM 20β-S for 2 to 3 min. The prediluted sperm was then diluted in activation solution containing the same concentrations of kepone and 20β-S. Immediately after activation, the motility was videotaped at 400x magnification for 1 min and the sperm motility parameters were calculated using a motion analysis system.

A high percentage of the untreated sperm were motile in the assay system, and a significant decrease on motility was observed after 2 to 3 min incuba-tion with the higher concentrations of kepone (Table 1.2). Sperm velocity and

TABLE 1.2

Effects of 2 to 3 min Exposure to Kepone on Croaker Sperm Motility

Conc. Kepone (mM)	% Motile	Speed (mm/sec)	Turning Rate (deg/sec)
0	84.3 ± 4.9	0.15 ± 0.01	455 ± 41
+ 100 nM 20β-S	87.2 ± 7.2	0.15 ± 0.01	449 ± 71
0.05	78.2 ± 5.2	0.14 ± 0.01	354 ± 29
+ 100 nM 20β-S	82.6 ± 5.0	0.14 ± 0.01	374 ± 31
0.2	35.7 ± 10[a]	0.10 ± 0.02	318 ± 21[a]
+ 100 nM 20β-S	43.4 ± 13[a]	0.12 ± 0.03	292 ± 32[a]
1.0	28.2 ± 9.3[a]	0.08 ± 0.02[a]	300 ± 29[a]
+ 100 nM 20β-S	18.7 ± 7.1[a]	0.13 ± 0.01	333 ± 45

[a] Significantly different from respective control groups.

the rate of turning were also significantly decreased at the high kepone concentrations. In this experiment, incubation of croaker sperm with 20β-S alone did not further increase sperm motility above the high percentage in untreated controls. This suggests that the sperm had previously been activated by exposure to 20β-S *in vivo*. Interestingly, coincubation with 100 nM 20β-S restored sperm velocity but did not restore the percent motile sperm or their rate of turning[32] (Table 1.2). Thus, inconsistent evidence of interactions between 20β-S and kepone concentrations to influence sperm motility were obtained under these assay conditions. Additional experiments will be required over a range of 20β-S and kepone concentrations to determine whether these compounds influence sperm motility by a common mechanism, that is by binding to the steroid membrane receptor. Decreases in sperm motility have been observed in fish exposed to a variety of xenobiotic compounds[102] and have been associated with declines in fertilization capacity. Interestingly, decreases in sperm motility and abnormal sperm have previously been reported in factory workers exposed to kepone, which was thought to be a primary cause of their decreased fertility.[11,103] Taken together, these studies on fish and humans suggest that sperm function may be particularly sensitive to disruption by xenobiotic estrogenic compounds. The experiments with croaker sperm probably provide the first evidence of binding of xenobiotic estrogens to a steroid membrane receptor on vertebrate sperm. Clearly, the progestin membrane receptor on vertebrate sperm is a potential site of interference by estrogenic xenobiotics and other endocrine-disrupting chemicals.

In conclusion, evidence has been obtained that a variety of xenobiotic estrogens are effective competitors for progestin plasma membrane receptors on both oocytes and sperm in a vertebrate model. Several of these xenobiotics can antagonize the actions of the progestin, 20β-S, thereby disrupting the processes of final gamete maturation. Localization of the receptor in the plasma membrane appears to be necessary for receptor binding to these lipophilic xenobiotic chemicals. However, further investigations of this mechanism of endocrine disruption are required to determine its toxicological significance.

1.3 Hypothalamic Monoaminergic Pathways

1.3.1 Hypothalamic Monoaminergic Function

1.3.1.1 Neuroendocrine Control of Gonadotropin Secretion in Atlantic Croaker

The neuroendocrine control of gonadotropin secretion in vertebrates is highly complex, involving multiple neural pathways and a wide variety of regulatory factors, including neurotransmitters, neuropeptides, amino acids, and steroids.[104-107] Considerable evidence has also been obtained for multifactorial control of gonadotropin secretion in croaker: a stimulatory influence of one or more GnRHs, a stimulatory influence of monoamine neurotransmitters, modulatory influences of gamma aminobutyric acid and melatonin, which vary seasonally, and negative and positive feedback control by gonadal steroids at different phases of the reproductive cycle.[108-113] In addition, other neuropeptides, such as neuropeptide Y, cholecystokinin and endogenous opioid peptides, and the amino acids β-alanine, glutamate, and taurine have been shown to influence gonadotropin secretion in other fish species.[107] Serotonin (5-HT) has a stimulatory influence on GnRH-induced gonadotropin secretion in croaker,[110] similar to the observation in mammals.[114] Furthermore, this potentiating effect of 5-HT appears to be mediated by 5-HT$_2$ receptors and is dependent on the time of day and reproductive state of the fish.[111] The results of these studies, along with the demonstration of the close proximity and overlapping of the 5-HT and GnRH systems in the preoptic-anterior hypothalamus (POAH) and the localization of the immunoreactive elements of the two systems in and around the gonadotropes,[115] indicate that 5-HT can alter gonadotropin secretion directly at the pituitary and can also act on the GnRH system at both the POAH and pituitary to influence gonadotropin secretion (unpublished observation).

1.3.1.2 Effect of Lead on Hypothalamic Monoaminergic Systems and Neuroendocrine Function

There is extensive literature on the reproductive toxicity and neurotoxicity of lead in vertebrates.[116,117] The effects of chronic lead exposure on reproductive endocrine function were investigated in Atlantic croaker. Administration of lead (0.5 and 1.5 mg/100 g body wt./d) in the diet for 30 d caused a marked suppression of ovarian steroidogenesis and ovarian growth.[118] The preliminary results suggested that the suppressive effects of lead were mediated in part by an impairment of gonadotropin secretion. Previous studies had shown that lead influences monoamine metabolism in both mammals and fish,[119,120] and the neuroendocrine axis is a major target of the metal in mammals.[21,27] Therefore, in a subsequent experiment, hypothalamic monoamine concentrations and gonadotropin secretion were measured in male croaker receiving the same lead treatment regime. Lead caused only minor changes in the hypothalamic concentrations of the biogenic amines epinephrine, norepinephrine, dopamine, and serotonin and their metabolites 3, 4 dihydroxyphenylacetic acid, 3-methoxytyramine, homovanillic acid, and 5-hydroxyindol acetic acid (5-HIAA).[14] The effects of the lead treatments on the concentrations of 5-HT and its metabolite 5-HIAA in the preoptic anterior and medial posterior hypothalamus are shown in Figure 1.7. There was a trend of a decrease in 5-HT concentrations and an increase in the content of its metabolite in both hypothalamic areas after lead exposure, but these changes were not significant. However, the hypothalamic 5-HIAA to 5-HT ratio, a measure of serotonin metabolism or turnover, was significantly elevated in the lead-treated fish (Figure 1.7). Chronic exposure to the higher dose of lead also significantly inhibited both basal and LHRHa-induced gonadotropin secretion from pituitary fragments *in vitro* (Figure 1.8). The attenuation of the gonadotropin response to LHRHa was similar to that observed after treatment with the 5-HT$_2$ receptor antagonist, Ketanserin.[110] Thus, these results provide preliminary evidence that the effects of lead on gonadotropin secretion may be partially mediated by decreases in hypothalamic serotonergic activity. The decrease in gonadotropin secretion after exposure to lead was accompanied by a dose-related inhibition of gonadal growth and decreased circulating levels of androgens.[14]

A dramatic decline in basal gonadotropin secretion and impairment of the response to LHRHa have also been demonstrated in croaker *in vivo* after chronic administration of Aroclor 1254 in the diet.[25] The PCB mixture caused a greater disturbance of hypothalamic neurotransmitter function than observed after treatment with lead. There was a significant decline in both 5-HT and dopamine concentrations as well as an increase in their metabolite-to-parent amine ratios in both the POAH and medial posterior hypothalamus (MPH) after PCB exposure.[25] In separate studies, PCBs have also been shown to interfere with monoamine metabolism in discrete brain areas of mammals[121] and to influence gonadotropin secretion.[122,123]

The studies with croaker suggest that the serotonergic system in hypothalamic areas of the brain controlling gonadotropin secretion is sensitive to interference by lead and Aroclor 1254, representatives of the different classes of neurotoxic and reproductive toxic chemicals. The toxic mechanisms of these two chemicals on the hypothalamic serotonergic system are thought to differ and are currently being investigated. Possible estrogenic actions of Aroclor 1254 metabolites mediated by nuclear estrogen receptors in the hypothalamus shall also be considered. A large body of evidence, mostly circumstantial, suggests that many other chemicals, including mercury, organochlorine and organophosphorous pesticides, xenobiotic estrogens,

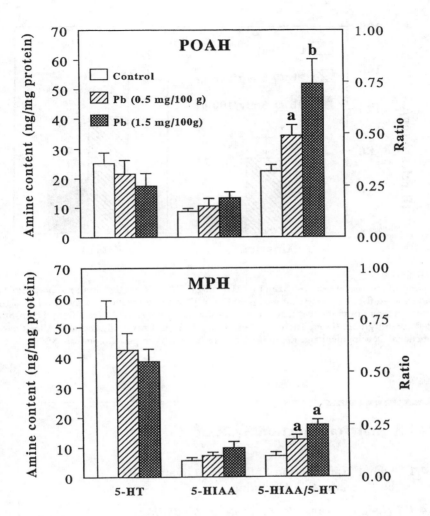

FIGURE 1.7
Lead-induced alterations in serotonin metabolism in the preoptic anterior hypothalamus (POAH) and medial posterior hypothalamus (MPH) of croaker brains. Bars represent means ± standard error of mean of 10-12 observations. a: significantly different from control group, b: significantly different from low dose group. 5-HIAA-5 hydroxy indolacetic acid. (From Thomas, P. and Khan, I. A., in Chemically Induced Alterations in Functional Development and Reproduction in Fish, 1997. With permission from SETAC.)

and central nervous system drugs, impair reproductive endocrine function at the hypothalamic level in vertebrates.[11,21,120,122,124,125] More comprehensive studies will be required, however, to determine whether alteration of neurotransmitter function is a widespread mechanism of neuroendocrine disruption by environmental chemicals.

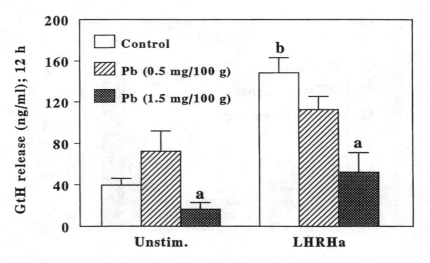

FIGURE 1.8

In vitro GtH release in response to an LHRH analog (LHRHa) from the pituitaries of control and lead-exposed fish. Bars represent means ± SEM of 10 to 12 observations; a: mean values significantly different from the respective control groups; b: significantly different from the unstimulated control group. (From Thomas, P. and Khan, I. A., in Chemically Induced Alterations in Functional Development and Reproduction in Fish, 1997. With permission from SETAC.)

1.4   Signal Transduction Systems

1.4.1   Signal Transduction Pathways Activated by Reproductive Hormones

1.4.1.1   Signal Transduction Systems Mediating Gonadotropin Secretion

The signal transduction systems involved in GnRH stimulation of gonadotropin secretion are broadly similar among the vertebrate groups.[126] Binding of GnRH to its receptor activates phospholipase C, resulting in the production of inositol phosphates and diacylglycerol. Diacylglycerol activates both calcium and phospholipid-dependent protein kinase C (PKC). Inositol 1, 4, 5-triphosphate releases calcium from intracellular stores in the rat pituitary, whereas it is thought that PKC may perform this function in the goldfish pituitary. However, in both vertebrate groups, mobilization of internal calcium stores and activation of PKC are important processes in GnRH stimulation of gonadotropin secretion. The increase in internal free calcium levels, in addition to causing further activation of PKC, probably also stimulates calmodulin-dependent events. PKC, calmodulin and arachidonic acid are all activated or mobilized during GnRH stimulation and are believed to be final mediators of gonadotropin secretion in both mammals and fish.[126] Voltage-sensitive calcium channels and extracellular calcium are also involved in mediating the gonadotropin response to GnRH. Activation of PKC results in opening of the calcium channels and influx of calcium, which is required for sustained release of gonadotropin in mammals, fish, and other vertebrates.[127,128] In goldfish and croaker, the calcium channel blocker, verapamil, blocks both initial and sustained secretion of gonadotropin in response to GnRH. Thus, calcium is important as a mediator of GnRH-induced gonadotropin secretion in vertebrates and is an ubiquitous second messenger of hormonal and other cellular responses.

Chemicals that interfere with calcium homeostasis, therefore, are likely to disrupt calcium-dependent hormonal responses. Lead, cadmium, and mercury are transported across cell membranes by calcium channels and interfere with calcium movement. In addition, they bind to calcium binding proteins such as calmodulin *in vitro*, substituting for calcium.[129] Pesticides such as DDT and lindane also alter calcium homeostasis, leading to egg shell thinning in birds, and cause neurotoxicity at high concentrations.

1.4.1.2 *Direct Effects of Cadmium on Gonadotropin Secretion from the Pituitary*

The direct effects of cadmium on gonadotropin secretion from croaker pituitaries were investigated in a pituitary fragment perifusion system.[28] Earlier *in vivo* studies had shown that chronic exposure to cadmium caused precocious ovarian recrudescence at the beginning of the reproductive season which was associated with dramatic increases in ovarian steroidogenesis and gonadotropin secretion from the pituitary.[125] Croaker pituitaries perifused with physiological saline alone secreted low amounts of gonadotropin (1–2 ng/ml). Infusion of GnRH caused a transient increase in gonadotropin secretion. The response to GnRH was dependent on the presence of calcium in the external medium and functional calcium channels, since it is blocked by the addition of verapamil. Gonadotropin secretion increased dramatically to 10-25 ng/ml within 20 min of infusion of cadmium (50 μM) at a rate of 1 ml/min (Figure 1.9). The croaker perifusion results corroborate earlier findings with rat pituitaries which demonstrate increases in gonadotropin secretion *in vitro* after exposure to perifusion buffers containing cadmium.[28] The croaker pituitary fragments maintained their responsiveness to GnRH stimulation after cadmium treatment and released large amounts of gonadotropin after GnRH infusion. Interestingly, both spontaneous and GnRH-stimulated secretion of gonadotropin from pituitary fragments in the cadmium-containing perifusion media were not dependent on the presence of calcium but were blocked in the presence of verapamil. These results suggest that cadmium acts via calcium channels in the gonadotropes to stimulate the calcium-dependent components of the GnRH signal transduction system which control gonadotropin secretion.

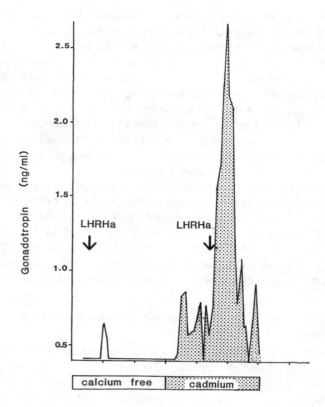

FIGURE 1.9
Representative profile of gonadotropin secretion from Atlantic croaker pituitaries perifused with calcium-free physiological saline with or without cadmium (20 μM) or LHRHa (100 ng/mL).

1.4.1.3 *Signal Transduction Systems Mediating Gonadal Steroid Secretion*

Overall, there is a remarkable degree of conservation among vertebrates in the signal transduction systems that mediate the actions of gonadotropins on gonadal tissues.[130] The involvement of cyclic AMP in the regulation of gonadal steroidogenesis has been clearly demonstrated in mammalian, avian, and teleost species.[131,132] In spotted seatrout ovaries, cyclic AMP levels increase dramatically within 15 min of stimulation by gonadotropin *in vitro* and precede the increase in steroid production.[132] Calcium from both intracellular and extracellular pools is also intimately involved in gonadotropin actions in vertebrate tissues.[130] Moreover, voltage-sensitive calcium channel blockers, such as verapamil, inhibit gonadotropin stimulation of gonadal steroidogenesis. In addition, other second messengers, such as inositol-1,4,5-triphosphate, diacylglycerol, and arachidonic acid and sodium and chloride ions appear to be involved in gonadotropin actions in certain target tissues.

Thus, xenobiotics could potentially interfere with a variety of signal transduction systems to modulate the actions of gonadotropin.

1.4.1.4 Direct Effects of Cadmium on Ovarian Steroidogenesis

An initial study showed that 40-d exposure of Atlantic croaker to 1 ppm cadmium in the water at the beginning of ovarian recrudescence significantly accelerated ovarian growth, which was associated with elevated circulating estradiol levels.[125] In addition, estradiol production from ovarian fragments of cadmium-treated fish incubated *in vitro* was increased and was accompanied by increases in ovarian cyclic AMP levels. It was not possible to determine from these *in vivo* studies whether the stimulation of ovarian growth and steroidogenesis was due to the increased gonadotropin secretion in the cadmium-treated fish or to direct actions of the metal at the ovarian level.

Direct effects of cadmium on steroidogenesis and cyclic AMP content in spotted seatrout ovaries were investigated in an *in vitro* incubation system.[14,132] Ovarian fragments from vitellogenic females were incubated in physiological media containing a range of cadmium concentrations (0.01 to 1000 ppm). Testosterone and estradiol concentrations were measured by radioimmunoassay in the media after 9 h and 18 h of incubation, respectively. Ovarian tissue was removed after 1-h incubation with cadmium for measurement of cAMP by a protein-binding method in a parallel experiment.

Cadmium caused a concentration-dependent stimulation of ovarian estradiol secretion and accumulation of cyclic AMP and also increased testosterone secretion (Figure 1.10). The steroid production was significantly increased by the lowest concentration of cadmium tested, 0.01 ppm. Cadmium over the range of concentrations of 0.1 to 100 ppm significantly elevated cyclic AMP and steroid production, but the response was attenuated at the highest concentration (1000 ppm).

The results suggest that cadmium stimulates steroidogenesis by elevating cyclic AMP levels. The mechanism of action of cadmium to influence cyclic AMP levels in steroidogenic tissues is unclear at present. Singhal demonstrated that cadmium treatment altered the activities of both phosphodiesterase and adenylate cyclase in mammalian tissues.[133] Cyclic AMP levels remained relatively constant in the rat testis after cadmium administration because the increase in adenylate cyclase activity was counteracted by an increase in cyclic AMP metabolism by phosphodiesterase. In contrast, the activity of only one of these enzymes was altered in the prostate after cadmium treatment resulting in an alteration of cyclic AMP levels. Differential effects of cadmium on the two enzymes regulating cyclic AMP levels could account for the increase in ovarian cyclic AMP observed in the present study. Cadmium also disrupts calcium homeostasis and calcium-dependent signal transduction systems.[30,134] Possible actions of cadmium on voltage-sensitive calcium channels, calmodulin, inositol-1, 4, 5-triphosphate, and mobilization of intracellular calcium stores to influence gonadal steroidogenesis also need to be investigated.

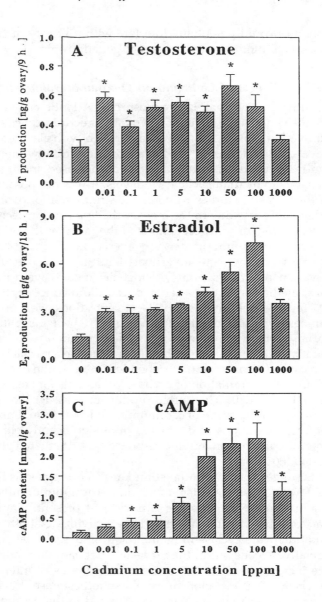

FIGURE 1.10

Effects of increasing concentrations of cadmium on *in vitro* production of (A) testosterone, (B) estradiol, and (C) cAMP accumulation by vitellogenic ovaries of spotted seatrout. Each bar represents the mean ± S.E.M. of six observations. Asterisks denote means significantly different from controls ($P < 0.05$, Newman Keul's multiple range 't' test). (From Thomas, P. and Khan, I. A., in *Chemically Induced Alterations in Functional Development and Reproduction in Fish*, 1997. With permission from SETAC.)

1.5 Concluding Remarks

Vertebrate reproduction is an intricate process involving extensive physiological coordination which is primarily controlled by the hormones secreted by the hypothalamus–pituitary–gonadal axis. The overall complexity of the reproductive endocrine system and the integrated nature of its response to environmental stimuli have complicated investigations of its disruption by xenobiotic chemicals. Chemicals potentially can exert their effects at multiple sites on the hypothalamus–pituitary–gonadal axis and by a variety of mechanisms to interfere with reproductive endocrine function.[21,22] In this chapter, evidence for endocrine disruption in the hypophysiotropic region of the hypothalamus, at the pituitary, ovary, oocytes, and sperm is discussed. Several novel mechanisms of endocrine disruption that warrant further investigation in different vertebrate models and target tissues are identified.

Our studies demonstrate binding of xenobiotic estrogens to MIS membrane receptors on fish oocytes and sperm and interference with MIS action. Watson and co-workers[135] have proposed studies on the interactions of environmental estrogens with an estrogen membrane receptor they have identified on prolactin cells in the rat pituitary. Experiments also are being conducted on possible interference by xenobiotic estrogens with binding of chemicals to membrane receptors on the nasal epithelium of fish, which mediate behavioral responses to MIS pheromones. These studies will further test the hypothesis that steroid membrane receptors are particularly susceptible to interference by xenobiotic chemicals. The likely discovery in the near future of new steroid membrane receptors on other target tissues will provide additional models to study this mechanism of endocrine disruption. However, currently, interference by xenobiotic estrogens with the steroid membrane receptor on vertebrate sperm and resulting loss in sperm function are of greatest concern and require additional study.

Evidence is also presented for chemical-induced alterations in hypothalamic serotonergic function, which were associated with impaired gonadotropin secretion. The neuroendocrine control of gonadotropin secretion is highly complex, involving a wide variety of neurotransmitters and other chemical messengers, and receives input via multiple neural pathways, including those emanating from sensory cells in the pineal, eyes, and olfactory organ. Therefore, any chemical that disrupts the normal functions of nerve cells, including neurosecretory cells, and glial cells and sensory cells has the potential to disrupt neuroendocrine function. Not surprisingly, there is a substantial amount of circumstantial evidence that representatives of different classes of toxic chemicals disrupt reproduction, primarily interfering with neuroendocrine function.[14,21-23,25,26,122] The neuroendocrine system is a likely major target of many lipophilic organic compounds, xenobiotic estrogens and antiandrogens, heavy metals, and neuropharmacological agents.[26,117,119-121] However, there are relatively few reports describing possible mechanisms of neuroendocrine disruptions induced by these chemicals.[25,27] Consequently, we have an incomplete understanding of the degree and nature of neuroendocrine disruption induced by exposure to xenobiotic chemicals.

Calcium, an ubiquitous intracellular messenger, is a component of many hormonal and other signal transduction mechanisms.[126,129,130,136] The toxicological consequences of chemical interference with calcium messenger systems in the neural, immune, cardiovascular, and renal systems have been considered.[129,136] The experiments reported here provide evidence that a heavy metal, cadmium, also causes endocrine disruption by interfering with the normal function of the calcium-dependent second messenger system in the pituitary-regulating gonadotropin secretion. Cadmium also interfered with the second messenger systems controlling gonadal steroidogenesis by increasing intracellular cyclic AMP levels. Disruption of calcium homeostasis by cadmium is also likely at the gonadal level, but the direct evidence is currently lacking. There is extensive evidence that lead also interferes with the regulation of internal calcium levels.[129,137] Calcium has important functions in both monoamine biosythesis and secretion in the central nervous system which appear to be regulated by calmodulin-dependent protein kinase.[138,139] Therefore it is possible that the effects of lead exposure on the serotonergic system in the croaker hypothalamus are also mediated by alterations in calcium regulation. Finally, it is well established that calcium channels and calcium influx have important roles in the activation of vertebrate sperm in response to steroids.[41,42] A more comprehensive knowledge of how chemicals disrupt calcium homeostasis and calcium-dependent signal transduction systems may be the key, therefore, to understanding many of the nontraditional mechanisms of endocrine disruption.

Acknowledgments

This research was supported by Public Health Service Grants ESO4214 and ESO7672 to Peter Thomas.

References

1. Colborn, T., Vom Saal, F. S. and Soto, A. M., Developmental effects of endocrine-disrupting chemicals in wildlife and humans, *Environ. Health Perspect.*, 101, 378, 1993.
2. Twonbly, R., Assault on the male, *Environ. Health Perspect.*, 103, 802, 1995.

3. Davis, W. P. and Bartone, S. A., Effects of kraft mill effluent on the sexuality of fish: an environmental early warning, in *Chemically-Induced Alterations in Sexual and Functional Development: The Wildlife/Human Connection,* Colborn, T. and Clement, C., Eds., Princeton Scientific Publishing Co., Princeton, NJ, 1992, 113.

4. Jobling, S. and Sumpter, J. P., Detergent components in sewage effluent are weakly oestrogenic to fish: an *in vitro* study using rainbow trout (*Oncorhynchus mykiss*) hepatocytes, *Aquat. Toxicol.,* 27, 361, 1993.

5. Raloff, J., The gender binders: are environmental hormones emasculating wildlife? *Sci. News,* 145, 24, 1994.

6. Davis, D. L., Bradlow, H. L., Wolff, M. W., Woodruff, T., Hoel, D. G., and Anton-Culver, H., Medical hypothesis: xenoestrogens as preventable causes of breast cancer, *Environ. Health Perspect.,* 101, 372, 1993.

7. Sharpe, R. and Skakkebaek, N. E., Are oestrogens involved in falling sperm counts and disorders of the male reproductive tract? *Lancet,* 341, 1392, 1993.

8. McLachlan, J. A., Functional toxicology: a new approach to detect biologically active xenobiotics, *Environ. Health Perspect.,* 101, 386, 1993.

9. Jobling, S., Reynolds, T., White, R., Porter, M. G., and Sumpter, J. P., A variety of environmentally persistent chemicals, including some phthalate plasticizers are weakly estrogenic, *Environ. Health Perspect.,* 103, 582, 1995.

10. Nelson, J. A., Effects of dichlorodiphenyltrichlorethane (DDT) analogs and polychlorinated biphenyl mixtures on $17\beta[^3H]$ estradiol binding to rat uterine receptor, *Biochem. Pharmacol.,* 23, 447, 1973.

11. Bulger, W. H. and Kupfer, D., Estrogenic activity of pesticides and other xenobiotics on the uterus and male reproductive tract, in *Endocrine Toxicity,* Thomas, J. A., Korach, K. S., and McLachlan, J. A., Eds., Raven Press, New York, 1985, 1.

12. Korach, K. S., Sarver, P., Chae, K., McLachlan, J. A., and McKinney, J. D., Estrogen receptor-binding activity of polychlorinated hydroxybiphenyls conformationally restricted structural probes, *Mol. Pharmacol.,* 37, 120, 1987.

13. Gray, E. L., Jr., Monosson, E., and Kelce, W. R., Emerging issues: the effects of endocrine disruptors on reproductive development, in *Interconnections Between Human and Ecosystem,* Guilio, R. T., and Monosson, E., Eds., Chapman and Hall, London, 1996, 46.

14. Thomas, P. and Khan, I. A., Mechanisms of chemical interference with reproductive endocrine function in sciaenid fish, in *Chemically-Induced Alterations in Functional Development and Reproduction of Fish,* Rolland, R. M., Gilbertson, M., and Peterson, R. E., Eds., SETAC Technical Publications Series, Pensacola, FL, 1997, 29.

15. Lee, A. V., Weng C-N., Jackson, J. G., and Yee, D., Activation of estrogen receptor-mediated gene transcription by IGF-1 in human breast cancer cells, *J. Endocrinol.,* 152, 39, 1997.

16. Ignar-Trowbridge, D. M., Pimentel, M., Parker, M. G., McLachlan, J. A., and Korach, K. S., Peptide growth factor cross-talk with the estrogen receptor requires the A/B domain and occurs independently of protein kinase C or estradiol, *Endocrinology,* 137, 1735, 1996.

17. Safe, S., Astroff, B., Harris, M., Zachorewski, T., Dickerson, R., Romkes, M., and Biegel, L., 2,3,7,8-tetracholorodibenzo-p-dioxin (TCDD) and related compounds as antiestrogens: characterization and mechanism of action, *Pharmacol. Toxicol.,* 64, 400, 1991.

18. Khara, I. and Saatcioglu, F., Antiestrogenic effects of 2,3,7,8-tetracholorodibenzo-*p*-dioxin are mediated by direct transcriptional interference with the liganded estrogen receptor, *J. Biol. Chem.,* 271, 10533, 1996.

19. Lundholm, C. E., The effects of DDE, PCB and chlordane on the binding of progesterone to its cytoplasmic receptor in eggshell gland mucosa of birds and the endometrium of mammalian uterus, *Comp. Biochem. Physiol.*, 89C, 361, 1988.

20. Kelce, W. R., Stone, C. R., Laws, S. C., Gray, L. E., Kemppainen, J. A., and Wilson, E. M., Persistent DDT metabolite *p,p'*-DDE is a potent androgen receptor antagonist, *Nature*, 375, 581, 1995.

21. Mattison, D. R., Gates, A. H., Leonards, A., Wide, M., Hemminki, K., and Copius Peereboom-Stegeman, J. H. J., Reproductive and developmental toxicity of metals: female reproductive system, in *Reproductive and Developmental Toxicity of Metals*, Clarkon, T. W., Norberg, G. N., Sager, P. R., Eds., Plenum Press, New York, 1983, 41.

22. Thomas, P., Teleost model for studying the effects of chemicals on female reproductive endocrine function, *J. Exp. Zool.*, 4, 126, 1990.

23. Uphouse, L., Effects of chlordecone on neuroendocrine function of female rats, *Neurotoxicology*, 6, 191, 1985.

24. Seegal, R. F., Brosch, C. O., and Bush, B., Regional alterations in serotonin metabolism induced by oral exposure of rats to polychlorinated biphenyls, *Neurotoxicology*, 7, 155, 1986.

25. Khan, I. A. and Thomas, P., Aroclor 1254-induced alterations in hypothalamic monoamine metabolism in the Atlantic croaker (*Micropogonias undulatus*): correlation with pituitary gonadotropin release, *Neurotoxicology*, 18, 553, 1997.

26. Cicero, T. J., Badger, T. M., Wilcox, C. E., Bell, R. D., and Meyer, E. R., Morphine decreases luteinizing hormone by an action on the hypothalamic-pituitary axis, *J. Pharmacol. Exp. Ther.*, 203, 548, 1977.

27. Klein, D., Wan, Y. Y., Kamyab, S., Okuda, H., and Sokol, R. Z., Effects of toxic levels of lead on gene regulation in the male axis: increase in messenger ribonucleic acids and intracellular stores of gonadotrops within the central nervous system, *Biol. Reprod.*, 50, 802, 1994.

28. Thomas, P., Effects of cadmium on gonadotropin secretion from Atlantic croaker pituitaries incubated *in vitro*, *Mar. Environ. Res.*, 35, 141, 1993.

29. Cooper, R. A., Goldman, J. M., Rehnberg, G. L., McElroy, W. K., and Hein, J. F., Effects of metal cations on pituitary hormone secretion *in vitro*, *J. Biochem. Toxicol.*, 2, 241, 1987.

30. Singhal, R. L., Vijayvargia, R., and Shukla, G. S., Toxic effects of cadmium and lead on reproductive functions, in *Endocrine Toxicology*, Thomas, J. A., Korach, K. S., McLachlan, J. A., Eds., Raven Press, New York, 1985, 149.

31. Ghosh, S. and Thomas, P., Antagonistic effects of xenobiotics on steroid-induced final maturation of Atlantic croaker oocytes *in vitro*, *Mar. Environ. Res.*, 39, 159, 1995.

32. Thomas, P., Breckenridge-Miller, D., and Detweiler, C., The teleost sperm membrane progestogen receptor: interactions with xenoestrogens, *Mar. Environ. Res.*, 46, 163-167, 1998.

33. Metzgan, D. A., Nontraditional sites of estrogen action, *Environ. Health Perspect.*, 5, 39, 1995.

34. Tsai, M. J. and O'Malley, B. W., Molecular mechanisms of action of steroid/thyroid receptor superfamily members, *Annu. Rev. Biochem.*, 63, 451, 1994.

35. Duval, D., Duront, S., and Homo-Delarche, F., Non-genomic effects of steroids. Interactions of steroid molecules with membrane structures and functions, *Biochim. Biophys. Acta*, 737, 409, 1983.

36. Haukkamaa, M., Membrane-associated steroid hormone receptors, in *Steroid Hormone Receptors: Their Intracellular Localization*, Clark, C. R., Ed., Ellis Horwood, Chichester, 1987, 155.
37. Touchette, N., Man bites dogma, a new role for steroid hormones, *J. NIH Res.*, 2, 71, 1990.
38. Pappas, T. C., Gametchu, B., Yannariello-Brown, J., Collins, T. J., and Watson, C. S., Membrane estrogen receptors in GH3/B6 cells are associated with rapid estrogen-induced release of prolactin, *Endocrine*, 2, 813, 1994.
39. Morley, P., Whitfield, J. F., Vanderhyden, B. C., Tsang, B. K., and Schwartz, J., A new, nongenomic estrogen action: the rapid release of intracellular calcium, *Endocrinology*, 131, 1305, 1992.
40. Nabekura, J., Oomura, Y., Minami, T., Mizuno, Y., and Fukudo, A., Mechanism of the rapid effect of 17β-estradiol on medial amygdala neurons, *Science*, 233, 226, 1986.
41. Thomas, P. and Meizel, S., Phophatidylinositol 4,5-biphosphate hydrolysis in human sperm stimulated with follicular fluid or progesterone is dependent upon Ca^{++} influx, *Biochem. J.*, 264, 539, 1989.
42. Blackmore, P. F., Neulen, J., Lattanzio, F., and Beebe, S. J., Cell surface-binding sites for progesterone mediate calcium uptake in human sperm, *J. Biol. Chem.*, 266, 18655, 1991.
43. Dluzen, D. E. and Ramirez, V. D., Progesterone effects upon dopamine release from the corpus striatum of female rats. II. Evidence for a membrane site of action and the role of albumin, *Brain Res.*, 476, 338, 1989.
44. Hua, S. Y. and Chen, Y. Z., Membrane receptor-mediated electrophysiological effects of glucocorticoid on mammalian neurons, *Endocrinology*, 124, 687, 1989.
45. Orchinik, M., Murray, T. F., and Moore, F. L., A corticosteroid receptor in neuronal membranes, *Science*, 252, 1848, 1991.
46. Gametchu, B., Glucocorticoid receptor-like antigen in lymphoma cell membranes: correlation to cell lysis, *Science*, 236, 456, 1987.
47. Pappas, T. C., Gametchu, B., and Watson, C. S., Membrane estrogen receptors identified by multiple antibody and impeded ligand labeling, *FASEB J.*, 9, 404, 1995.
48. Pietras, R. and Szego, C. M., Estrogen receptors in uterine plasma membrane, *J. Steroid Biochem.*, 2, 1471, 1979.
49. Suyemitsu, T. and Terayama, H., Specific binding sites for natural glucocorticoids in plasma membranes of rat liver, *Endocrinology*, 96, 1499, 1975.
50. Ke, F-C. and Ramirez, V. D., Binding of progesterone to nerve cell membranes of rat brain using progesterone conjugated to ^{125}I-bovine serum albumin as a ligand, *J. Neurochem.*, 54, 467, 1990.
51. Lan, N. C., Chen, J-S., Belelli, D., Pritchett, D. B., Seeburg, P. H., and Gee, K. W., A steroid recognition site is functionally coupled to an expressed $GABA_A$-benzodiazepene receptor, *Eur. J. Pharmacol.*, 188, 403, 1994.
52. Masui, Y. and Clarke, H. J., Oocyte maturation, *Int. Rev. Cytol.*, 57, 185, 1979.
53. Sadler, S. E. and Maller, J. L., Identification of a steroid receptor on the surface of *Xenopus* oocytes by photoaffinity labeling, *J. Biol. Chem.*, 257, 355, 1982.
54. Goetz, F. W., Hormonal control of oocyte final maturation and ovulation in fish, in *Fish Physiology*, Vol. IXB, Hoar, W. S., Randall, D. J., and Donaldson, E. M., Eds., Academic Press, New York, 1983, 117.
55. Masui, Y. and Markert, C. L., Cytoplasmic control of nuclear behavior during meiotic maturation of frog oocytes, *J. Exp. Zool.*, 177, 129, 1971.

56. Smith, L. D. and Ecker, R. E., The interaction of the steroids with *Rana pipens* oocytes in the induction of maturation, *Dev. Biol.*, 25, 232, 1971.

57. Ishikawa, K., Hanaoka, Y., Kondo, Y., and Imai, K., Primary action of steroid hormone at the surface of amphibian oocyte in the induction of germinal vesicle breakdown, *Mol. Cell. Endocrinol.*, 9, 91, 1977.

58. Godeau, J. F., Scharder-Slatkine, S., Hubert, P., and Baulieu, F. F., Induction of maturation in *Xenopus laevis* oocytes by a steroid linked to a polymer, in *Proc. Natl. Acad. Sci. U.S.A.*, 75, 2353, 1978.

59. Nagahama, Y., 17α,20β-dihydroxy-4-pregnen-3-one: a teleost maturation-inducing hormone, *Dev. Growth Diff.*, 29, 1, 1987.

60. Nagahama, Y., Yoshikuni, M., Yamashita, M., and Tanaka, M., Regulation of oocyte maturation in fish, in *Fish Physiology*, Vol. XIII, Molecular Endocrinology of Fish, Sherwood, N. M. and Hew, C. L., Eds., Academic Press, San Diego, 1994, 393.

61. Sadler, S. E., Bower, M. A., and Maller, J. L., Studies of a plasma membrane steroid receptor in *Xenopus* oocytes using the synthetic progestin RU486, *J. Steroid Biochem.*, 22, 419, 1985.

62. Blondeau, J. P. and Baulieu, E. E., Progesterone receptor characterized by photoaffinity labeling in the plasma membrane of *Xenopus laevis* oocytes, *Biochem. J.*, 219, 785, 1984.

63. Kostellow, A. B., Weinstein, S. P., and Morill, G. A., Specific binding of progesterone to the cell surface and its role in the meiotic divisions in *Rana* oocytes, *Biochim. Biophys. Acta*, 720, 356, 1982.

64. Liu, Z. and Patiño, R., High-affinity binding of progesterone to the plasma membrane of *Xenopus* oocytes: characteristics of binding and hormonal and developmental control, *Biol. Reprod.*, 78, 980, 1993.

65. Patiño, R. and Thomas, P., Characterization of membrane receptor activity for 17α,20β,21-trihydroxy-4-pregnen-3-one in ovaries of spotted seatrout (*Cynoscion nebulosus*), *Gen. Comp. Endocrinol.*, 78, 204, 1990.

66. Thomas, P. and Trant, J. M., Evidence that 17α,20β,21-trihydroxy-4-pregnen-3-one is a maturation-inducing steroid in spotted seatrout, *Fish Physiol. Biochem.*, 7, 185, 1989.

67. Maneckjee, A., Idler, D. R., and Weisbart, M., Demonstration of putative membrane and cytosol steroid receptors for 17α,20β-dihydroxy-4-pregnen-3-one in brook trout, *Salvelinus fontinalis*, during terminal stages of oocyte maturation, *Fish Physiol. Biochem.*, 6, 19, 1991.

68. Yoshikuni, M., Shibata, N., and Nagahama, S., Specific binding of [³H]17α,20β-dihydroxy-4-pregnen-3-one to oocyte cortices of rainbow trout (*Oncorhynchus kisutch*), *Fish Physiol. Biochem.*, 1, 15, 1993.

69. King, W. V., Ghosh, S., Thomas, P., and Sullivan, C. V., A receptor for the oocyte maturation-inducing hormone, 17α,20β,21-trihydroxy-4-pregnen-3-one on ovarian membranes of striped bass, *Biol. Reprod.*, 56, 266, 1997.

70. Thomas, P. and Das, S., Correlation between binding affinities of C21 steroids for the maturation-inducing steroid membrane receptor in spotted seatrout ovaries and their agonist and antagonist activities in an oocyte maturation bioassay, *Biol. Reprod.*, 57, 999, 1997.

71. Trant, J. M. and Thomas, P., Structure-activity relationships of steroids in inducing germinal vesicle breakdown of Atlantic croaker oocytes *in vitro*, *Gen. Comp. Endocrinol.*, 71, 307, 1988.

72. Towle, A. C. and Sze, P. Y., Steroid binding to synaptic plasma membrane: differential binding of glucocorticoids and gonadal steroids, *J. Steroid Biochem.*, 18, 135, 1983.

73. Pinter, J. and Thomas, P., Characterization of a progestogen receptor in the ovary of the spotted seatrout *Cynoscion nebulosus*, *Biol. Reprod.*, 52, 667, 1995a.

74. Pinter, J. and Thomas, P., The ovarian progestogen receptor in the spotted seatrout, *Cynoscion nebulosus*, demonstrates steroid specificity intermediate between progesterone and glucocorticoid receptors in other vertebrates, *J. Steroid Biochem. Mol. Biol.*, 60, 113, 1997.

75. Scatchard, G., The attractions of proteins for small molecules and ions, *Ann. N.Y. Acad. Sci.*, 51, 660, 1949.

76. Patiño, R. and Thomas, P., Effects of gonadotropin on ovarian intrafollicular processes during the development of oocyte maturational competence in a teleost, the Atlantic croaker: evidence for two distinct stages of gonadotropic control of final oocyte maturation, *Biol. Reprod.*, 43, 818, 1990b.

77. Thomas, P. and Patiño, R., Changes in 17α,20β,21-trihydroxy-4-pregnen-3-one membrane receptor concentrations in ovaries of spotted seatrout during final oocyte maturation, in *Proc. 4th Int. Symp. Reproductive Physiology of Fish*, Scott, A. P., Sumpter, J., Kime, D., and Rolge, M. S., Eds., University of East Anglia, 1991, 122.

78. Thomas, P., Hormonal control of final oocyte maturation in sciaenid fish, in *Perspectives in Comparative Endocrinology*, Davey, K. G., Peter, R. E., and Tobe, S. S., Eds., Nat. Res. Council Can., 1994, 619.

79. Birnbaum, C. S., The role of structure in the disposition of halogenated aromatic xenobiotics, *Environ. Health Perspect.*, G1, 11, 1985.

80. Antunes-Madeira, M. C., Almeida, L. M., and Madeira, V. M. C., Depth-dependent effects of DDT and lindane on the fluidity of native membranes and extracted lipids. Implications for mechanisms of toxicity, *Bull. Environ. Contam. Toxicol.*, 51, 787, 1993.

81. Osman, R. A., Andria, M. L., Jones, A. D., and Meizel, S., Steroid induced exocytosis: the human sperm acrosome reaction, *Biochem. Biophys. Res. Commun.*, 168, 828, 1989.

82. Sueldo, C. E., Oehinger, S., Subias, E., Mahony, M., Alexander, N. J., Burkman, L. J., and Acosta, A. A., Effect of progesterone on human zona pellucida sperm binding and oocyte penetrating capacity, *Fertil. Steril.*, 60, 137, 1993.

83. Blackmore, P. F., Fisher, J. F., Spilman, C. H., and Bleasdale, J. E., Unusual steroid specificity of the cell surface progesterone receptor on human sperm, *Mol. Pharmacol.*, 49, 727, 1996.

84. Baldi, E., Casano, R., Falseti, C., Krausz, C., Maggi, M., and Forti, G., Intracellular calcium accumulation and responsiveness to progesterone in capacitating human spermatozoa, *J. Androl.*, 12, 323, 1991.

85. Sabeur, K., Edwards, D. P., and Meizel, S., Human sperm plasma membrane progesterone receptor(s) and the acrosome reaction, *Biol. Reprod.*, 54, 993, 1996.

86. Baldi, E., Falsetti, C., Krausz, C., Gervasi, G., Carloni, V., Casano, R., and Forti, G., Stimulation of platelet-activating factor synthesis by progesterone and A23187 in human spermatozoa, *Biochem. J.*, 292, 209, 1993.

87. Blackmore, P. F., Rapid non-genomic actions of progesterone stimulate Ca^{2+} influx and the acrosome reaction in human sperm, *Cell. Signal.*, 5, 531, 1993.

88. Suarez, S. S. and Pollard, J. W., Capacitation, the acrosome reaction, and motility in mammalian sperm, in *Controls of Sperm Motility: Biological and Clinical Aspects*, Gagnon, C., Ed., CRC Press, Boca Raton, FL, 1990, 77.

89. Aitken, R. J., Buckingham, D. W., and Irvine, D. S., The extragenomic action of progesterone on human spermatozoa: evidence for a ubiquitous response that is down-regulated, *Endocrinology*, 137, 3999, 1996.

90. Meizel, S. and Turner, K. O., Progesterone acts at the plasma membrane of human sperm, *Mol. Cell. Endocrinol.*, 11, R1, 1991.

91. Blackmore, P. F. and Lattanzio, F. A., Cell surface localization of a novel non-genomic progesterone receptor on the head of human sperm, *Biochem. Biophys. Res. Commun.*, 181, 331, 1991.

92. Tesarik, J., Mendoza, C., Moos, J., and Carreras, A., Selective expression of a progesterone receptor on the human sperm surface, *Fertil. Steril.*, 58, 784, 1992.

93. Uhler, M. L., Leung, A., Chan, S. Y. W., and Wang, C., Direct effects of progesterone and antiprogesterone on human sperm hyperactivated motility and acrosome reaction, *Fertil. Steril.*, 58, 1191, 1992.

94. Yang, J., Serres, C., Philibert, D., Robel, P., Baulieu, E. E., and Jouannet, P., Progesterone and RU486: opposing effects on human sperm, *Proc. Natl. Acad. Sci. U.S.A.*, 1994, 529.

95. Thomas, P., Breckenridge-Miller, D., and Detweiler, C., Binding characteristics and regulation of the 17,20β, 21-trihydroxy-4-pregnen-3-one (20β-S) receptor on testicular and sperm plasma membranes of spotted seatrout (*Cynoscion nebulosus*), *Fish Physiol. Biochem.*, 17, 109, 1997.

96. Thomas, P., Das, S., Breckenridge-Miller, D., and Detweiler, C., Characterization and regulation of a progestin receptor on Atlantic croaker sperm membranes, in *Advances in Comparative Endocrinology*, Vol. II, Kawashima, S. and Kikuyama, S., Eds., Monduzzi Editore S.p.A., 1997, 1381.

97. Billard, R. and Cosson, M. P., The energetics of fish sperm motility, in *Controls of Sperm Motility: Biological and Clinical Aspects*, Gagnon, C., Ed., CRC Press, Boca Raton, FL, 1990, 153.

98. Miura, T., Yamauchi, K., Takahashi, H., and Nagahama, Y., The role of hormones in the acquisition of sperm motility in salmonid fish, *J. Exp. Zool.*, 261, 359, 1992.

99. Billard, R. and Cosson, M. P., Some problems related to the assessment of sperm motility in freshwater fish, *J. Exp. Zool.*, 261, 122, 1992.

100. Cosson, M. P., Billard, R., and Letellier, L., Rise of internal Ca^{2+} accompanies the initiation of trout sperm motility, *Cell. Motil. Cytoskel.*, 14, 424, 1989.

101. Detweiler, C. and Thomas, P., The role of ions and ion channels in the regulation of Atlantic croaker sperm motility, *J. Exp. Zool.*, 281, 139-148, 1998.

102. Donaldson, E. M. and Scherer, E., Methods to test and assess effects of chemicals on reproduction in fish, in *Methods for Assessing the Effects of Chemicals on Reproductive Functions*, Vouk, V. B. and Shelton, P. J., Eds., John Wiley & Sons, Chichester, 1983, 354.

103. Barlow, S. M. and Sullivan, F. M., *Reproductive Hazards of Industrial Chemicals*, Academic Press, London, 1982.

104. Kordon, C. and Drouva, S. V., Interplay between hypothalamic hormones and sex steroids in the control of neuroendocrine reproductive functions, in *Neuroendocrine Regulation of Reproduction*, Yen, S. S. C. and Vale, W. W., Eds., Serono Symposia, Norwell, MA, 1990, 259.

105. Kah, O., Anglade, I., Leperte, E., Dubourg, P., and de Monbrison, D., The reproductive brain in fish, *Fish Physiol. Biochem.*, 11, 85, 1993.

106. Malven, P. V., Gonadotropins in the female, in *Mammalian Neuroendocrinology*, CRC Press, Boca Raton, FL, 1993, chap. 11, 181.

107. Trudeau, V. L. and Peter, R. E., Functional interactions between neuroendocrine systems regulating GtH II release, in *Proc. Fifth Int. Symp. Reproductive Physiology of Fish*, Goetz, F. W. and Thomas, P., Eds., The University of Texas at Austin, Printing Department, Austin, 1995, 44.

108. Copeland, P. A. and Thomas, P. Control of gonadotropin release in the Atlantic croaker: evidence for lack of dopaminergic inhibition, *Gen. Comp. Endocrinol.*, 74, 474, 1989.

109. Copeland, P. A. and Thomas, P., Purification of maturational gonadotropin from Atlantic croaker (*Micropogonias undulatus*) and development of a homologous radioimmunoassay. *Gen. Comp. Endocrinol.*, 73, 425, 1989.

110. Khan, I. A. and Thomas, P., Stimulatory effects of serotonin on maturational gonadotropin release in the Atlantic croaker, *Micropogonias undulatus*, *Gen. Comp. Endocrinol.*, 88, 388, 1992.

111. Khan, I. A. and Thomas, P., Seasonal and daily variations in the plasma gonadotropin II response to a LHRH analog and serotonin in Atlantic croaker (*Micropogonias undulatus*): evidence for mediation by $5\text{-}HT_2$ receptors, *J. Exp. Zool.*, 269, 531, 1994.

112. Khan, I. A. and Thomas, P., Neuroendocrine control of gonadotropin II release in the Atlantic croaker: involvement of gamma-aminobutyric acid, in *Proc. Fifth Symp. Int. Reproductive Physiology of Fish*, Goetz, F. W. and Thomas, P., Eds., The University of Texas at Austin, Printing Department, Austin, 1995, 73.

113. Khan, I. A. and Thomas, P., Melatonin influences gonadotropin II secretion in the Atlantic croaker *(Micropogonias undulatus)*, *Gen. Comp. Endocrinol.*, 104, 231, 1996.

114. Vitale, M. L., Parisi, M. N., Chiocchio, S. R., and Tramezzani, J. H., Serotonin induces gonadotropin release through stimulation of LHRH release from the median eminence, *J. Endocrinol.*, 24, 309, 1986.

115. Khan, I. A. and Thomas, P., Immunocytochemical localization of serotonin and gonadotropin-releasing hormone in the brain and pituitary gland of the Atlantic croaker, *Micropogonias undulatus*, *Gen. Comp. Endocrinol.*, 91, 167, 1993.

116. Abel, E. L., *Lead and Reproduction, a Comprehensive Bibliography*, Greenwood Press, London, Conn., 1984, 117.

117. Pounds, J. G., Cory-Slechta, D. A., and Cranmer, J. M., Eds., *New Dimensions of Lead Neurotoxicity: Redefining Mechanisms and Effects*, Intox Press, Little Rock, Ark., 1993.

118. Thomas, P., Reproductive endocrine function in female Atlantic croaker exposed to xenobiotics, *Mar. Environ. Res.*, 24, 179, 1988.

119. Singh, A. and Ashraf, M., Neurotoxicity in rats sub-chronically exposed to low levels of lead, *Vet. Hum. Toxicol.*, 31, 21, 1989.

120. Katti, S. R. and Sathyanesan, A. G., Lead nitrate induces changes in brain constituents of the freshwater fish *Clarias batrachus* (L), *Neurotoxicology*, 7, 45, 1986.

121. Seegal, R. F., Bush, B., and Shain, W., Lightly chlorinated *ortho*-substituted PCB congeners decrease dopamine in nonhuman primate brain and in tissue culture, *Toxicol. Appl. Pharmacol.*, 106, 136, 1990.

122. Müller, W. F., Hobson, W., Fuller, G. B., Knauf, W., Coulston, F., and Konte, F., Endocrine effects of chlorinated hydrocarbons in rhesus monkeys, *Ecotox. Environ. Saf.*, 2, 161, 1978.

123. Jansen, H. T., Cooke, P. S., Porcelli, J., Liu, T-C., and Hansen, L. G., Estrogenic and antiestrogenic actions of PCBs in the female rat: *in vitro* and *in vivo* studies, *Reprod. Toxicol.*, 7, 237, 1993.
124. Wilson, C. A. and Leigh, A. J., Endocrine toxicology of the female reproductive system, in *Endocrine Toxicology*, Atterwill, C. K. and Flack, J. D., Eds., Cambridge University Press, 1992, 313.
125. Thomas, P., Effects of Aroclor 1254 and cadmium on reproductive endocrine function and ovarian growth in Atlantic croaker, *Mar. Environ. Res.*, 28, 499, 1989.
126. Chang, J. P. and Jobin, R. M., Regulation of gonadotropin release in vertebrates: a comparison of GnRH mechanisms of action, in *Perspectives in Comparative Endocrinology*, Davey, K. G., Peter, R. E., Tobe, S. S., Eds., National Research Council of Canada, Ottawa, 1994, 41.
127. Naor, Z., Signal transduction mechanisms of Ca^{2+} mobilization hormones: the case of gonadotropin releasing hormone, *Endocrinol. Rev.*, 11, 326, 1990.
128. Chang, J. P., Jobin, R. M., and Wong, A. O. L., Intracellular mechanisms mediating gonadotropin and growth hormone release in goldfish, *Carassius auratus*, *Fish Physiol. Biochem.*, 11, 25, 1993.
129. Pounds, J. G. The role of all calcium in current approaches to toxicology, *Environ. Health Perspect.*, 84, 7, 1990.
130. Van der Kraak, G. and Wade, M. G., Comparison of signal transduction pathways mediating gonadotropin actions in vertebrates, in *Perspectives in Comparative Endocrinology*, Davey, K. G., Peter, R. E., and Tobe, S. S., Eds., National Research Council of Canada, 1994, 59.
131. Adashi, E. Y. and Resnick, C. E., 3',5'-Cyclic monophosphate as an intracellular second messenger of luteinizing hormone: application of the forskolin criteria, *J. Cell. Biochem.*, 31, 317, 1986.
132. Singh, H. and Thomas, P., Mechanism of stimulatory action of growth hormone on ovarian steroidogenesis in spotted seatrout *Cynoscion nebulosus*, *Gen. Comp. Endocrinol.*, 89, 341, 1993.
133. Singhal, R. L., Testicular cyclic nucleotide and adrenal catecholamine metabolism following chronic exposure to cadmium, *Environ. Health Perspect.*, 38, 111, 1981.
134. Viarengo, A. and Nicotera, R., Possible role of Ca^{++} in heavy metal cytotoxicity, *Comp. Biochem. Physiol.*, 100E, 81, 1991.
135. Watson, C. S., Pappas, T. C., and Gametchu, B., The other estrogen receptor in the plasma membrane — implications for the actions of environmental estrogens, *Environ. Health Perspect.*, 103, Suppl. 7, 41, 1995.
136. Ramussen, H., Barrett, P., Smallwood, J., Bollag, W., and Isales, C., Calcium ion as intracellular messenger and cellular toxin, *Environ. Health Perspect.*, 84, 17, 1990.
137. Simons, T. J. B., Cellular interaction between lead and calcium, *Br. Med. Bull.*, 42, 431, 1986.
138. Fujusawa, H., Yamauchi, J. Nakata, H., and Okuno, S., Role of calmodulin in neurotransmitter synthesis, *Fed. Proc.*, 43, 3011, 1984.
139. Miller, J. J., Multiple calcium channels and neuronal function, *Science*, 235, 46, 1987.

2

Diethylstilbestrol (DES) and Environmental Estrogens Influence the Developing Female Reproductive System

Retha R. Newbold

CONTENTS

2.1 Introduction

Concern has increased that widespread adverse effects are occurring in humans, domestic animals, and wildlife populations as a result of exposure to environmental chemicals that possess endocrine disrupting activity.[1-3] Adverse long-term health consequences in women have been proposed to be linked to exposure to these endocrine-modulating chemicals; increased cancer rates in the breast, ovary, and uterus, as well as other reproductive tract abnormalities (endometriosis and subfertility/infertility) have been reported. Similarly, concerns regarding adverse effects in wildlife and

0-8493-3164-1/99/$0.00+$.50
© 1999 by CRC Press LLC

domestic animals have focused on observations regarding reproductive disorders involving the following endpoints: reduced fertility, reduced egg hatchability, reduced viability of offspring, slow growth rates, wasting and lower rates of activity in neonates, impaired hormone activity, and modified adult sexual behavior observed in various species, including birds, fish, alligators, panthers, and mink. Possible immune dysfunction has also been reported in dolphins, whales, and turtles.[3] All of these abnormalities may be caused by disruption of normal endocrine function in animals as a result of exposure to environmental chemicals that mimic the actions of naturally occurring hormones.[4-5]

In mammals and other vertebrates, hormones provide an essential role in regulating normal reproductive tract development and function.[6] For example, during differentiation and periods of high mitotic activity, hormones aide cell-to-cell communications; in addition, specific and coordinated cellular responses are directed by hormones in target tissues. In fact, it has long been known that hormones produced by one group of cells have the ability to direct and signal the course of development and response of another group of cells. Thus, steriod hormones have been identified as major players in regulating developmental processes in many tissues, in particular, the reproductive tract. Hormones accomplish their function of stimulating or inhibiting various pathways in cells by binding with receptor molecules. The hormone/receptor complex then interacts with DNA and with second-messenger systems to produce specific actions, such as protein synthesis and cAMP turnover. Environmental chemicals that mimic hormones can (a) duplicate the normal hormone process, or (b) they may also interact with the receptor causing an aberrant function, (c) they may interact synergistically or additively with natural hormones causing an exaggerated response, or (d) they may interact with the receptor and block hormone/receptor interactions, resulting in no function.

Disruption of normal endocrine function has been at the center of many toxicological studies focusing on reproductive toxicants for many years. However, a key issue involved with the recent concern regarding adverse effects of environmental endocrine-disrupting chemicals is that such effects may be caused by exposure to relatively small doses during a "unique window of vulnerability" for the fetus or neonate during development; these effects may not show up until much later in life.[7] Developmental exposures, in particular, are very difficult to monitor, since chemicals may exert their effects only at a specific time in differentiation and then disappear. So, using even the most sophisticated analytical procedures to detect minute amounts of chemicals may not associate a particular chemical exposure with an adverse outcome. Further difficulty in identifying suspect chemicals is complicated by the vast number of compounds that have been reported to have endocrine-disrupting effects.[4] For example, many man-made or generated chemicals used in industrial and household products, including pesticides and plasticizers, pharmaceuticals, and dietary supplements, as well as some naturally occurring substances such as phytoestrogens found in plants have endocrine-modulating activity.

Although difficulties in identifying chemicals and in showing an association with specific long-term effects still exist, ample concern remains that chemicals with endocrine-modulating activity are adversely affecting reproductive tract development and function. Although it has been assumed that after maturity exposure to endocrine disrupters does not permanently alter the function of hormone-responsive tissues, experimental animals studies have demonstrated permanent changes in brain[8] and vaginal tissues[9] in mature females after administration of estrogenic chemicals. Thus, chronic, low level exposure to estrogenic chemicals in the environment, even after maturity, can also have adverse effects in humans similar to those observed in estrogen-treated laboratory animals and, therefore, present a health risk. However, exposure of the fetus and/or neonate is of the utmost concern because of the increased susceptibility of this stage of development to environmental insults. Considering what is currently known about chemicals that can disrupt the endocrine system, their effects (1) may be manifested differently, and with permanent consequences, in the embryo, fetus, and neonate as compared to effects resulting from exposure to adults; (2) can alter the course of development for the exposed organism, with the outcome dependent on the specific developmental exposure periods; and (3) are often delayed and not recognized until the organism reaches maturity or perhaps even later in life, although the critical period of exposure occurred during embryonic, fetal, or neonatal life.

As an example, the profound effects of estrogens on the developing reproductive tract have been demonstrated by prenatal exposure to the synthetic estrogen, diethylstilbestrol (DES).[10]

2.2 The DES Paradigm for Adverse Effects of Developmental Exposure to Environmental Estrogens

While it is an increasing concern that chemicals in the environment like kepone, methoxychlor, DDT, and its metabolites that have hormonal activity may be exerting adverse effects at low levels of environmental exposure, the scientific community has had a long history with teratogenic and carcinogenic effects of synthetic estrogenic compounds. For centuries, it has been recognized that the ovary controlled the estrous cycle but not until the early twentieth century were the biologically active substances produced by the ovary described. The term "estrogens" was coined for these substances because of their ability to induce estrus in animals. The physiological, biochemical, and pharmacological properties of estrogens were extensively studied by many laboratories, and the search for a synthetic substitute immediately followed. Diethylstilbestrol (DES), a nonsteroidal compound with properties similar to the natural female sex hormone, estradiol, was synthesized in 1938. This potent synthetic estrogen was specifically designed for its estrogenic activity. Like many of today's environmental estrogens, DES was not structurally similar to the natural estrogens.[4] In fact, early research with DES demonstrated that compounds with diverse structures could exhibit similar biological functions associated with estrogens. A historical account of the development and use of DES and the early search for compounds with estrogenic activity has been summarized.[11] DES also demonstrated another significant point, the potential toxic effects of estrogens. These well-documented effects in DES-exposed humans justify the concern regarding developmental exposure to other environmental estrogens and endocrine disruptors.

For almost 30 years, physicians prescribed DES to women with high risk pregnancies to prevent spontaneous abortions and other complications of pregnancy. Unfortunately, in 1971, a report associated DES with a rare form of reproductive tract cancer termed "vaginal adenocarcinoma," which was detected in a small number of adolescent daughters of women who had taken the drug while pregnant. DES also was linked to more frequent benign reproductive tract problems in an estimated 95% of the DES-exposed daughters; reproductive organ dysfunction, abnormal pregnancies, reduction in fertility, immune system disorders, and periods of depression were reported. Similarly, the DES-exposed male offspring demonstrated structural, functional, and cellular abnormalities following prenatal exposure; hypospadias, microphallus, retained testes, inflammation, and decreased fertility were reported.[10] DES became one of the first examples of an estrogenic toxicant in humans; it was shown to cross the placenta and induce a direct effect on the developing fetus. Although DES is no longer used clinically to prevent miscarriage, a major concern remains that when DES-exposed women age and reach the time at which the incidence of reproductive organ cancers normally increase, they will show a much higher incidence of cancer than unexposed individuals. Further, the possibility of second generation effects has been suggested,[12-14] which puts still another generation at risk for developing problems associated with the DES treatment of their grandmothers. Thus, the DES episode continues to be a serious health concern and remains a reminder of the potential toxicities that can be caused by hormonally active chemicals.

Questions about the mechanisms involved in DES-induced teratogenic and carcinogenic effects prompted us to develop an experimental animal model to study the adverse effects of estrogens and other endocrine-disrupting chemicals on reproductive tract development and differentiation. The murine animal model has successfully replicated and predicted many adverse effects observed in women with similar DES exposure (Table 2.1). Some of the most significant effects are discussed with the expectation that

TABLE 2.1

Some Comparative Effects of DES in Women and Mice
Following Developmental Exposure

- Structural malformation of the oviduct, uterus, cervix, and vagina
- Salpingitis isthmica nodosa (SIN) of the oviduct
- Paraovarian cysts (mesonephric origin)
- Vaginal adenocarcinoma

these findings might provide useful information pertinent to the evaluation of the possible adverse effects of other environmental estrogenic compounds.

2.3 The DES Animal Model to Study Human Disease

The prenatal DES exposure model uses pregnant, outbred CD-1 mice that are treated subcutaneously with DES dissolved in corn oil on days 9 through 16 of gestation. The doses of DES range from 0.01 to 100 µg/kg maternal body weight. The highest dose of DES is equal to or less than that given therapeutically to pregnant women, and the lower DES doses are comparable to exposure to weak estrogenic compounds found in the environment. Pregnant mice deliver their young on day 19 of gestation, and their offspring are followed for up to 24 months of age. The time of *in utero* DES exposure for the offspring encompasses the major period of organogenesis of the genital tract in the mouse. While many developmental events in the genital tract continue into neonatal life for the mouse, similar differentiation events occur entirely prenatally in humans.[15] In both species, however, early in the normal development of the reproductive tract of an embryo, there is an undifferentiated stage in which the sex of the embryo cannot be determined. At this stage, the gonads have not developed into either testis or ovary, and all embryos have a double set of genital ducts, Müllerian (paramesonephric) and Wolffian (mesonephric) ducts. In the female, as sex differentiation occurs, the Müllerian ducts differentiate into the oviduct, uterus, cervix, and upper vagina, while the mesonephric duct regresses. In the male, under the influence of testicular secretions, the mesonephric ducts form the epididymis, vas deferens, and other tissues such as the seminal vesicles, while the Müllerian ducts regress. Exposure to DES during this critical period of sex differentiation resulted in alterations in both the female and male reproductive tract, including the partial or complete retention of the opposite duct system in both sexes. Although adverse effects are demonstrated in both sexes, only changes in developmentally DES-exposed females will be further discussed. Resulting abnormalities in the females include structural, functional, and long-term changes throughout all regions of the reproductive tract.[16,17]

TABLE 2.2

Effect of Prenatal Exposure to DES on the Fertility
of Female Offspring[a]

Treatment (μg/kg/d)	Number of Females	Total # of Young Per Mouse Over Breeding Period[b]
Control	83	73.8 ± 2.5[c]
DES-0.01	64	66.5 ± 2.7
DES-1.0	61	55.4 ± 2.6
DES-2.5	21	39.9 ± 4.3
DES-5.0	20	18.3 ± 4.4
DES-10	67	3.1 ± 0.8
DES-100	40	1.8 ± 0.7

[a] Female mice exposed prenatally to DES (0.01–100 μg/kg maternal body weight/d) on days 9-16 of gestation were bred when they were sexually mature to control male mice.

[b] Breeding period was for 32 weeks.

[c] Mean ± standard error.

From McLachlan, J. A., Newbold, R. R., Shah, H. C., Hogan, M. D., and Dixon, R., *Fertil. Steril.*, 38(3), 364, 1982. With permission.

2.3.1   Reproductive Tract Dysfunction

Poor reproductive outcome has been reported in humans,[10] and subfertility and infertility have been reported in animals[18] following developmental exposure to DES. For mice, reproductive tract dysfunction was assessed in the DES-exposed animal model by breeding prenatal DES-exposed female mice to control untreated male mice using a continuous breeding protocol.[18] The breeding study showed that prenatal exposure to varying doses of DES (0.01 to 100 μg/kg maternal body weight) resulted in a striking dose-related decrease in the fertility of the offspring (Table 2.2). Over the 32-week breeding period, the effects ranged from minimal subfertility (90% of controls at the lowest DES dose) to essential sterility at the two highest DES doses (10 and 100 μg/kg). It was interesting to note that exposure to DES at the lowest dose (0.01 μg/kg maternal body weight), which was chosen as an environmentally relative dose, showed a decrease in fertility approximately midway through the study.[18] This may represent an example of early reproductive senescence at low dose exposures. The mechanisms responsible for the subfertility in the female mice exposed to DES *in utero* were the result of multiple factors: oviductal malformation; ovarian dysfunction; altered uterine environment and reproductive tract secretions; uterine, cervical, and vaginal structural alterations. Taken together, these alterations establish the fact that exposure to DES, even at relatively low levels, impairs reproductive capacity throughout the animal's lifetime. Numerous reports of altered pregnancy outcomes in young women exposed *in utero* to DES, as well as accidental exposure of wildlife to DES, resulting in infertility, demonstrate the importance of these similar findings in the DES-exposed mouse model, and suggest that other environmental estrogens may also play a role in decreased female fertility. Specific alterations in reproductive tract tissues are further discussed in more detail.

2.3.2 Ovary

Unquestionably, the ovary is a target for perturbation by DES and other environmental estrogenic compounds. While the ovary is itself a direct target for these toxicants,[19,20] the hypothalamic/pituitary axis also may be disturbed by exposure to DES, which may manifest as ovarian/reproductive tract dysfunction. Increased inflammation, early depletion of follicles, multi-ovular follicles, decreased number of corpora lutea, altered gonadotropin levels, increased number of ovarian cysts, increased interstitial compartment, and ovarian tumors were observed in the developmentally exposed DES mice and were likely contributors to reproductive dysfunction in this animal model. These data of ovarian toxicity in the prenatal DES experimental animal model support the contention that chemical endocrine disrupters may indeed be related to decreases in fertility later in life. It also suggests that an association with developmental exposure to endocrine-disrupting chemicals and ovarian tumors reported to be on the rise in the general population is a possibility.

2.3.3 Oviduct

The association of prenatal exposure to DES and the development of abnormalities in the oviduct was a common finding. For example, a teratogenic defect noticeable at birth in the DES-exposed offspring was a malformation of the oviduct observed in 100% of the high dose DES animals.[21]

Marked differences in structural development were observed when oviductal differentiation in prenatal DES-exposed animals was compared to control animals. The oviductal segment of the Müllerian duct normally differentiated late on gestational day 16 for this strain of mouse with a narrowing of the cranial portion of the duct. On day 17 of gestation, the Müllerian duct developed slight undulations in the oviductal region and then a series of loose, wavy folds followed by deep coils. Following birth (day 19 of gestation), the oviduct was identifiable as a discrete region of the Müllerian duct, and its caudal limits were demarcated by an enlargement of the uterine segment by day 1 of neonatal life. By postnatal day 10, the ovary rotated into the position it occupied in adult life, and the oviduct increased in length and diameter, resulting in tightly packed coils.

In contrast, DES treatment retarded oviductal morphogenesis in mice exposed *in utero*. Differences were readily apparent by neonatal day 1 when normal Müllerian duct coiling was absent in DES-treated female offspring.

Differences became more obvious during postnatal development of the reproductive tract because the oviduct in DES-treated mice failed to lengthen or coil and retained a fetal-like appearance. In those animals exposed to DES *in utero*, the ovary did not rotate, and there was little or no demarcation between the oviduct and the uterus. Also, the angle of entry of the oviduct into the uterus was altered; the oviduct appeared to join the uterus at its apex and formed a straight tube. This oviductal malformation was observed in all of the females treated prenatally with 100 µg/kg maternal body weight of DES but was never observed in any control animals. Animals exposed to doses less than 100 µg/kg showed less extensive malformation with fewer coils being the most prominent feature; the lowest DES dose did not result in any apparent structural changes in the oviduct.

Oviductal malformations observed in DES-dosed animals persisted throughout the lifetime of the animal and permanently distorted the anatomical relationship with the uterus, oviduct, and ovary. The retention of this fetal anatomical location suggested the term "developmentally arrested oviduct," which was used to describe this phenomenon.[21] The use of this term was supported by the relative lack of growth of the oviductal segment of the reproductive tract. Although body weights of the prenatal DES-treated and control mice were similar at maturity (38 g vs. 36 g, respectively), the average length of the oviducts from DES-treated females was only about half that of control females.

The experimental DES-exposed animal model clearly established the oviduct as a target for the teratogenic effects of DES. Moreover, the arrest in development resulting from prenatal exposure to DES suggests a role for estrogens in the normal morphogenesis of the oviduct. It is possible that an increase in estrogen levels during oviductal development may play a role in the ultimate structural or functional integrity of this tissue in humans, as well as mice. In fact, some of the more important features of the "developmentally-arrested oviduct" in mice exposed prenatally to DES, such as decreased oviductal length, relative lack of fimbriae, and abnormal anatomical location, have been described in women exposed to DES during gestation.[22] Thus, altered or arrested development of the mammalian oviduct appears to be a general biological consequence of prenatal exposure to DES. A recent report has described molecular mechanisms associated with this developmental arrest.[23] Estrogens were shown to regulate the expression of important homeobox genes during development; expression of the homeobox gene Hoxa-9 corresponds to oviductal, Hoxa-10 corresponds to cervical, and Hoxa-11 corresponds to uterine differentiation events. DES was demonstrated to downregulate the expression of these homeobox genes during Mullerian duct differentiation, resulting in malformed reproductive structures.[23] Other environmental estrogens may similarly downregulate these specific genes if exposure occurs during critical stages of differentiation, leading to malformations and dysfunction of the reproductive tract.

Functional alterations were also characteristic of the malformed oviducts.[21] Dye injected into the uterine lumen of DES-treated females could pass readily into the oviduct and ovarian bursa. However, when dye was injected into the uterus of control mice, a uterotubal valve inhibited the retrograde flow of dye back into the lumen of the oviduct. This experiment indicated that the uterotubal junction was not functioning in DES-exposed mice to retain the dye in the uterus. Considering the extensive malformation of the oviduct and uterus in the mice exposed prenatally to high doses of DES, the passage of dye readily from the lumen of the uterus to the oviduct was not surprising. This missing barrier for the mouse may be a factor in the increased inflammation observed in the ovary and oviduct as the mice aged.[19] Although structural variation exists among species in the uterotubal junction region, malformations have also been reported in DES-exposed women.

In addition, cellular defects in the oviduct of DES-exposed mice likely contributed to functional abnormalities. Microscopic alterations in oviductal epithelium accompanied the structural teratogenicity associated with prenatal DES treatment.[24] In control mice, histological differentiation of the oviduct coincided with morphogenic development; the epithelium showed increased cell height, pseudostratification, and evidence of secretory activity. In contrast, histological differentiation was halted in DES-treated mice; one example was the fimbriae, which developed only minimally. In the ampulla of the oviduct of both control and DES-treated animals, ciliated and secretory columnar cells were commonly observed. However, in DES-treated animals, the arrangement of the columnar cells lining the oviductal lumen and the mucosal folds were very irregular. Further, "gland formation" was observed in the oviduct of DES-exposed animals, which extended through the muscularis, a histological feature never observed in control mice.[24] Epithelial hyperplasia was often noted, and inflammatory changes were more prevalent in all segments of the oviduct of DES-treated animals as compared to controls.

The histologic changes in DES-exposed mice, i.e., epithelial hyperplasia and gland formation (diverticuli) of the oviductal mucosa that extend into the muscle wall, resemble the clinically described lesion, salpingitis isthmica nodosa (SIN). Since its description in the late 1800s, the etiology and pathogenesis of salpingitis isthmica nodosa had been the subject of much debate. Clinically, this lesion had been related to ectopic tubal pregnancy and infertility. The data obtained from the experimental DES-exposed animal model raise the possibility that clinically noted cases of salpingitis isthmica nodosa can result from an altered hormonal environment during early development. This is supported by the report describing salpingitis isthmica nodosa in the oviduct of young women exposed prenatally to DES.[25]

While the mechanisms for regulating normal differentiation and development of the reproductive tract remain largely unknown, the alterations observed in the oviduct following developmental exposure to DES provide an excellent opportunity to study factors involved in the regulation and differentiation of Müllerian duct-derived epithelium. Although the observed changes appear to reside in the epithelium, it is not clear whether the epithelium is responding independently or in combination with factors from the underlying stroma. Since the connective tissue in these DES-treated mice is relatively thin and hypoplastic, it may have been a defect in the stromal compartment that modified the epithelial response.

Finally, considering these observations in the oviduct of DES-treated mice, it is possible that the proliferative capacity of the epithelium in Müllerian duct-derived tissues (oviduct, uterus, cervix, and upper vagina) may be determined by hormonal exposure during development. If estrogen levels are significantly elevated, as with prenatal DES treatment of animals and humans, the proliferative capacity of the reproductive tract epithelium may be permanently altered. The clinical lesion of salpingitis isthmica nodosa, where the oviductal epithelium possesses an increased capacity for proliferation and forming "gland-like structures" capable of penetrating the muscle layer, may be an example.

2.3.4 Mesonephric Duct Remnants

The mesonephric system, which normally regresses during differentiation of the female reproductive tract,[15] was also affected by prenatal DES exposure. Cystic paraovarian structures between the ovary and oviduct were often observed, especially in the high dose DES-exposed animals. The cysts were predominantly localized in the region of the ovarian hilus, which was consistent with the location of mesonephric remnants. Mesonephric cysts of the magnitude observed in DES-exposed animals were never observed in control animals. The arrangement and location of the multiple cysts often observed in the DES animal model were similar to the multiple cysts described in a woman prenatally exposed to DES.[26] Whether adverse effects on the mesonephric system are specific for DES or are a common finding for other hormonally active compounds merits further study.

2.3.5 Uterus, Cervix, and Vagina

In addition to the oviduct, structural changes were observed in other regions of the reproductive tract. The uterus was a frequent target of DES-induced toxic effects. Following prenatal exposure to the high DES dose (100 µg/kg), the uterus of immature animals was smaller in diameter and length as compared to control untreated females of the same age. Histological changes in the immature DES-exposed uterus included a poorly organized muscle compartment and decreased gland formation. In response to estrogen stimulation, immature mice exposed to high doses of DES during prenatal development displayed decreased uterine growth response, decreased uterine luminal fluid quantity and protein concentration, alterations in specific uterine luminal proteins, and altered cellular differentiation (squamous metaplasia). Altered cellular responses were also observed in lower DES dose groups, but the responses were different. Structural hypoplasia of the uterus and decreased responsiveness of the uterus to an estrogen challenge remained common features throughout the life of the high dose prenatally DES-exposed animals. In aged prenatal DES-exposed females, cystic endometrial hyperplasia and squamous metaplasia in hypoplastic uterine structures were frequently found. Also, a low incidence of benign (leiomyomas) and malignant (adenocarcinoma, stromal cell sarcoma) tumors was observed in prenatally DES-exposed mice.[27] The low incidence of malignant uterine tumors following prenatal DES exposure is in contrast to the high prevalence seen after exposure to DES on neonatal days 1-5; modifying the DES animal model to test for sensitivity in the neonatal period, a time which corresponds to developmental events that are still occurring prenatally in humans, results in ~95% of the mice (≥18 months of age) developing uterine adenocarcinoma. These two exposure periods (prenatal and neonatal) for the mouse point out the unique sensitivity of the uterus to perturbation with estrogenic substances if exposure occurs during critical stages of differentiation.

In the cervico-vaginal region of the prenatally DES-exposed animals, striking structural abnormalities were also observed. All of the prenatal DES animals (100 µg/kg) showed enlargement in the cervical area of the reproductive tract. Further, in some of the severely affected cases, the Müllerian ducts did not fuse in the cervix to form a common cervical canal. In other less severe cases, the cervix was short cranio-caudally, but it still had an enlarged diameter, both internal and external, with increased stromal elements. The epithelial mucosa of the cervix had fewer folds, and those that were present were less convoluted and shallower than the folds observed in control tissues. Also, the vaginal fornix was shallower in prenatally DES-exposed animals as compared to controls; in a low percentage of prenatal DES-exposed animals, the fornix was entirely absent.[28] Prominent mesonephric remnants also were observed in the cervico-vaginal region as described in the oviduct.[28]

In addition to oviductal, uterine, and cervical abnormalities, the vagina demonstrated multiple alterations following prenatal DES exposure. Aged prenatal DES-treated animals (100 µg/kg) had excessive vaginal keratinization that often extended into the cervix. The vaginal epithelium of these DES animals was composed of many layers of immature and mature cells covered by sheets of keratin. Leukocytes were seen in the superficial layers of the vagina of many animals. In some animals, increased keratinization combined with basal cell hyperplasia resulted in irregular pegs of epithelium, which extended into the subadjacent stroma. In 25% of the 12- to 18-month-old prenatal DES-exposed mice, epidermoid tumors of the vagina were observed. Excessive keratinization, epithelial pegs, and epidermoid tumors were not usually observed in the vagina of animals exposed to doses of DES lower than 100 µg/kg and were never observed in control untreated animals.

The benign lesion, vaginal adenosis, was seen in 75% of the mice exposed to DES on days 1–5 of neonatal life, but it was not a common finding in mice treated prenatally with DES.[28] The often-cited DES-associated neoplastic lesion, vaginal adenocarcinoma, was observed after prenatal DES exposure but not after neonatal exposure. Although vaginal adenocarcinoma is an extremely rare tumor in both animals and humans, it is considered a hallmark lesion of DES exposure.[10] The development of vaginal adenocarcinoma has been thought to originate from an alteration in the cellular differentiation of the Müllerian duct epithelium. However, the relationship of vaginal adenosis and adenocarcinoma remains unclear. Since neonatal mouse studies show a high incidence of vaginal adenosis but no cases of vaginal adenocarcinoma, the demonstration of vaginal adenocarcinoma in the prenatal DES-exposed animal model that shows a low incidence of adenosis suggests that the stage of cellular differentiation at the time of DES exposure may be the most critical event in the final expression of these abnormalities. By necessity, experimental animal models that are developed to study toxicity of various chemicals should encompass both prenatal and neonatal reproductive tract differentiation, especially since the corresponding developmental events occur entirely prenatally in humans.

Additional structural malformations were observed in the lower reproductive tract. Urethral openings, abnormally located anterior to the vulva (persistent urogenital sinus) were seen in some of the animals exposed prenatally to 100 µg/kg of DES (female hypospadias). "Gland-like structures" associated with this abnormality were assumed to be of urothelial origin. Female hypospadias have also been reported in the DES-exposed human population.

Taken together, the alterations observed throughout all regions of the murine reproductive tract demonstrate that exposure to estrogenic compounds during critical stages of sex differentiation results in adverse structural, functional, and long-term consequences. The long-term changes in these tissues include various lesions, some of which are neoplastic. The natural history and the mechanisms involved in the induction and progression of the lesions are critical issues for continued study.

In summary, the developmentally DES-exposed mouse model has provided some useful comparisons to similarly DES-exposed women.[17] The finding of the extremely rare lesion, vaginal adenocarcinoma, in prenatally DES-exposed mice alone recommends the mouse model for the study of human disease. Continued investigation into the range of DES-induced abnormalities observed in the mouse model using prenatal and/or neonatal exposures will offer a better understanding of the developmental events and the mechanisms involved in the chemical disruption of reproductive tract differentiation and resulting toxicities.

2.4 Potential Mechanisms

Numerous studies have demonstrated that developmental exposure to DES interferes with the normal differentiation of the Müllerian duct and the regression of the Wolffian duct. Although the mechanisms are not completely understood, a molecular component in the malformation of the tissues and perhaps in the cellular changes may be responsible. Recent studies by Maas et al.,[23] discussed earlier, suggest a molecular mechanism responsible for the structural alterations observed in oviduct, uterus, cervix, and vagina. Cellular changes also may be closely linked to these structural alterations. Furthermore, permanent abnormal gene imprinting has been described,[29] in which neonatal exposure to DES causes demethylation of an estrogen-responsive gene in the mouse uterus. The relationship of this finding to tumor induction is being investigated.

The role of the estrogen receptor (ER) in the induction of abnormalities and tumors following developmental exposure to DES has also been studied by using transgenic mice which overexpress ER (MT-mER). Transgenic ER mice were treated with DES during neonatal life and were followed as they aged. It was hypothesized that because of the abnormal expression of the ER, the reproductive tract tissues of the MT-mER mice may be more susceptible to tumors after neonatal exposure to DES. In fact, it is interesting to note that mice overexpressing the ER were at a higher risk of developing abnormalities, including uterine adenocarcinoma, in response to neonatal DES as compared to DES-treated wild type mice; at 8 months, 73% of the DES-treated MT-mER mice compared to 46% of the DES-treated wild type mice had uterine adenocarcinoma. Further, these abnormalities occurred at an earlier age as compared to wild type DES mice.[30] The transgenic mouse studies suggest that the level of ER present in a tissue may be a determining factor in the development of estrogen-related tumors. The specific role in the induction and progression of the lesions requires additional study. Additional transgenic mouse models that express variant forms of the ER or the ER knockout, as well as, experimental models contructed with the new ERβ, will also aid in determining the role of the ER in the development of these reproductive lesions. Since various estrogenic compounds have been reported to bind preferentially to either ERα or ERβ, these models will be essential in extrapolating human health risks to environmental estrogen exposures.

2.5 Summary and Conclusions

Sufficient evidence has been accumulated through the years by many laboratories to show that exposure of the developing fetus to exogenous estrogens adversely affects the differentiation of the genital tract. Data demonstrate that reproductive tract structure and function are altered, and long-term changes occur, including both benign and malignant cellular abnormalities. Cellular changes were seen in aged DES-exposed females at all doses examined; the degree of severity of specific lesions was dose related. Although fertility was decreased in mice in a dose-dependent manner after developmental estrogen exposure at all doses tested, a decrease in fertility was observed in low dose estrogen-exposed animals only later in life. These data suggest that fertility may not be a sensitive marker of reproductive toxicants in mice exposed to low levels of endocrine disrupters until they age. Similarly, male offspring exposed developmentally to low doses of DES did not show altered fertility early in life but were still susceptible to increased reproductive tract tumors later in life.[31] In combination, these data suggest that estrogenic substances occurring in the environment at low levels may adversely affect fertility later in life, but of further concern, they may have additional long-term consequences, including neoplasia, that warrant attention. While reports of inverted dose-response curves, which suggest enhanced response at low dose levels, remain in debate,[32] the DES animal model provides the opportunity to test this possibility. Low dose DES exposure was associated with reproductive tract dysfunction and long-term abnormalities.

While animal studies must be considered carefully if extrapolation to humans is to follow, the DES-exposed mouse model has provided some interesting comparisons to similarly exposed humans. The model has replicated and predicted many of the lesions observed in DES-exposed women. Although DES is a potent estrogen, it continues to provide markers of the adverse effects of exposure to estrogenic and other endocrine-disrupting substances during development, whether these exposures come from naturally occurring chemicals, synthetic or environmental contaminants, or pharmaceutical agents. Although chemicals not associated with hormone-mimicking activity may be involved indirectly or directly in reproductive tract toxicities, by far the most common culprits are those substances demonstrating endocrine-modulating effects. Further, mature animals may experience adverse effects to these chemicals, but the developing organism is particularly sensitive to perturbation by these compounds and often experiences permanent, long-lasting consequences. Ongoing mechanistic studies will help identify potential female reproductive toxicants and will help to better assess the risks of exposure to endocrine-disrupting chemicals in the environment if chemical exposures occur during critical stages of development.

Acknowledgments

The author is greatly indebted to Ms. Wendy Jefferson and Elizabeth Padilla-Burgos for skillful technical expertise in the conduct of the DES experiments and their critical editorial comments in the preparation of this paper. The author also thanks Dr. Michael Shelby for his helpful comments and his review of the paper. Finally, the long-standing association with Dr. John McLachlan and his invaluable contribution to the field of environmental estrogens is gratefully acknowledged.

References

1. Colborn, T. and Clement, C., *Chemically-Induced Alterations in Sexual and Functional Development: The Wildlife/Human Connection*, Princeton Scientific Publishing Co., Princeton, NJ, 1992.
2. Colborn, T., vom Saal, F. S., and Soto, A. M., Developmental effects of endocrine-disrupting chemicals in wildlife and humans, *Environ. Health Perspect.*, 101, 378, 1993.
3. Colborn, T., Dumanski, D., and Myers, J. P., *Our Stolen Future*, Penguin Books, Inc., New York, 1996.
4. McLachlan, J. A., *Estrogens in the Environment*, Elsevier Science Publ. Co., New York, 1985.
5. McLachlan, J. A., Functional toxicology: a new approach to detect biologically active xenobiotics. *Environ. Health Perspect.*, 101, 386, 1993.
6. George, F. W. and Wilson, J. D., Sex determination and differentiation, in *The Physiology of Reproduction*, Knobil, E., Neil, J. D., Ewing, L. L., Greenwald, G. S., Markert, C. L., Pfaff, D. W., Eds., Raven Press, New York, 1988, 3.
7. Bern, H., The fragile fetus, in *Chemically-Induced Alterations in Sexual and Functional Development: The Wildlife/Human Connection*, Colborn, T. and Clement, C., Eds., Princeton Scientific Publ., Princeton, NJ, 1992, 9.
8. Brawer, J. R., Naftolin, F., Martin, J., and Sonnenschein, C., Effects of a single injection of estradiol valerate on the hypothalamic arcuate nucleus and on reproductive tract function in the rat, *Endocrinology*, 103, 501, 1978.
9. Adler, A. J. and Nelson, J. F., Aging and chronic estradiol exposure impair estradiol-induced cornification but not proliferation of vaginal epithelium in C57Bl/6J mice, *Biol. Reprod.*, 38, 175, 1988.
10. Herbst, A. L. and Bern, H. A., *Developmental Effects of Diethylstilbestrol (DES) in Pregnancy*, Thieme-Stratton, New York, 1981.
11. Newbold, R. R. and McLachlan, J. A., Transplacental hormonal carcinogenesis: diethylstilbestrol as an example, in *Cellular and Molecular Mechanisms of Hormonal Carcinogenesis*, Huff, J., Boyd, J., and Barrett, J. C., Eds., Wiley-Liss, New York, 1996, 131.
12. Turusov, V. S., Trukhanova, L. S., Parfenov, Y. D., and Tomatis, L., Occurrence of tumors in descendants of CBA male mice prenatally treated with diethylstilbestrol, *Intl. J. Cancer*, 50, 131, 1992.
13. Walker, B. E., Intensity of multigenerational carcinogenesis from diethylstilbestrol in mice, *Carcinogenesis*, 18, 791, 1997.
14. Newbold, R. R., Hanson, R. B., Jefferson, W. N., Bullock, B. C., Haseman, J., and McLachlan, J. A., Increased tumors but uncompromised fertility in the female descendants of mice exposed developmentally to diethylstilbestrol, *Carcinogenesis*, 19(9), 1655, 1998.

15. Tuchmann-Duplessis, H. and Haegel, P., *Illustrated Human Embryology,* Springer Verlag, New York, 1982.
16. Newbold, R. R. and McLachlan, J. A., Diethylstilbestrol associated defects in murine genital tract development, in *Estrogens in the Environment,* McLachlan, J. A., Ed., Elsevier Science Publ. Co., New York, 1985, 288.
17. Newbold, R. R., Cellular and molecular effects of developmental exposure to diethylstilbestrol: implications for other environmental estrogens, *Environ. Health Perspect.,* 103, 83, 1995.
18. McLachlan, J. A., Newbold, R. R., Shah, H. C., Hogan, M. D., and Dixon, R. L., Reduced fertility in female mice exposed transplacentally to diethylstilbestrol (DES), *Fertil. Steril.,* 38(3), 364, 1982.
19. Newbold, R. R., Bullock, B. C., and McLachlan, J. A., Exposure to diethylstilbestrol during pregnancy permanently alters the ovary and oviduct, *Biol. Reprod.,* 28, 735, 1983.
20. Haney, A. F., Newbold, R. R., and McLachlan, J. A., Prenatal DES exposure in the mouse; effects on ovarian histology and steroidogenesis *in vitro, Biol. Reprod.,* 30, 471, 1984.
21. Newbold, R. R., Tyrey, S., Haney, A. F., and McLachlan, J. A., Developmentally arrested oviduct: a structural and functional defect in mice following prenatal exposure to diethylstilbestrol, *Teratology,* 27, 417, 1983.
22. DeCherney, A. H., Cholst, I., and Naftolin, F., Structure and function of the fallopian tubes following exposure to diethylstilbestrol (DES) during gestation, *Fertil. Steril.,* 36, 741, 1981.
23. Ma, L., Benson, G., Lim, H., Dey, S. K., and Maas, R. L., Abdominal B(AbdB) Hoxa genes: regulation in adult uterus by estrogen and progesterone and repression in mullerian duct by the synthetic estrogen DES, *Biol. Reprod.,* 1972(2), 141, 1998.
24. Newbold, R. R., Bullock, B. C., and McLachlan, J. A., Animal model of human disease: diverticulosis and salpingitis isthmica nodosa (SIN) of the fallopian tube: estrogen-induced diverticulosis and SIN of the mouse oviduct, *Am. J. Pathol.,* 117, 333, 1984.
25. Shen, S. C., Bansal, M., Purrazzella, R., Malviya, V., and Stiauss, L., Benign glandular inclusions in lymph nodes, endosalpingiosis, and salpingitis isthmica nodosa in a young girl with clear cell adenocarcinoma of the cervix, *Am. J. Surg. Pathol.,* 1, 293, 1983.
26. Haney, A. F., Newbold, R. R., Fetter, B. F., and McLachlan, J. A., Paraovarian cysts associated with prenatal diethylstilbestrol exposure: comparison of the human with a mouse model, *Am. J. Pathol.,* 124, 405, 1986.
27. McLachlan, J. A., Newbold, R. R., and Bullock, B. C., Long-term effects on the female mouse genital tract associated with prenatal exposure to diethylstilbestrol, *Cancer Res.,* 40, 3988, 1980.
28. Newbold, R. R. and McLachlan, J. A., Vaginal adenosis and adenocarcinoma in mice exposed prenatally or neonatally to diethylstilbestrol, *Cancer Res.,* 42, 2003, 1982.
29. Li, S., Washburn, K. A., Moore, R., Uno, T., Teng, C., Newbold, R. R., McLachlan, J. A., and Negishi, M., Developmental exposure to diethylstilbestrol elicits demethylation of the estrogen responsive lactoferrin gene in the mouse uterus, *Cancer Res.,* 57(19), 4356, 1997.

30. Couse, J. F., Davis, V. L., Hanson, R. B., Jefferson, W. N., McLachlan, J. A., Bullock, B. C., Newbold, R. R., and Korach, K. S., Accelerated onset of uterine tumors in transgenic mice with aberrant expression of the estrogen receptor after neonatal exposure to diethylstilbestrol, *Mol. Carcinogenesis*, 19, 230, 1997.
31. Newbold, R. R., Hanson, R. B., Jefferson, W. N., Bullock, B. C., Haseman, J., and McLachlan, J. A., Increased tumors in the male descendants of mice exposed developmentally to diethylstilbestrol, *Intl. J. Canc.*, (submitted).
32. Sheehan, D. M. and vom Saal, F. S., Low dose effects of endocrine disruptors — a challenge for risk assessment, *Risk Policy Report*, September 19, 1997.

3

Ovotoxic Environmental Chemicals: Indirect Endocrine Disruptors

Patricia B. Hoyer

CONTENTS

0-8493-3164-1/99/$0.00+$.50

3.1   Introduction

Reproductive function in women can be compromised by exposure to toxic chemicals.[1] Recently many couples have postponed the start of a family because of the women pursuing careers. This trend has enhanced an awareness of chemicals in the workplace and environment and their impact on the life span of reproductive function. A variety of considerations can affect fertility in women who are older when they begin a family, and women with fertility problems may not discover them until their reproductive life span is waning. In addition to a generally reduced quality of oocytes with age, more years of exposure to environmental influences can also have a potential effect. In considering the risk of environmental exposures on reproductive function and women's health, special attention should be paid to those chemicals with the potential to impair ovarian function, because the ovary is critical to normal reproduction. The ovary performs two important roles, development and delivery of the female gamete (oocyte) and production of ovarian hormones, such as inhibin and the female sex steroids, estrogens and progesterone.[2,3] Whereas the oocyte is required for fertilization, ovarian hormone output is required for oocyte development, feedback signaling to the hypothalamus and pituitary, and establishment and early maintenance of pregnancy.

Reproductive toxicants can affect ovarian function in a variety of ways. Indirect effects on ovarian function might result from altered pituitary output of gonadotropins (follicle stimulating hormone, FSH, and luteinizing hormone, LH). Such alterations could be caused by chemicals that disrupt neuroendocrine feedback by estrogen and progesterone. Alternatively, reproductive toxicants can have direct ovarian effects on steroid hormone production. The estrogens are responsible for oocyte development, whereas progesterone is required for implantation and early maintenance of pregnancy. Therefore, xenobiotic exposure that alters ovarian steroid hormone production could affect oocyte development and ovulation, as well as neuroendocrine feedback, reproductive tract function, and pregnancy. By a different route, reproductive toxicants can affect ovarian function through destruction of ooctyes. Extensive destruction of oocytes damages ovarian follicles, which also destroys steroid hormone production. The ultimate result of complete follicular destruction in a woman is ovarian failure (menopause). Following ovarian failure, neuroendocrine feedback is disrupted, and circulating levels of gonadotropins rise. Therefore, oocyte destruction ultimately disrupts endocrine balance by causing a reduction in estrogen and progesterone and an elevation in FSH and LH.

In summary, endocrine disruptions can be caused by reproductive toxicants via direct alterations in steroid hormone production (ovary) or by interference with steroid hormone action (hypothalamus, pituitary, reproductive tract). Alternatively, endocrine disruption can be indirect, resulting from ovarian failure caused by extensive oocyte destruction. In addition to an increased risk of osteoporosis and cardiovascular disease in menopause, there is a known increase in the incidence of ovarian cancer.[4] This observation has been well supported in animal studies.[5] Therefore, in addition to reduced fertility resulting from ovotoxicity in females, there are the health risks associated with premature ovarian failure (early menopause). Because of these health risks, the subject of this chapter is chemicals that destroy ovarian follicles.

3.2   Ovarian Function

3.2.1   Follicular Development

3.2.1.1   Fetal Development

Development and maturation of oocytes occur within ovarian follicles. Successful ovulation requires appropriate follicular development, during which the follicle has passed through a number of distinct developmental stages.[3] Throughout the life of a female, preceding each menstrual cycle, some follicles are selected to develop to maturity for ovulation and potential fertilization. The most immature stage of follicular development is termed primordial. This is the stage at which follicles first appear in the ovary of a developing female fetus. Primordial follicles provide the pool for recruitment of developing follicles; therefore, they are the fundamental reproductive unit of the ovary.

Because of the nature of fetal development of ovarian follicles, women are born with a finite number of primordial oocytes, which cannot be regenerated later in life. During fetal development of the ovaries, primordial germ cells that are formed invade the indifferent gonad and undergo rapid hyperplasia. By one month of embryonic life, primordial germ cells have become established in the genital ridge, and oogonia are proliferating by mitosis.[3] During the period of mitotic proliferation of germ cells, somatic cells (granulosa, theca, endothelial cells) and supporting connective tissue develop and gradually become interspersed among the oogonia.[3] Oogonia develop into oocytes in synchronous waves, once they stop dividing and enter into the first meiotic division. During this period, oocytes grow slowly and proceed to the diplotene stage of the meiotic prophase. The oocyte does not fully complete the first meiotic division at this time but becomes arrested until ovulation, if this should occur. Therefore, the pool of oocytes at the time of birth is finite and comprises the total germ cells available throughout life. Around the time of birth, small individual oocytes within the ovary become surrounded by a few flattened somatic cells (pregranulosa cells) and a basement membrane to form primordial follicles.[3] Association of the granulosa cells with the oocyte at all times is critical for maintenance of viability and follicle growth and development.[6]

3.2.1.2   Primordial Follicles

In humans, one to two preovulatory follicles develop approximately every 28 d, whereas, in rats, 6 to 12 follicles develop every 4 to 5 d.[2] The primordial follicles from which these follicles develop are located primarily near the ovarian cortex and represent the pool for recruitment. Regular waves of the onset of development of primordial follicles is a continuous process from birth, until ovarian failure occurs.[2] However, throughout the reproductive life span, the total number of primordial follicles selected to develop for ovulation is small compared to the total population. Instead, the vast majority of follicles are lost to attrition in various early stages of development by a process called atresia. The exact mechanism for selection of a preovulatory follicle is not understood but is believed to be under intraovarian control.[2]

3.2.1.3   Primary Follicles

Some primordial follicles leave the quiescent state as soon as they are formed, and some are dormant for months or years.[3] The first sign of oocyte growth in primordial follicles is alteration of surrounding squamous (flattened) granulosa cells into cuboidal shaped cells.[3] Once the follicle makes this transition from primordial to primary, other structural changes occur such as development of the zona pellucida and acquisition of the theca layer. The zona pellucida is composed of a glycoprotein matrix to provide protection for the oocyte as well as to provide attachments for the specialized inner layer of granulosa cells, known as cumulus cells.[2,3] At this stage, another layer of specialized somatic cells begins to form as the cells proliferate and form a shell outside the basement membrane enclosing the oocyte and granulosa cell layer. These cells appear in concentric rings surrounding the follicle and are designated theca interna cells. Theca cells provide two important functions: (1) attachment of arterioles for the development of an independent blood supply and (2) secretion of progestins and androgens to regulate follicle development.[3]

3.2.1.4 Growing Follicles

The oocyte contained in an early growing follicle has a large, spherical nucleus (germinal vesicle) that grows in proportion to the growth of the oocyte, and the follicular cells continue to proliferate and form a second layer around the oocyte.[2,3] As the follicle continues to develop, the layers of granulosa cells surrounding the oocyte increase rapidly to reach follicular diameters of up to 250 μm. Gap junctions are formed between individual cells in the granulosa cell layer to facilitate intercellular transport of nutrients and metabolites to the oocyte.[2] Additionally, a number of autocrine, paracrine, and endocrine signals begin to influence follicular development. The somatic cells acquire receptors for FSH to enhance follicle growth, and they develop steroidogenic capacity for synthesis of androgens, estrogens, and progesterone.

3.2.1.5 Antral Follicles

The number of follicles that reach the final stage of development is quite small compared to those that began development from the primordial pool. In women, only one follicle per menstrual cycle is usually chosen as the dominant follicle destined for ovulation. As the follicle develops, it acquires a fluid-filled cavity, antrum, formed by separations within the granulosa cell layers. During the final period of development, a preovulatory follicle becomes more sensitive to the gonadotropins FSH and LH than were smaller antral and growing follicles.[2] Theca cells within the follicle contain receptors for LH and respond to hormonal input with synthesis and secretion of androgens. Conversely, granulosa cells contain receptors for FSH and respond to hormonal input with expression of the enzyme aromatase. In this capacity, granulosa cells can directly convert the androgens secreted by theca cells to estrogens. Prior to ovulation, granulosa cells also begin to express receptors for LH in readiness for receiving the LH surge as a trigger for ovulation and luteinization.[3] Prior to ovulation and after the LH surge, the oocyte will be signaled to continue meiotic progression through metaphase, anaphase, telophase, and arrest in metaphase of the second meiotic division. The second meiotic division is only completed if fertilization of the oocyte occurs.

3.2.2 Atresia

Ovarian content of oocytes is dynamic and fluctuates with age. As a female ages, the number of primordial follicles selected to develop decreases, suggesting a relationship between the number of primordial follicles remaining and ovulatory recruitment.[2] The total number of oocytes peaks during embryonic development. In humans, the peak number of oocytes ever present, about seven million, occurs at five months gestation, at birth the number has dropped to two million; it falls to 250,000 to 400,000 at puberty and to essentially none at menopause.[3,7] During the lifetime of a woman, ovulation only accounts for 400 to 600 oocytes. Therefore, the others have been lost at various stages of development by a process called atresia.

3.2.3 Cell Death

The ultimate event associated with follicular atresia is cell death. This is the natural fate of the majority of ovarian follicles because only a select few follicles that develop will ever be ovulated.[3] Follicular atresia in rats has been shown to occur via a mechanism of physiological cell death, apoptosis.[8] Apoptosis is used by many tissues to delete unwanted cells by a nontraumatic mechanism.[9,10] Therefore, this form of cell death is physiological and likely to go undetected by the organism. This is in distinct contrast to cell death by necrosis, which usually occurs in response to injury and which elicits an inflammatory response in the surrounding tissue. The distinction between apoptosis and necrosis is based upon morphological characteristics.[9] The earliest definitive changes of a cell undergoing apoptosis is compaction of chromatin into dense masses (margination) along the nuclear membrane, condensation of the cytoplasm, and reduction in nuclear size. Shrinkage of the total cellular volume leads to an increase in cell density and compaction of cytoplasmic organelles, which retain their membrane integrity. As the condensation continues, nuclear and plasma membranes begin to separate into multiple apoptotic bodies and nuclear and cytoplasmic blebbing are observed. Following release from the dying cell, these apoptotic bodies are quickly phagocytosed by healthy neighboring cells. On the other hand, necrosis is a passive form of cell death that results following exposure of cells to traumatic influences. In contrast to the shrinkage involved in apoptosis, necrosis involves organelle and cytoplasmic swelling caused by a destruction of plasma membrane integrity. This leads to the release of lysosomal enzymes, which accelerate membrane disintegrations and lead to an inflammatory response. Apoptosis and necrosis can also be distinguished by certain biochemical features. Specifically, in apoptosis, genomic DNA is degraded in a specific pattern of internucleosomal degradation to produce low molecular weight fragments that are multiples of approximately 185 base pairs and appear on agarose gel electrophoresis as a characteristic "ladder" formation.[10] However, this pattern of DNA fragmentation is not uniformly observed in all cells undergoing apoptosis.[11] For example, it was recently reported in rats that the specific endonuclease required for internucleosomal fragmentation of DNA (laddering) is not expressed in granulosa cells from immature (small preantral) ovarian follicles.[12] Therefore, even though these cells can undergo apoptosis, DNA will be degraded in a nonspecific, random pattern.[13] Therefore, the most reliable distinction between apoptotic and necrotic mechanisms of cell death still resides in morphological evaluation.[11]

3.2.4 Menopause

Once the ovary is depleted of primordial follicles, ovarian failure (menopause) occurs. Menopause has been associated with a variety of health problems in women. These include increased rates of osteoporosis, cardiovascular disease, arthritis, urinary tract infections, and depression.[14] Additionally, in laboratory animals, premature ovarian failure is associated in the long term with an increased incidence of ovarian neoplasms.[5] A variety of environmental factors have been highly correlated with premature or early menopause. As an example, active or passive exposure to cigarette smoke significantly accelerates the onset of menopause.[15,16] Therefore, as a woman ages, her overall health is significantly affected by the onset of menopause, which can be impacted further by environmental factors to which she has been exposed.

3.3 Effects of Ovotoxicants

Reproductive toxicants can compromise ovarian function via destruction of oocyte-containing follicles.[1,5] The ovary contains enzymes responsible for biotransformation and detoxification of many xenobiotics. Both the rat and mouse ovary contain epoxide hydrolase, glutathione-S-transferases, and cytochromes P-450, which metabolize known ovarian toxicants.[17,18] Therefore, biotransformation of a chemical within the ovary could occur within selected compartments, thereby providing exposure of certain classes of oocytes to highly concentrated bioactive forms of ovotoxicants.

The level of exposure to an environmental chemical required to produce ovarian damage is of particular importance. It is under rare, accidental circumstances that individuals are exposed acutely to toxic levels of reproductive toxicants, and the effects of these exposures can usually be detected and evaluated. However, the possible effects of chronic exposure to low levels of reproductive toxicants are more difficult to determine. Therefore, fertility problems caused by low levels of ongoing environmental exposures may go unrecognized for years because of the potential for additive or cumulative effects that might be produced. These types of exposures might manifest as early menopause and/or still later development of ovarian cancer. Because of their insidious nature, these types of exposures can cause 'silent' damage and are of the utmost concern.

Another factor related to the effect of exposure of a woman to a reproductive toxicant is the developmental stage in her reproductive life span at the time of exposure (Figure 3.1). Temporary infertility may be manifest in the adult cyclic woman, but exposure during childhood can delay or accelerate puberty. Sterility might be produced by a chemical-induced destruction of germ cells during fetal development or in childhood. In adults, sterility

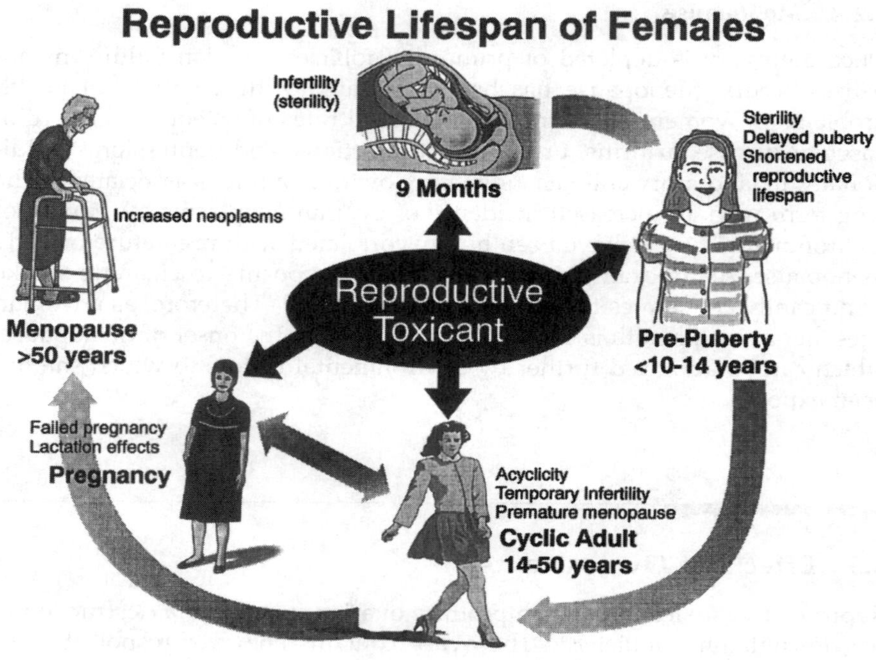

Reproductive Lifespan of Females

FIGURE 3.1

Potential effects of reproductive toxicants on the reproductive lifespan in females. Exposure to reproductive toxicants can have long-term impact on female reproductive capacity. The effect can vary depending upon whether the damage occurred during fetal development, childhood, regular adulthood, or pregnancy. One possible result can be premature ovarian failure (menopause). (From Hoyer, P. B., *Comprehensive Toxicology*, Vol. 10, Elsevier Publishing, Oxford, 1997, 253. With permission.)

might also be produced in the form of premature menopause resulting from chemical-induced ovarian failure. In children and adults this could result from the extensive destruction of oocytes.

For chemicals that destroy oocytes, the stage of development at which the follicle is destroyed determines the impact that exposure to the chemical will have on reproduction. Chemicals that selectively damage large growing or antral follicles only temporarily interrupt reproductive function because these follicles can be replaced by recruitment from the greater pool of primordial follicles. Thus, these chemicals produce a readily reversible form of infertility that is manifest relatively soon after exposure.[19-21] Conversely, chemicals that extensively destroy oocytes contained in primordial and primary follicles cause permanent infertility and precocious ovarian failure (premature menopause in humans), since once a primordial follicle is destroyed, it cannot be replaced. Destruction of oocytes contained in primordial follicles may have a delayed effect on reproduction until such a time that recruitment for the number of growing and antral follicles can no longer be supported.[19,22]

TABLE 3.1

Long-term Effects of 30-d Dosing of Female B6C3F1 Mice
with VCH[a]

Day[b]	Small Follicles (% control)	Serum FSH (% above control)	Estrous Cyclicity[c]
30	11%*	30%	yes
120	3%*	50%	yes
240	<1%*	130%*	yes
360	0%*	160%*	no*

[a] Data expressed as % control mice.
[b] Day after onset of dosing (30 d)
[c] Determined by vaginal cytology
* Different from control mice, p < 0.05
Reprinted with permission from *Annu. Rev. Pharmacol. Toxicol.*, 36,
307, 1996; summarized from Hooser, S. B., Douds, D. A., Hoyer, P. B.,
and Sipes, I. G., *Reprod. Toxicol.*, 8, 315, 1994. With permission.

Although direct destruction of ovarian follicles may not immediately alter circulating hormone levels, the long-term result is disruption of negative feedback at the level of the hypothalamus and pituitary in response to loss of ovarian hormone regulation. FSH produced in the anterior pituitary regulates follicular development and is under a negative feedback regulation of release by ovarian hormones, such as estrogen, progesterone, and inhibin.[23] The mechanism by which chemicals are ovotoxic could disrupt this feedback loop of endocrine regulation by a direct effect at the level of the hypothalamus and/or pituitary. Conversely, a primary effect at the ovarian level might cause a later disruption of this regulatory axis. In the latter case, ovarian failure would produce rather than result from changes in circulating FSH levels, and FSH levels should increase due to loss of negative feedback from the ovarian hormones. In a long-term study, female B6C3F1 mice were treated with the occupational chemical, 4-vinyl-cyclohexene (VCH) for 30 d (age 28 to 58 d) and then observed for 1 year (Table 3.1).[22] Although a greater than 90% loss of oocytes in small follicles was measured by 30 d, FSH levels were only first observed to be increased above control animals at 240 d. Therefore, ovarian changes preceded the rise in circulating FSH levels. Also at 240 d, vaginal cytology still displayed evidence of ovarian cyclicity in VCH-treated mice. However, by 360 d (from the onset of 30 d of dosing), unlike control animals, complete ovarian failure had resulted in VCH-treated mice, as determined by increased circulating levels of FSH, lack of cyclicity, the complete absence of ovarian follicular or luteal structures, and marked ovarian atrophy. Furthermore, at 360 d there was histological evidence of preneoplastic changes in ovaries of treated mice. From this study, it was concluded that the ovarian failure and preneoplastic changes that occur long after cessation of dosing with VCH are indirect consequences resulting from the depletion of small, preantral follicles.

3.4   Ovotoxic Chemicals

3.4.1   Preantral Follicle Damage

Chemicals that extensively destroy primordial and primary follicles can cause irreversible infertility (premature menopause in humans), since once destroyed they cannot be replaced. Furthermore, destruction of primordial follicles will have a delayed effect on cyclicity that is undetected until there are no follicles left to be recruited for development.[19,22]

3.4.1.1   Ionizing Radiation

Rapidly dividing primordial germ cells and oogonia present during fetal development in all species are highly sensitive to destruction.[24] Destruction of oocytes contained in ovarian primordial follicles can be caused by a variety of environmental chemicals.[5] Additionally, exposure to irradiation is known to produce rapid destruction of oocytes contained in primordial follicles, followed by increased follicular atresia, stromal hypertrophy, and loss of ovarian weight.[24] These effects are suspected in humans because of reports of amenorrhea and sterility in women undergoing therapeutic irradiation.[25,26] In animal studies, Mattison and Schulman[7] noted that prenatal exposure to ionizing radiation also affects the number of oocytes and reproductive capacity of female offspring.

3.4.1.2   Chemotherapeutic Agents

Now that cancer patients are living longer, the toxic effects of chemotherapeutic drugs on the health and quality of life of these survivors have become important issues. Since the beginning of antineoplastic therapy to treat a variety of diseases and malignancies, the ability of these agents to produce ovarian failure has been documented. Nitrogen mustard, chlorambucil, and vinblastine have all been reported to cause sterility in women.[25-27] Cyclophosphamide (CPA), an alkylating agent in cancer chemotherapy has also been shown to cause premature ovarian failure and secondary tumors in women.[28,29] These observations in humans have motivated a variety of studies with CPA in rodents to better elucidate its mechanism of ovotoxicity. Miller and Cole[30] studied the ovaries in mice treated with CPA in low doses for 1 year and found reduced numbers of oocytes (especially primordial) and corpora lutea with no effect on other tissues such as the kidney, spleen, thymus, or lymph nodes. Estrous cyclicity was destroyed, and cysts/tumors were observed in the ovarian germinal epithelium. In a short-term study, susceptibility to CPA was greatest in primordial follicles in exposed C57BL/6N and D2 mice and SD rats.[31] These results were in contrast to a report in which loss of antral follicles was not associated with a loss of primordial follicles in SD rats injected with CPA.[32] However, in the first study, follicle loss was only observed in rats at concentrations high enough to cause overall toxicity. Plowchalk and Mattison[33] observed a time- and dose-dependent relationship between CPA and ovarian toxicity by looking at changes in ovarian structure and function. In C57BL/6N mice given a single intraperitoneal (i.p.) injection of CPA (75, 200, or 500 mg/kg), primordial follicle numbers were significantly reduced to 73%, 42%, and 38% of controls, respectively. The loss of primordial follicles was essentially complete at 3 d, and the estimated ED_{50} (concentration that produced 50% follicle loss) was 122 mg/kg body weight. From these results it appears that premature ovarian failure in women treated with CPA is likely to be via destruction of primordial follicles.

3.4.1.3 Cigarette Smoking

Epidemiological studies conducted over the last four decades have demonstrated a relationship between smoking and impaired fertility. Cigarette smoke is a well-known reproductive toxicant. One study reported that rates of pregnancy were reduced to 57% in heavy smokers and 75% in light smokers when compared with nonsmokers; furthermore, smokers required 1 year longer to conceive than did nonsmokers.[34] Women smokers have also been reported to experience a 1- to 4-year earlier age for the onset of menopause.[16,35] Thus, a significant amount of data exist to demonstrate a relationship between smoking and reduced fertility, but the mechanism is not well understood. Along with the impact on fertility, there are also effects of cigarette smoke on pregnancy and the fetus. Prenatal exposure to cigarette smoke has been associated with retarded intrauterine growth and premature deliveries.[36] Additionally, conception in women whose mothers smoked while pregnant was significantly reduced when compared with women whose mothers did not smoke.[37] In animal studies, exposure of mice *in utero* to cigarette smoke resulted in a reduced number of ovarian primordial follicles in female offspring.[38]

There are several possible mechanisms by which cigarette smoke might be involved in the earlier onset of menopause among smokers. Cigarette smoke is a complex mixture of alkaloids (nicotine), polycyclic aromatic hydrocarbons (PAH), nitroso compounds, aromatic amines, and protein pyrolysates, many of which are carcinogenic.[39] Nicotine acting on the central nervous system might affect secretion of hormones involved in regulation of ovarian function.[35] Smoking women have been shown to have significantly decreased follicular levels of estradiol when compared with nonsmokers.[40] Furthermore, extracts of cigarette smoke significantly decreased estradiol secretion by human granulosa cells in culture.[41] Alternatively, cigarette smoke can induce certain liver metabolizing enzymes, which may also accelerate metabolism of steroid hormones.[35,42] However, because of the logical association between early menopause and oocyte destruction, some of the effects of cigarette smoke on fertility are likely to be due to ovotoxicity.

3.4.1.4 Polycyclic Aromatic Hydrocarbons

Many animal studies have demonstrated ovotoxic effects of PAHs. Cigarette smoke contains high levels of the PAHs, benzo[a]pyrene (BaP), 3-methyl-cholanthrene (3-MC), and 9:10-dimethyl-1:2-benzanthracene [DMBA; 16]. Krarup[43,44] reported that 9:10-dimethyl-1:2-benzanthracene (DMBA) depletes oocytes and produces ovarian tumors in mice. Subsequently, these effects have also been reported in a number of studies for 3-MC and BaP.

The three PAHs destroyed oocytes in small follicles in Sprague Dawley rats and in D2 and B6 mice within 14 d following a single i.p. injection.[45] Yet, under these conditions, mice were more susceptible to ovotoxicity than rats. Related to the mechanisms of these effects, BaP produced chromosomal aberrations in Chinese hampster ovarian (CHO) cells and mouse oocytes,[46] and 3-MC produced a destruction of oocytes that ultrastructurally resemble the physiological process of atresia.[47] Oocyte destruction in primordial and primary follicles was observed in mice treated with DMBA, BaP, and 3-MC.[48] The relative toxicities for primordial follicles were DMBA > 3-MC > BaP. Daily oral exposure during pregnancy in mice between 7 and 16 d of gestation with high doses of BaP caused complete sterility of the female offspring.[49] Pregnant mice exposed to a lower dose (10 mg BaP per kilogram) gave birth to offspring with severely compromised fertility.[49] In both studies the litters of exposed mothers were smaller in number and size when compared with controls. A direct relationship between the dose of PAHs and destruction of primordial follicles has been shown in the mouse ovary.[48] In a subsequent study, mice given single i.p. doses ranging from 1 to 100 mg/kg of BaP demonstrated an ED_{50} of 15 mg/kg for oocyte destruction in B6 mice.[50] Interestingly, significant oocyte destruction was demonstrated following a single high dose of BaP (100 mg/kg), whereas, the same level of oocyte loss was observed with a low dose (10 mg/kg) given daily for 10 d.[51] This observation provides support for a cumulative ovotoxic effect of chronic exposures to low doses.

3.4.1.5 Occupational Chemicals

1,3-butadiene (BD) and the related olefins, isoprene and styrene, are released during the manufacture of synthetic rubber and thermoplastic resins, and the estimated annual occupational exposure of U.S. employees is 3,700–1,000,000 people.[52] These chemicals have also been reported in cigarette smoke and automobile exhaust.[52,53] Chronic inhalation studies have shown that carcinogenesis for BD is higher in mice than in rats.[54] Animals exposed to BD and its metabolites by inhalation at concentrations of 62.5 ppm demonstrated that target tissues in mice (heart, lung, fat, spleen, and thymus) contained significantly greater amounts of BD epoxides than those same tissues in rats.[54] At lower doses, female mice exposed daily by inhalation for up to 2 years exhibited ovarian atrophy, granulosa cell hyperplasia, and benign and malignant granulosa cell tumors.[55] Therefore, reproductive effects were observed following chronic exposure to low doses.

Because of the potential for epoxidation of these compounds, they have the potential to be ovotoxic and carcinogenic. In one study, the metabolite of BD in female B6C3F1 mice dosed daily for 30 d, 1,3-butadiene monoepoxide (1.43 mmole/kg) depleted small follicles by 98% and growing follicles by 87%, compared with control animals.[56] At a much lower dose, 0.14 mmole/kg, the diepoxide of 1,3-butadiene depleted small follicles by 85% and growing follicles by 63%. The results of this study support that a diepoxide formed in the metabolism of BD is more potent at inducing follicle loss. Additionally, isoprene was reported to be ovotoxic, whereas styrene and its monoepoxide did not reduce mouse ovarian follicle numbers.[56]

There are mixed opinions as to the risk of human exposure to BD-induced toxicity. According to Bond et al.,[57] there is not enough evidence for an association between occupational exposure and human lymphatic and hematopoietic cancers. They have shown that the metabolic activation of the carcinogenic form occurs to a greater extent in mice than in rats and humans. Furthermore, they concluded that because concentrations likely to be encountered in the environment or workplace are usually below 2 ppm, thus there is not likely a carcinogenic risk to humans. However, the potential cumulative effect of long-term exposure to low concentrations over the course of years was not discussed. This is particularly important when the target cells are of a nonrenewing type (for instance, ovarian follicles).

The dimerization of 1,3-butadiene forms 4-vinylcyclohexene, VCH. The VCH family of compounds are occupational chemicals released at low concentrations during the manufacture of rubber tires, placticizers, and pesticides.[52,58] VCH and its diepoxide metabolite, 4-vinylcyclohexene diepoxide (VCD), have been shown in mice and rats to (1) produce extensive destruction of primordial and primary follicles,[59] (2) cause premature ovarian failure,[22] (3) increase the risk for development of ovarian tumors,[60] and (4) affect normal ovarian development of female offspring exposed *in utero*.[61] Because no significant effects on other tissues have been reported in studies with this class of compounds, the damage they produce appears to be highly specific and does not involve widespread toxicity. Ovarian damage caused by VCH and its related epoxide metabolites has been demonstrated by a variety of exposure routes, including dermal,[62] oral,[61] inhalation,[63] and i.p. injection.[59] It is, therefore, important to understand the mechanism(s) by which this damage, shown to have such far-reaching effects, is initiated. The overall sequence of events associated with VCH-induced ovarian toxicity is shown in Figure 3.2. Logically, gaining a detailed understanding of the mechanisms of ovotoxicity requires focusing on the primary events associated with the destruction of primordial and primary follicles. Dosing of mice with VCH (800 mg/kg) or VCD (80 mg/kg) for 30 d destroyed about 90% of the ovarian small preantral (primordial and primary) follicles.[22,59] Follicle loss was not seen at 10 d, but was significant following 15 d of daily dosing.[59] The loss of follicles within 30 d of daily dosing was sufficient to cause premature ovarian failure within 1 year, as evidenced by loss of cyclicity, ovarian atrophy, and preneoplastic changes in ovarian cells.[22] In the longer term, 2 years of dosing

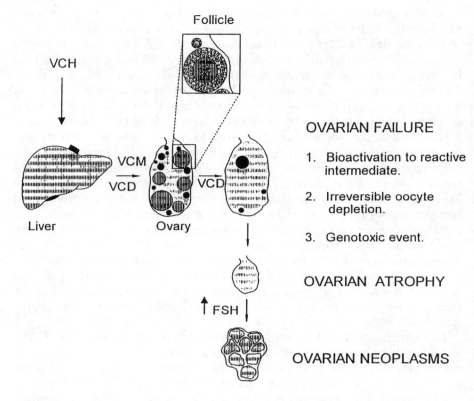

FIGURE 3.2
Model of ovotoxicity in mice produced by VCH. The liver is the primary site of bioactivation of VCH to its epoxide metabolites, VCM (4-vinyl-cyclohexene monepoxides) and VCD (4-vinyl-cyclohexene diepoxide). VCD produces destruction of ovarian small preantral follicles, producing extensive, irreversible ovotoxicity. After time, due to follicular destruction, atrophy and premature ovarian failure result, and FSH levels rise. These events can lead to development of ovarian neoplasms. (From Hoyer, P. B. and Sipes, I. G., *Annu. Rev. Pharmacol. Toxicol.*, 36, 325, 1996. With permission.)

with VCH resulted in development of ovarian tumors in female mice.[60] These were described as: (1) mixed germinal epithelial and granulosa cells neoplasms; (2) granulosa cell-derived neoplasms; or (3) tubular adenomas on the outer surface of the ovary.[60] Another study evaluated the effects of a 2-year dermal application of VCD.[62] These results showed an increase in neoplasms of the skin in male and female mice at the site of application and an additional increase in the development of ovarian follicular atrophy and tubular hyperplasia in female mice.

3.4.1.6   *Other Ovotoxic Agents*

The alkylating agents 1,4-di(methanesulfonoxy)-butane (Myleran), trimethylenemelamin (TEM), and isopropyl methanesulfonate (IMS) have been shown to destroy oocytes in small follicles in SECXC57BLF1 mice following a single i.p. injection.[19] This destruction was observed within 3 d of dosing with TEM and IMS and within 14 d with Myleran. Daily oral administration of nitrofurazone over 2 years caused ovarian lesions, including development of benign mixed tumors and granulosa cell tumors in mice.[64] The results of an *in vitro* mutagenicity study in *E. coli* using a number of industrial and laboratory chemicals demonstrated a high correlation between alkylating activity and increased mutagenicity.[65] In addition to the chemicals discussed so far, Dobson and Felton[24] reported a variety of other compounds that were capable of producing significant primordial follicle loss in mice. These chemicals included methyl and ethyl methanesulfonate, busulfan, and urethane. Additionally, of a number of fungal toxins and antibiotics tested, procarbazine HCl, and 4-nitroquinoline-1-oxide were ovotoxic. Finally, dibromochloropropane, urethane, N-ethyl-N-nitrosourea, and bleomycin demonstrated primordial follicle killing, with bleomycin being the most potent. In general, all of these ovotoxic chemicals are also known to possess mutagenic-carcinogenic effects. Thus, these studies have provided a further correlation between ovotoxicity and subsequent development of tumorigenesis. How these two events are linked is not clearly understood at this time. Hexachlorobenzene (HCB), a persistent halogenated hydrocarbon in the environment, has been identified as a contaminant in human follicular fluid.[66] This is of particular concern in view of the ability of HCB to destroy primordial follicles in Rhesus and cynomolgus monkeys.

3.4.2 Antral Follicle Damage

Damage to large growing or antral follicles causes reversible interruption of cyclicity by impacting on ovarian steroid production and ovulation. This effect is generally reversible because more follicles can ultimately be recruited for development from the pool of primordial follicles that remains.

3.4.2.1 *Chemotherapeutic Agents*

In addition to widespread destruction of primordial follicles by cyclophosphamide in ovaries of rats and mice, large antral follicles are also affected. Under conditions that completely destroyed primordial follicles in mice, only partial destruction of antral follicles could be observed.[33] This demonstrated the greater sensitivity of primordial germ cells to this compound in mice. Conversely, in rats, dosing with CPA caused destruction of antral follicles at doses that did not affect primordial follicles.[32] However, in both studies, other reproductive effects in response to dosing, such as lower ovarian weight, reduced follicular and corpus luteum volume, and lower circulating 17-β estradiol levels, were most highly associated with the loss of antral follicles.[32,33] Additionally, the effect on antral follicle numbers in both studies was reversible. Thus, whereas ovotoxicity that impacts the primordial follicle pool causes irreversible effects, damage to larger follicles has a temporary impact on cyclicity. The immediate precursors of phosphoramide mustard (bioactive form of CPA) were given in mice and were also observed to reduce antral follicle numbers and cause loss of ovarian volume and uterine weight.[67]

3.4.2.2   Polycyclic Aromatic Hydrocarbons

An effect of DMBA and BaP on antral follicles has been reported in mice. DMBA was reported to decrease small follicles initially, with a secondary effect on large follicles.[68] In a morphological assessment of ovaries collected from mice that were dosed with PAHs, Mattison[69] reported that BaP, 3-MC, and DMBA all destroyed primordial follicles; however, only DMBA decreased antral follicles. Yet, in a subsequent study in mice, BaP decreased numbers of corpora lutea, and this effect was reversible.[70] These observations are consistent with disrupted ovulation and targeting of BaP to antral follicles, which were reduced in number at the higher doses. The discrepancy in findings between the two studies is not easily understood; however, it is apparent that under certain conditions, PAH damage to antral follicles can occur.

3.4.2.3   Phthalates

Di-(2-ethylhexyl)phthalate (DEHP) is widely used in the production of many polyvinyl chloride-based plastics, including medical and food packages. Because it is not covalently linked to the plastic resin, DEHP can contaminate the surrounding environment.[21] Chronic occupational exposure of Russian women to phthalates has been associated with decreased rates of pregnancy, increased rates of miscarriage, and anovulation. A recent study in female SD rats reported that repeated oral exposure to DEHP caused disruptions of reproductive function.[21] These disruptions included delayed ovulations, reduced granulosa cell size in antral follicles, decreased circulating estradiol, progesterone, and LH levels, and increased FSH. These observations provide evidence that this class of chemicals has a specific effect on preovulatory (large antral) follicles, and the authors concluded that this was due specifically to suppression of granulosa cell estradiol production.

3.4.2.4   Halogenated Aryl Hydrocarbons

Endocrine disrupters that display estrogenic/antiestrogenic effects have been studied actively in their ability to target developmental and uterine sites of action. The intracellular mechanisms of these disruptions are only beginning to be understood. The pesticide, 2,3,7,8-tetrachlorodibenzo-*p*-dioxin (TCDD) has been the subject of many studies related to sexual development and fertility.[71] However, a few recent studies have reported that TCDD also apparently causes direct ovarian effects. The effect of a single oral dose of TCDD on a number of oocytes ovulated and estrous cyclicity was observed in female rats.[72] Treatment with TCDD prolonged the diestrus stage and reduced the time in proestrus and estrus. Additionally, there was a reduction in the number of oocytes ovulated in treated rats. These findings provide strong evidence that ovulations have been reduced. This observation was further studied as the effect of TCDD on hormone-induced follicular development and ovulation.[73] The data from this study were consistent with reduced ovulation via a hypothalamic-pituitary effect. However, ovulation was also reduced in hypophysectomized animals, suggesting a direct ovarian effect as well. As regards to the mechanisms by which this ovarian effect might occur, an *in vitro* study observed that TCDD significantly reduced 17-β-estradiol production by human luteinized granulosa cells in culture.[74] Further investigation of intracellular mechanisms involved suggested that TCDD produced these effects via interactions with the epidermal growth factor (EGF) linked-mitotic signaling pathway involving mitogen-activated protein kinases and protein kinase A.

The polychlorinated biphenyl, 3,3′,4,4′-tetrachlorobiphenyl (TCB), has been shown to have teratogenic effects in the mouse[75] and to be embryolethal in the rat.[76] A transplacental effect of TCB on ovarian development in fetal mice has also been reported.[77] When mice were exposed on day 13 of gestation, a 40 to 50% loss of follicles in all stages of development was observed in female offspring at 28 d of age. However, this reduction did not adversely affect reproductive capacity during a 5-month period of testing.

Thus, it appears that direct endocrine disrupters may exert their reproductive and developmental effects at a variety of different sites. Even though an initial impact on endocrine balance may cause some of the observed effects, there is growing evidence to suggest that direct ovarian effects are produced as well.

3.5 Ovarian Metabolism

3.5.1 Bioactivation

Many xenobiotic chemicals are metabolized once they have been taken into the body. In some cases, the chemical form that is introduced must be metabolized to a more reactive intermediate to produce toxic effects. There is good evidence for bioactivation of many of the ovotoxic chemicals that have been discussed. This conversion represents bioactivation of the parent compound and is catalyzed by Phase I classes of enzymes, such as the family of cytochrome P450-associated enzymes. Microsomal cytochrome P-450 content increased in rat ovaries as the animals developed toward puberty, with even greater increases in pregnant rats.[18] This suggests that expression of these enzymes may be under hormonal control. Whether bioactivation of various parent compounds occurs directly in the ovary or in other metabolically active tissues such as liver is generally not well known. However, the capabilities for ovarian metabolism are available.

3.5.2   Detoxification

The second phase of xenobiotic metabolism relates to detoxification and involves Phase II classes of enzymes. This formation of nontoxic metabolites usually also enhances their solubility for excretion. Major enzymatic pathways for detoxification of xenobiotic epoxides are hydration to corresponding diols (catalyzed by microsomal epoxide hydrolase, EH), and conjugation with glutathione (catalyzed by glutathione-S-transferase, GST). Detoxification reactions catalyzed by EH and GST occur in many tissues, including the ovary.[18,78] Activities of these enzymes in rats were elevated right after birth and decreased by two weeks of age, then increased slowly and reached a maximum near puberty. Additionally, ovarian GST activity was even further elevated in pregnant rats.[18] Thus, these data provide evidence for hormonal induction of ovarian detoxification enzymes.

3.5.3   Metabolism

3.5.3.1   Cyclophosphamide

Cyclophosphamide given as a chemotheraputic agent induces widespread loss of primordial follicles and can cause sterility. However, it has been determined that the antineoplastic and ovotoxic form of this chemical is phosphoramide mustard.[67,79] Phosphoramide mustard cyclohexylamine salt (PMC) and trans-4-phenylcyclophosphamide (T4P) both can be enzymatically converted to phosphoramide mustard, whereas didechlorocyclophosphamide (DCPA) and allyl alcohol (AA) are precursors for inactive acrolein. These compounds were used to investigate ovarian toxicity in female C57BL/6N mice.[67] Only PMC and T4P produced ovarian toxicity. Moreover, these reactive intermediates were more effective at lower concentrations than was CPA. Thus, it was concluded that phosphoramide mustard is the bioactive form of the parent compound, cyclophosphamide. The ovary does not appear to metabolize cyclophosphamide; rather, metabolism is thought to occur in the liver with uptake of the reactive metabolites from the blood.[79] The greater potency of PMC and T4P compared to CPA in mice was explained as these compounds bypassing important detoxification steps, allowing more toxic metabolite to reach the ovary.[67]

3.5.3.2   Polycyclic Aromatic Hydrocarbons

Polycyclic aromatic hydrocarbons are not directly ovotoxic but require metabolic activation to reactive metabolites. Ovarian enzymes involved in the biotransformation (i.e., aryl hydrocarbon hydroxylase and epoxide hydrolase) of PAHs have been identified in mice and rats,[80] monkeys,[81] and humans.[82] Therefore, oocyte destruction by PAHs may involve distribution of the parent compound to the ovary where ovarian enzymes metabolize the compound to reactive intermediates.[80] These metabolites are capable of covalent binding to macromolecules such as DNA, RNA, and protein.[83] However, the direct intracellular target for ovotoxicity has not been determined. B6 mice were more susceptible to BaP than D2 mice;[51] yet, both strains were equally susceptible to the arene oxide metabolite of BaP.[83] Furthermore, inhibition of PAH metabolism with α naphthoflavone prevented oocyte destruction observed in mice.[80] These observations indicate that the PAHs must undergo bioactivation to arene oxides to produce their ovotoxic effects.

Oocyte destruction by PAHs involves distribution of the parent compound to the ovary where enzymes metabolize the chemicals to reactive intermediates.[51] BaP, for example, is metabolized initially by microsomal cytochrome P450 enzymes to arene oxides.[84] Once formed, the arene oxides may spontaneously form phenols, which can be converted to their corresponding trans-dihydrodiol by epoxide hydrolase. It is the diol epoxide, 7,8-dihydrodiol-9,10-epoxide, that demonstrates the greatest degree of mutagenicity, carcinogenicity, and ovotoxicity.[50] Detoxification involves conjugation with glutathione by glutathione-S-transferase or further hydrolysis to the tetrol. Alternatively, the dihydrodiols formed from the arene oxides can be conjugated to inactive glucuronides or sulfate esters for excretion, prior to formation of the reactive intermediates. Other PAHs, DMBA and 3-MC, follow similar metabolic pathways.[84] The requirement for bioactivation has been shown by treating mice with a known competitive inhibitor of PAH metabolism, α-naphthoflavone.[48] This treatment reversed oocyte destruction caused by BaP, 3-MC, and DMBA.

The involvement of ovarian enzymes for bioactivation was demonstrated in studies that employed intraovarian injections of BaP.[85] The enzyme responsible for the initiation of PAH metabolism is a cytochrome P450-dependent microsomal monoxygenase, aryl hydrocarbon hydroxylase (AHH).[83] AHH has been studied in detail to determine the relationship between metabolism of PAHs and ovotoxicity.[50] Treatment of B6 mice with 3-MC increased ovarian AHH activity.[47] In murine studies, the extent of ovarian toxicity caused by PAHs has been correlated with the levels or inducibility of AHH activity.[50] DMBA metabolism by cytochrome P450-dependent DMBA mono-oxygenase activity has been measured in enriched granulosa/theca cell fractions isolated from ovaries collected from rats,[86] monkeys,[81] and humans.[82] In general, this activity was higher in follicular cells from unstimulated rats, or in cells collected following hormonal stimulation in monkeys and humans. Increased ovarian DMBA hydroxylase activity was measured during proestrus and estrus in rats, suggesting induction of enzyme expression by estradiol and/or gonadotropins. Taken together, these data provide evidence that bioactivation of the PAHs can be performed directly within the ovary.

3.5.3.3   4-Vinylcyclohexene

Several lines of evidence have established the role of biotransformation in VCH-induced ovarian toxicity. Following 30 d of daily dosing of female B6C3F1 mice and Fischer 344 rats with VCH, small preantral follicles (primordial and primary) were reduced in ovaries of mice but not rats

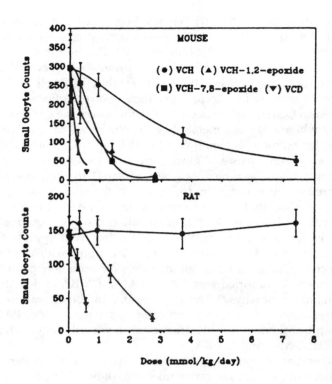

FIGURE 3.3
Comparison of the dose-response relationship in the reduction in small oocyte counts in the ovaries of rats and mice treated i.p. with VCH or VCH epoxides for 30 d. The standard deviations are indicated by bars. (From Smith, B.J., Mattison, D.R., and Sipes, I.G., *Toxicol. Appl. Pharmacol.*, 105, 372, 1990. With permission.)

(Figure 3.3).[59] Through the activity of cyotchrome P450 enzymes, VCH can be converted to two possible monoepoxides [4-vinylcyclohexene monepoxide, VCME], 1,2-VCME, and 7,8-VCME. Ultimately, each of these can be further metabolized to the diepoxide, VCD. When mice and rats were dosed daily with VCME and VCD in this study, unlike VCH, ovotoxic effects were observed in both mice and rats. Furthermore, the compound with the lowest ED50 for follicular destruction in both species was VCD. Thus, it was concluded that the species variation in susceptibility to VCH was, in part, due to differences in the capacity of mice and rats to form the epoxide metabolites. In support of this, measurable amounts of 1,2-VCME were detected in mouse but not rat blood up to 6 h following administration of VCH.[87] Subsequent *in vitro* studies revealed that metabolism of VCH in hepatic microsomes collected from mice converted VCH to 1,2-VCME at a rate four to six times greater than that in rats.[88] These results have provided evidence that epoxidation of VCH represents bioactivation and differing rates in these reactions underlie the observed species variation in VCH-induced ovotoxicity. Structure-activity studies have supported this conclusion and provided evidence that the diepoxide, VCD, is the ultimate ovarian toxicant.[56]

3.5.3.4   Vinylcyclohexene Diepoxide

Enhanced susceptibility of mice as compared with rats to VCH-induced ovotoxicity, therefore, appears to result from a greater rate of bioactivation. Although VCD produced follicular loss in rats, higher doses of VCD were required than in mice. This suggested that detoxification of VCD may also play a role in VCH-induced ovarian toxicity. Subsequently, it was shown that the mouse, as compared with the rat, has a reduced capacity to convert VCD to its inactive tetrol derivative.[89] Similar results have been reported for epoxides of butadiene.[90] Therefore, mice appear to be deficient in a major detoxification pathway for this class of compounds, and the greater susceptibility of mice relates to both enhanced bioactivation and reduced detoxification of the ovotoxic epoxides.

Microsomal epoxide hydrolase as well as cytosolic GST, likely to be involved in metabolism of VCD, are present in the ovary.[18] Evidence that the diepoxide of VCH and VCD is metabolized by epoxide hydrolase has been provided in studies with rabbit liver microsomes.[91] Additionally, although direct metabolism of VCD by conjugation with glutathione (GSH) as evidence of GST activity has not been reported, injection of mice with VCD depleted hepatic GSH levels by 96% within 2 h.[92] This reduction in GSH was thought to reflect its increased conjugation with VCD. Many studies have shown that the ovary is a primary target tissue for VCD; however, the role of the ovary in metabolism of VCD has not been widely studied.

In vitro studies have investigated the role of EH in detoxification of VCD. Hydrolysis of VCD was detected in hepatic microsomes prepared from mice and rats; however, the rate of conversion was greater in rat compared with mouse tissue.[93] Furthermore, hydrolysis was measured in microsomes prepared from rat but not mouse ovaries. Therefore, in addition to enhanced rates of bioactivation of VCH, mice also demonstrate reduced rates of detoxification of VCD when compared with rats. These differences in metabolic capabilities may contribute to the greater susceptibility of mice to VCH-induced ovotoxicity.

Using isolated preantral follicles prepared from rat ovaries, experiments were performed to identify the direct ability of the ovary to metabolize VCD [Figure 3.4].[94] Following *in vitro* incubation, the smallest follicles (fractions 1a and 1b; primordial, primary, and early growing) displayed a lower capacity to convert VCD to the tetrol than did larger preantral follicles (fractions 1c and 2). These results provide evidence that the rat ovary can directly detoxify VCD to the tetrol but that diminished capacity may reside in those smallest follicles that are physiologically targeted for ovotoxicity.

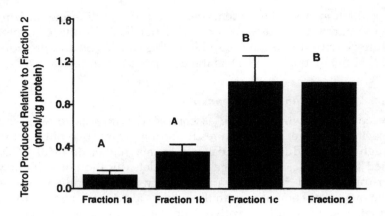

Follicles Prepared by Elutriation

FIGURE 3.4
Metabolism of VCD to tetrol by adult rat preantral follicles. Preantral follicles were separated into distinct fractions as primary and primordial (1a), primary and small growing (1b), small and large growing (1c), and large growing (2) preantral stages of development. Follicular fractions were incubated 1 h with [^{14}C]-VCD (76 μM). Following incubation, media were collected and [^{14}C]-tetrol content was measured by HPLC. Bars with different letters are significantly different from each other, n = 3, p<0.05. (From Flaws, J.A., Salyers, K.L., Sipes, I.G., and Hoyer, P.B., *Toxicol. Appl. Pharmacol,* 126, 286, 1994. With permission.)

3.6   Mechanisms of Ovotoxicity

How ovotoxic effects of environmental chemicals are produced is generally not well understood but might be due to one of several possible mechanisms. Oocyte destruction can result from a toxic chemical directly impairing oocyte viability. Conversely, because oocytes at all stages of follicular development are surrounded by granulosa cells, these mechanisms might also be indirect, involving alterations within the granulosa cell, which compromise its ability to maintain viability in the oocyte.[6] Lastly, environmental chemicals might cause follicle loss by accelerating the overall rate of atresia, the normal mechanism by which the majority of follicles degenerate during development.

3.6.1   Cell Death

Only a select few follicles in the ovary will ever develop fully and be ovulated.[3] Instead, the vast majority of ovarian follicles begin development but are lost by a process of cell death, called atresia. Atretic follicles at all stages of development can be distinguished morphologically from healthy follicles.

Follicular atresia in rats has been shown to occur via a mechanism of physiological cell death, apoptosis.[8] Thus, morphological changes of a cell undergoing atresia are those characteristic of apoptosis.

It has been proposed that most forms of xenobiotic-induced premature ovarian failure are due to increased rates of atresia.[1] However, there appears to be a relationship between the dose given of a chemical, the duration of treatment, and the type of cell death that follows. Whereas low doses induce apoptosis, higher doses often cause necrosis.[95,96] Furthermore, a temporal relationship between apoptosis and necrosis has also been reported. Following a single dose of the hepatotoxin dimethylnitrosamine, apoptosis was rapidly induced (1-7 h), whereas necrosis was reported at a later time (12–24 h).[97,98] Taken together, these results suggest that mild cellular damage can induce a program for death, apoptosis, whereas more severe damage results in passive cell death, necrosis.[99]

In studies investigating ovotoxicity in rats and mice, morphological evidence consistent with both types of cell death have been reported. Ovaries collected from mice given a relatively high dose of CPA, 500 mg/kg demonstrated necrotic damage in oocytes contained in primordial follicles.[33,70] This effect was specific for the oocyte because surrounding granulosa cells appeared unchanged. Conversely, atretic changes in primordial follicles were reported at lower doses (100 mg/kg). In antral follicles, there was evidence of atresia at the higher dose (500 mg/kg).[33] This was similar to the effect observed in antral follicles in rats dosed with 150 mg/kg CPA.[32]

In mice treated with PAHs (80 mg/kg BaP, 3-MC, or DMBA), oocyte morphology consistent with necrosis was observed in primordial follicles.[69] These changes caused by 3-MC and BaP were seen in the absence of visible effects in the associated granulosa cells. However, DMBA produced more visible toxicity by destroying oocytes and follicles more extensively and disrupting ovarian architecture. Morphological evidence consistent with increased atresia in small preantral follicles was also reported in ovaries collected from rats dosed daily for 10 days with the occupational chemical, VCD, 80 mg/kg.[13] In rats treated with the phthalate, DEHP, antral follicle damage was observed in association with retarded ovulation.[21] The morphological changes in these follicles were also consistent with atresia.

In recent years there has been an increase in the investigation of apoptotic cell death following treatment with toxic chemicals.[99] Hepatotoxicants, such as thioacetamide, acetaminophen, and dimethylnitrosamine, induce apoptosis *in vivo* and *in vitro*.[100,101] The halogenated aromatic hydrocarbon, tetrachlorodibenzo-p-dioxin (TCCD), can induce apoptosis in immature thymocytes.[102] The PAH, DMBA, induced internucleosomal cleavage (apoptosis) in mouse thymocytes and spleen cells.[103] Therefore, a number of reports have provided examples of xenobiotic-induced apoptosis. Although there are examples of morphological evidence of ovotoxicity consistent with atresia, few reports have classified the specific type of cell death induced by reproductive toxicants in the ovary as apoptosis. Distinguishing characteristics associated with apoptosis were observed in primordial and primary follicles

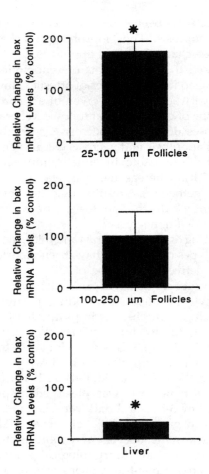

FIGURE 3.5

Effect of VCD dosing on *bax* mRNA levels. Total RNA was prepared from isolated small ovarian preantral follicles (primordial, primary, small growing, 25–100 mm), large growing ovarian preantral follicles (100–250 mm), or liver cells collected from rats dosed daily for 10 d with vehicle control (control) or VCD (80 mg/kg, i.p.). mRNA encoding *bax* was measured using RT-PCR, and normalized to RP-L19 mRNA levels. Data are expressed as effect of VCD treatment versus control, $^*p < 0.05$, VCD different from control. (From Springer, L.N., Tilly, J.L., Sipes I.G., and Hoyer, P.B., *Toxicol. Appl. Pharmacol.*, 139, 402, 1996. With permission.)

in ovaries from rats dosed with the occupational chemical, VCD.[13] Furthermore, there was no evidence of necrosis, such as cellular swelling or infiltration of macrophages in ovaries from treated rats. In additional support that ovotoxicity is via apoptosis, elevated levels of mRNA encoding the cell death enhancer gene, *bax* (elevated in apoptosis) were measured in isolated fractions of small preantral follicles collected from VCD-dosed rats

(Figure 3.5).[104] This effect was specific for the small follicles targeted by VCD and was not seen in large preantral follicles or hepatocytes (nontarget tissues).

3.6.2 Sites of Cellular Damage

In general, intracellular sites targeted by ovotoxic chemicals have not been identified. Many ovotoxic compounds also cause an increased incidence of ovarian tumors.[5] Many epoxidated compounds have been associated with increased mutagenicity in *in vitro* bacterial assays.[105] The ability of epoxides to produce DNA adducts and induce sister chromatin exchanges has also demonstrated effects at the molecular level.[106,107] However, whether DNA damage is the event that initiates ovotoxicity has not been determined for these chemicals. It has been proposed that plasma membrane damage is more highly correlated with ovotoxicity that DNA damage.[24] This observation was supported by comparing alkylating properties with genetic activity in a variety of epoxide-containing chemicals.[108] Thus, the cellular event(s) initiated directly by ovotoxic chemicals may be at the level of proteins involved in signaling pathways or regulatory mechanisms associated with cell death/viability determination, rather than as a direct result of DNA damage.

3.6.3 Gene Expression

The effect of ovotoxic exposures on ovarian gene expression has not been widely studied to date. Xenobiotic exposure is well known to induce expression of metabolizing enzymes in liver. Several chemicals have demonstrated a similar capacity in ovarian tissue. For example, ovarian AHH activity can be induced by the PAH, 3-MC, and the halogenated hydrocarbon, TCDD.[109] Induction of bioactivation and detoxification enzyme activities by PAHs were compared in ovary, adrenal, and liver.[17] Ovarian induction of AHH was observed with 3-MC and DMBA, whereas glutathione-S-transferase and epoxide hydrolase activities were not induced. These results demonstrated that regulation of the ovarian and adrenal systems are closely related, and those in liver are different. A different type of evidence for induction of ovarian metabolizing enzymes was reported in ovaries from rats dosed for 10 d with the occupational chemical, VCD.[104] Following treatment, mRNA encoding epoxide hydrolase was increased in isolated small preantral follicles from dosed rats. This increase was specific in small follicles (targeted by VCD) when compared with larger growing follicles and liver (nontarget tissues). Because of the evidence for ovarian involvement in regulating a response to ovotoxic chemicals, there is bound to be more emphasis in the future on understanding the regulation of gene expression as exposure to these agents progresses.

3.7   Summary

In summary, environmental chemicals that impact ovarian function can directly disrupt endocrine balance by decreasing production of ovarian hormones and interfering with ovulation. These effects are rather immediate, target large antral follicles, and can be reversed once there is no longer exposure to the chemical. On the other hand, ovarian function can be impaired by exposure to chemicals that destroy small preantral follicles. This produces an indirect disruption of endocrine balance once hormonal feedback mechanisms have been affected. The manifestation of this type of ovarian toxicity is delayed until irreversible ovarian failure has occurred. This particular type of ovotoxicity is of particular concern in women because of the health risks known to be associated with menopause. Future research should be aimed at understanding specific mechanisms of ovotoxicity and improving our ability to predict human risk from the wide variety of exposures to these chemicals in the environment.

References

1. Mattison, D. R., *Reproductive Toxicology,* Raven Press, New York, 1985, 109.
2. Richards, J. S., Maturation of ovarian follicles: actions and interactions of pituitary and ovarian hormones on follicular cell differentiation, *Physiol. Rev.,* 60, 51, 1980.
3. Hirshfield, A. N., Development of follicles in the mammalian ovary, *Int. Rev. Cytol.,* 124, 43, 1991.
4. Mant, J. W. F. and Vessey, M. P., *Trends in Cancer Incidence and Mortality,* Cold Spring Harbor Laboratory Press, Plainview, NY, 19, 287, 1994.
5. Hoyer, P. B. and Sipes, I. G., Assessment of follicle destruction in chemical-induced ovarian toxicity, *Annu. Rev. Pharmacol. Toxicol.,* 36, 307, 1996.
6. Buccione, R., Schroeder, A. S., and Eppig, J. J., Interactions between somatic cells and germ cells throughout mammalian oogenesis, *Biol. Reprod.,* 43, 543, 1990.
7. Mattison, D. R. and Schulman, J. D., How xenobiotic compounds can destroy oocytes, *Contemp. Obstet. Gynecol.,* 15, 157, 1980.
8. Tilly, J. L., Kowalski, K. I., Johnson, A. L., and Hsueh, A. J. W., Involvement of apoptosis in ovarian follicular atresia and postovulatory regression, *Endocrinology,* 129, 2799, 1991.
9. Wyllie, A. H., Kerr, J. F. R., and Currie, A. R., Cell death: the significance of apoptosis, *Int. Rev. Cytol.,* 68, 251, 1980.
10. Compton, M. M., A biochemical hallmark of apoptosis: internucleosomal degradation of the genome, *Canc. Metastasis Rev.,* 11, 105, 1992.
11. Payne, C. M., Bernstein, C., and Bernstein, H., Apoptosis overview emphasizing the role of oxidative stress, DNA damage and signal-transduction pathways, *Leukemia Lymphoma,* 19, 43, 1995.

12. Boone, D. L., Yan, W., and Tsang B. K., Identification of a deoxyribonuclease I-like endonuclease in rat granulosa and luteal cell nuclei, *Biol. Reprod.*, 53, 1057, 1995.

13. Springer, L. N., McAsey, M. E., Flaws, J. A., Tilly, J. L., Sipes, I. G., and Hoyer, P. B., Involvement of apoptosis in 4-vinylcyclohexene diepoxide-induced ovotoxicity in rats, *Toxicol. Appl. Pharmacol.*, 139, 394, 1996.

14. Sowers, M. F. R. and LaPietra, M. T., Menopause: its epidemiology and potential association with chronic diseases, *Epidemiol. Rev.*, 17, 287, 1995.

15. Cooper, G. S., Baird, D. D., Hulka, B. S., Weinberg, C. R., Savitz, D. A., and Hughes, C. L., Follicle stimulating hormone concentrations in relation to active and passive smoking, *Obstet. Gynecol.*, 85, 407, 1995.

16. Beverson, R. B., Sandler, D. P., Wilcox, A. J., Schreinemachhers, D., Shore, D. L., and Weinberg, C., Effect of passive exposure to smoking on age at natural menopause, *Br. Med. J.*, 293, 792, 1986.

17. Bengtsson, M. and Rydstrom, J., Regulation of carcinogen metabolism in the rat ovary by the estrous cycle and gonadotropin, *Science*, 219, 1437, 1983.

18. Mukhtar, H., Philpot, R. M., and Bend, J. B., The postnatal development of microsomal epoxide hydrase, cytosolic glutathione S-transferase, and mitochondrial and mircrosomal cytochrome P-450 in adrenals and ovaries of female rats, *Drug Metab. Disp.*, 6, 577, 1978.

19. Generoso, W., Stout, S. K., and Huff, S. W., Effects of alkylating chemicals on reproductive capacity of adult female mice, *Mut. Res.*, 13, 171, 1971.

20. Jarrell, J. F., Bodo, L., Young Lai, E. V., Barr, R. D., and O'Connell, G. J., The short-term reproductive toxicity of cylcophosphamide in the female rat, *Reprod. Toxicol.*, 5, 481, 1991.

21. Davis, B. J., Maronpot, R. R., and Heindel, J. J., Di-(2-ethylhexyl)phthalate suppresses estradiol and ovulation in cycling rats, *Toxicol. Appl. Pharmacol.*, 128, 216, 1994.

22. Hooser, S. B., Douds, D. A., Hoyer, P. B., and Sipes, I. G., Long term ovarian and hormonal alterations due to the ovotoxin, 4-vinylcyclohexene, *Reprod. Toxicol.*, 8, 315, 1994.

23. Hedge, G. A., Colby, H. D., and Goodman, R. L., *Clinical Endocrine Physiology*, Saunders, Philadelphia, 1987, 189.

24. Dobson, R. L. and Felton, J. S., Female germ cell loss from radiation and chemical exposures, *Am. J. Ind. Med.*, 4, 175, 1983.

25. Chapman, R. M., Gonadal injury resulting from chemotherapy, *Am. J. Ind. Med.*, 4, 149, 1983.

26. Damewood, M. D. and Grochow, L. B., Prospects for fertility after chemotherapy or daiation for neoplastic disease, *Fertil. Steril.*, 45, 443, 1986.

27. Sobrinho, L. G., Levine, R. A., and DeConti, R. C., Amenorrhea in patients with Hodgkins disease treated with antineoplastic agents, *Am. J. OB Gyn.*, 109, 135, 1971.

28. Warne, G. L., Fairley, K. F., Hobbs, J. B., and Martin, F. I. R., Cyclophosphamide-induced ovarian failure, *New Engl. J. Med.*, 289, 1159, 1973.

29. Koyama, H., Wada, T., Nishizawa, Y., Iwanaga, T., Aoki, Y., Terasawa, T., Kosaki, G., Yamamoto, T., and Wada, A., Cyclophosphamide-induced ovarian failure and its therapeutic significance in patients with breast cancer, *Cancer*, 39, 1403, 1977.

30. Miller, J. J., III and Cole, L. J., Changes in mouse ovaries after prolonged treatment with cyclophosphamide, *Proc. Soc. Exp. Biol. Med.*, 133, 190, 1970.

31. Shiromizu, K., Thorgeirsson, S. S., and Mattison, D. R., Effect of cyclophospha-mide on oocyte and follicle number in Sprague Dawley rats, C57BL/6N and DBA/2N mice, *Ped. Pharm.*, 4, 213, 1984.

32. Jarrell, J., Young Lai, E. V., Barr, R., McMahon, A., Belbeck, L., and O'Connell, G., Ovarian toxicity of cyclophosphamide alone and in combination with ova-rian irradiation in the rat, *Canc. Res.*, 47, 2340, 1987.

33. Plowchalk, D. R. and Mattison, D. R., Reproductive toxicity of cyclophospha-mide in the C57BL/6N mouse. 1. Effects on ovarian structure and function, *Reprod. Toxicol.*, 6, 411, 1992.

34. Baird, D. D. and Wilcox, A. J. Cigarette smoking associated with delayed conception, *J. Am. Med. Assoc.*, 253, 2979, 1985.

35. Jick, H., Porter, J., and Morrison, A. S., Relation between smoking and age of natural menopause, *Lancet*, 1, 1354, 1977.

36. Mattison, D. R., Plowchalk, B. S., Meadows, M. J., Miller, M. M., Malek, A., and London, S., The effect of smoking on oogenesis, fertilization, and implantation, *Semin. Reprod. Endocrinol.*, 7, 291, 1989.

37. Weinberg, C. R., Wilcox, A. J., and Baird, D. D., Reduced fecundability in women with prenatal exposure to cigarette smoking, *Am. J. Epidemiol.*, 125, 1072, 1989.

38. Vahakangas, K., Rajaniemi, H., and Pelkonen, O., Ovarian toxicity of cigarette smoke exposure during pregnancy in mice, *Toxicol. Lett.*, 25, 75, 1985.

39. Stedman, R. L., The chemical composition of tobacco and tobacco smoke, *Chem. Rev.*, 68, 153, 1968.

40. VanVoorhis, B. J., Syrop, C. H., Hammit, D. G., Dunn, M. S., and Snyder, G. D., Effects of smoking on ovulation induction for assisted reproductive techniques, *Fertil. Steril.*, 58, 981, 1992.

41. Barbieri, R. L., McShane, P. M., and Ryan, K. J., Constituents of cigarette smoke inhibit human granulosa cell aromatase, *Fertil. Steril.*, 46, 232, 1986.

42. Yeh, J. and Barbierei, R. L., Effects of smoking on steroid production, metabo-lism, and estrogen related diseases, *Semin. Reprod. Endocrinol.*, 7, 326, 1989.

43. Krarup, T., 9:10-dimethyl-1:2-benozanthracene induced ovarian tumors in mice, *Acta Path. Micro. Scand.*, 70, 241, 1967.

44. Krarup, T., Oocyte destruction and ovarian tumorigenesis after direct applica-tion of a chemical carcinogen (9:10-dimethyl-1:2-benzanthrene) to the mouse ovary, *Int. J. Canc.*, 4, 61, 1969.

45. Mattison, D. R., Difference in sensitivity of rat and mouse primordial oocytes to destruction by polycyclic aromatic hydrocarbons, *Chem.-Biol. Interact.*, 28, 133, 1979.

46. Basler, A. and Rohrborn, G., Chromosome aberrations in oocytes of NMR1 mice and bone marrow cells of chinese hamsters induced with 3,4 benzpyrene, *Mut. Res.*, 38, 327, 1976.

47. Gulyas, B. J., and Mattison, D. R., Degeneration of mouse oocytes in response to polycyclic aromatic hydrocarbons, *Anat. Rec.*, 193, 863, 1979.

48. Mattison, D. R. and Thorgeirsson, S. S., Ovarian aryl hydrocarbon hydroxylase acitivity and primordial oocyte toxicity of polycyclic aromatic hydrocarbons in mice, *Canc. Res.*, 39, 3471, 1979.

49. Mackenzie, K. M. and Angevine, D. M., Infertility in mice exposed *in utero* to benzo(a)pyrene, *Biol. Reprod.*, 24, 183, 1981.

50. Mattison, D. R., Shiromizu, K., and Nightingale, M. S., Oocyte destruction by polycyclic aromatic hydrocarbons, *Am. J. Ind. Med.*, 4, 191, 1983.

51. Mattison, D. R. and Nightingale, M. R., The biochemical and genetic characteristics of murine ovarian aryl hydrocarbon (Benzo(a)pyrene)hydroxylase activity and its relationship to primoridal oocyte destruction by polycyclic aromatic hydrocarbons, *Toxicol. Appl. Pharmacol.*, 56, 399, 1980.

52. IARC (International Agency for Research on Cancer), *IARC Monographs on the Evaluation of Carcinogenic Risks to Humans: Some Industrial Chemicals*, Lyon, France, 1994, 60.

53. Melnick, R. L. and Huff J., 1,3-Butadiene: Toxicity and carcinogenicity in laboratory animals and in humans, *Rev. Environ. Contam. Toxicol.*, 124, 111, 1992.

54. Thornton-Manning, J. R., Dahl, A. R., Bechtold, W. E., Griffith, W. C., Jr., and Henderson, R. F., Disposition of butadiene monoepoxide and butadiene diepoxide in various tissues of rats and mice following a low level inhalation exposure 1,3-butadiene, *Carcinogenesis*, 16, 1723, 1995.

55. Melnick, R. L., Huff, J., Chou, B. J., and Miller, R. A., Carcinogenicity of 1,3-butadiene in C57BL/6 X C3HF1 mice at low exposure concentrations, *Canc. Res.*, 50, 6592, 1990.

56. Doerr, J. K., Hooser, S. B., Smith, B. J., and Sipes, I. G., Ovarian toxicity of 4-vinylcyclohexene and related olefins in B6C3F1 mice: role of diepoxides, *Chem. Res. Toxicol.*, 8, 963, 1995.

57. Bond, J. A., Recio, L., and Andjelkovich, D., Epidemiological and mechanistic data suggest that 1,3-butadiene will not be carcinogenic to humans at exposures likely to be encountered in the environment or workplace, *Carcinogenesis*, 16, 165, 1995.

58. Rappaport, S. M. and Fraser, D. A., Air sampling and analysis in rubber vulcanization area. *Am. Hyg. Assoc. J.*, 38, 205, 1977.

59. Smith, B. J., Mattison, D. R., and Sipes, I. G., The role of epoxidation in 4-vinylcyclohexene-induced ovarian toxicity, *Toxicol. Appl. Pharmacol.*, 105, 372, 1990.

60. National Toxicology Program (NTP), NTP Technical Report No. 303. U.S. Department of Health and Human Services, Public Health Service, National Institutes of Health, Public Information, National Toxicology Program, Research Triangle Park, NC, 1986.

61. Grizzle, T. B., George, J. D., Fail, P. A., Seely, J. C., and Heindel, J. J., Reproductive effects of 4-vinylcyclohexene in swiss mice assessed by a continuous breeding protocol, *Fund. Appl. Toxicol.*, 22, 122, 1994.

62. National Toxicology Program (NTP), NTP Technical Report No. 362, U.S. Department of Health and Human Services, Public Health Service, National Institutes of Health, Public Information, National Toxicology Program, Research Triangle Park, NC, 1989.

63. Bevan, C., Stadler, J. C., Elliott, G. S., Frame, S. R., Baldwin, J. K., Leung, H.-W., Moran, E., and Panepinto, A. S., Subchronic toxicity of 4-vinylcyclohexene in rats and mice by inhalation exposure, *Fund. Appl. Toxicol.*, 32, 1, 1996.

64. Kari, F. W., Huff, J. E., Leininger, J., Haseman, J. K., and Eustis, S. L., Toxicity and carcinogenicity of nitrofurazone in F344/N rats and B6C3F1 mice, *Food Chem. Tox.*, 27, 129, 1989.

65. Hemminki, K., Falck, K., and Vainio, H., Comparison of alkylation rates and mutagenicity of directly acting industrial and laboratory chemicals, *Arch. Toxicol.*, 46, 277, 1980.

66. Sevcik, M. L. and Jarrell, J. F., *Comprehensive Toxicology*, Elsevier Press, Oxford, 1997, 10, 369.

67. Plowchalk, D. R. and Mattison, D. R., Phosphoramide mustard is responsible for the ovarian toxicity of cylcophosphamide, *Toxicol. Appl. Pharmacol.*, 107, 472, 1991.

68. Krarup, T., Oocyte survival in the mouse ovary after treatment with 9,10-1,2-benzanthracene, *J. Endocrinol.*, 46, 483, 1970.

69. Mattison, D. R., Morphology of oocyte and follicle destruction by polycyclic aromatic hydrocarbons in mice, *Toxicol. Appl. Pharmacol.*, 53, 249, 1980.

70. Swartz, W. J. and Mattison, D. R., Benzo(a)pyrene inhibits ovulation in C57BL/6N mice, *Anat. Rec.*, 212, 268, 1985.

71. Safe, S. and Krishnan, V., Chlorinated hydrocarbons: estrogens and antiestrogens, *Toxicol. Lett.*, 82, 731, 1995.

72. Li, X., Johnson, D. C., and Rozman, K. K., Effects of 2,3,7,8-tetrachlorodibenzo-*p*-dioxin (TCDD) on estrous cyclicity and ovulation in female Sprague-Dawley rats, *Toxicol. Lett.*, 78, 219, 1995.

73. Li, X., Johnson, D. C., and Rozman, K. K., Reproductive effects of 2,3,7,8-tetrachlorodibenzo-*p*-dioxin (TCDD) in female rats: ovulation, hormonal regulation, and possible mechanism(s), *Toxicol. Appl. Pharmacol.*, 133, 321, 1995.

74. Moran, F. M., Enan, E., Vandevoort, C. A., Stewart, D. R., Conley, A. J., Overstreet, J. W., and Lasley, B. L., 2,3,7,8-tetrachlorodibenzo-p-dioxin (TCDD) effects on steroidogenesis of human luteinized granulosa cell *in vitro, Biol. Reprod. Suppl. 1*, 56, 65, 1997.

75. Lucier, G. W., Davis, G. J., and McLachlan, J. A., 17th Hanford Biol. Symp. Monograph, Oak Ridge Tech. Inform. Centre, 1977, 188.

76. Wardell, R. E., Seegmiller, R. E., and Bradshaw, W. S., Induction of prenatal toxicity in the rat by diethylstilbesterol, zeranol, 3,4,3′,4′-tetrachlorobiphenyl, cadmium and lead, *Teratol.*, 226, 229, 1982.

77. Ronnback, C., Effect of 3,3′4,4′-tetrachlorobiphenyl (TCB) on ovaries of fetal mice, *Pharmacol. Toxicol.*, 69, 340, 1991.

78. Heinrichs, W. L. and Juchau, M. R., *Extrahepatic Metabolism of Drugs and Other Foreign Compounds*, SP Medical and Scientific Books, New York, 1980, 1, 319.

79. Anderson, D., Bishop, J. B., Garner, R. C., Ostrodky-Wegman, P., and Selby, P. B., Cyclophosphamide: review of its mutagenicity for an assessment of potential germ cell risks, *Mut. Res.*, 330, 115, 1995.

80. Mattison, D. R., Oocyte destruction by polycyclic aromatic hydrocarbons, *Am. J. Ind. Med.*, 4, 191, 1983.

81. Bengtsson, M. and Mattison, D. R., Gondatropin-dependent metabolism of 7,12-dimethylbenz(a)anthracene in the ovary of rhesus monkey, *Biochem. Pharmacol.*, 38, 1869, 1989.

82. Bengtsson, M., Hamberger, L., and Rydstrom, J., Metabolism of 7,12-dimethylbenz(a)anthracene by different types of cells in the human ovary, *Xenobiotica*, 18, 1255, 1988.

83. Sims, P. and Grover, P. L., Epoxides in PAH metabolism and carcinogenesis, *Adv. Canc. Res.*, 20, 165, 1974.

84. Mumatz, M. M., George, J. D., Gold, K. W., Cibulas, W., and Derosa, C. T., ASTDR evaluation of health effects of chemicals. IV. Polycyclic aromatic hydrocarbons (PAHs): understanding a complex problem, *Toxicol. Ind. Health*, 12, 742, 1996.

85. Shiromizu, K. and Mattison, D. R., The effect of intraovarian injection of benzo(a)pyrene on primordial oocyte number and ovarian aryl hydrocarbon [benzo(a)pyrene] hydroxylase activity, *Toxicol. Appl. Pharmacol.*, 76, 18, 1984.

86. Bengtsson, M., Reinholt, F. P., and Rydstrom, J., Cellular localization and hormonal regulation of 7,12-dimethylbenz[a]anthracene mono-oxygenase activity in the rat ovary, *Toxicology*, 71, 203, 1992.

87. Smith, B. J., Carter, D. E., and Sipes, I. G., Comparison of the disposition and *in vitro* metabolism of 4-vinylcyclohexene in the female mouse and rat, *Toxicol. Appl. Pharmacol.*, 105, 364, 1990.

88. Smith, B. J., Mattison, D. R., and Sipes, I. G., *Biological Reactive Intermediates IV*, Plenum Press, New York, 1990, 465.

89. Salyers, K. L., Zheng, W., and Sipes, I. G., Disposition and toxicokinetics of 4-vinyl-1-cyclohexene diepoxide in female F344 rats and B6C3F1 mice, *ISSX Proc.*, 4, 169, 1993.

90. Csanady, G. A., Guengerich, F. P., and Bond, J. A., Comparison of the biotransformation of 1,3-butadiene and its metabolite, butadiene monoepoxide by hepatic and pulmonary tissues from humans, rats and mice, *Carcinogenesis*, 13, 1143, 1992.

91. Watabe, T., Hiratsuka, A., Isobe, M., and Ozawa, N., Metabolism of d-limonene by hepatic microsomes to non-mutagenic epoxides toward Salmonella typhimurium, *Biochem. Pharmacol.*, 29, 1068, 1980.

92. Giannarini, C., Citti, L., Gervasi, P. G., and Turchi G., Effects of 4-vinylcylcohexene and its main oxirane metabolite on mouse hepatic microsomal enzymes and glutathione levels, *Toxicol. Lett.*, 8, 115, 1981.

93. Carpenter, S. C. and Keller, D. A., Species differences in metabolism of 4-vinylcyclohexene (VCH) and its epoxide metabolites *in vitro*, *Toxicologist*, 14, 338, 1994.

94. Flaws, J. A., Salyers, K. L., Sipes, I. G., and Hoyer, P. B., Reduced ability of rat preantral ovarian follicles to metabolize 4-vinyl-1-cyclohexene diepoxide *in vitro*, *Toxicol. Appl. Pharmacol.*, 126, 286, 1994.

95. Ray, S. D., Sorger, C. L., Raucy, J. L., and Corcoran, G. B., Early loss of large genomic DNA *in vivo* with accumulation of Ca2+ in the nucleus during acetominophen-induced liver injury, *Toxicol. Appl. Pharmacol.*, 106, 346, 1990.

96. Collins, R. J., Harmon, B. V., Gobe, G. C., and Kerr, J. F. R., Internucleosomal DNA cleavage should not be the sole criterion for identifying apoptosis, *Int. J. Radiat. Biol.*, 61, 451, 1992.

97. Pritchard, D. J. and Butler, W. H., Apoptosis — the mechanism of cell death in dimethylnitrosamine-induced hepatotoxicity, *J. Pathol.*, 158, 253, 1989.

98. Hirata, K., Ogata, I., Ohta, Y., and Fujiwara, K., Hepatic sinusoidal cell destruction in the development of intravascular coagulation in acute liver failure of rats, *J. Pathol.*, 158, 157, 1989.

99. Corcoran, G. B., Fix, L., Jones, D. P., Moslen, M. T., Oberhammer, F. A., and Buttyan, R., Apoptosis: molecular control points in toxicology, *Toxicol. Appl. Pharmacol.*, 128, 169, 1994.

100. Shen, W., Kamendulis, L. M., Ray, S. D., Corcoran, G. B., Acetaminophen-induced cytotoxicity in cultured mouse hepatocytes: correlation of nuclear Ca2+ accumulation and early DNA fragmentation with cell death, *Toxicol. Appl. Pharmacol.*, 111, 242, 1991.

101. Faa, G., Ambu, R., Congiu, T., Costa, V., Ledda-Columbano, G. M., Coni, P., Curto, M., Giacomini, L., and Columbano, A., Early ultrastructural changes during thioacetamide-induced apoptosis in rat liver, *J. Submicroscop. Cytol. Pathol.*, 24, 417, 1992.

102. McConkey, D. J., Hartzell, P., Nicotera, P., Wyllie, A. H., and Orrenius, S., Stimulation of endogenous endonuclease activity in hepatocytes exposed to oxidative stress, *Toxicol. Lett.*, 42, 123, 1988.

103. Burchiel, S. W., Davis, D. A. P., Ray, S. D., Archuleta, M. M., Thilsted, J. P., and Corcoran, G. B., DMBA-induced cytotoxicity in lymphoid and non lymphoid organs of B6C3F1 mice: relation of cell death to target cell intracellular calcium and DNA damage, *Toxicol. Appl. Pharmacol.*, 113, 126, 1992.

104. Springer, L. N., Tilly, J. L., Sipes, I. G., and Hoyer, P. B., Enhanced expression of bax in small preantral follicles during 4-vinylcyclohexene diepoxide-induced ovotoxicity in the rat, *Toxicol. Appl. Pharmacol.*, 139, 402, 1996.

105. Wade, M. J., Moyer, J. W., and Hine, C. H., Mutagenic action of a series of epoxides, *Mut. Res.*, 66, 367, 1979.

106. Citti, L., Gervasi, P. G., Turchi, G., Bellucci, G., and Bianchini, R., The reaction of 3,4-epoxy-1-butene with deoxyguanosine and DNA *in vitro*: synthesis and characterization of the main adducts, *Carcinogenesis*, 5, 47, 1984.

107. deRaat, W. K., Induction of sister chromatid exchanges by styrene and its presumed metabolite styrene oxide in the presence of rat liver homogenate, *Chem.-Biol. Interact.*, 20, 163, 1978.

108. Turchi, G., Bonatti, S., Citti, L., Gervasi, P. G., and Abbondandolo, A., Alkylating properties and genetic activity of 4-vinylcyclohexene metabolites and structurally related epoxides, *Mut. Res.*, 83, 419, 1981.

109. Mattison, D. R. and Thorgeirsson, S. S., Genetic differences in mouse ovarian metabolism of benzo(a)pyrene and oocyte toxicity, *Biochem. Pharmacol.*, 26, 909, 1977.

4

Dietary Phytoestrogens

Heather B. Patisaul and Patricia L. Whitten

CONTENTS

4.1 Introduction

Phytoestrogens, a group of estrogenic compounds found in plants, are particularly interesting to compare to other environmental substances with

0-8493-3164-1/99/$0.00+$.50
© 1999 by CRC Press LLC

endocrine action. These naturally occurring substances gain access to body tissues and fluids, often in concentrations considerably in excess of endogenous steroids. Although they are weak estrogens compared to estradiol, their potencies are rather similar to the *in vivo* and *in vitro* ranges reported for endocrine disruptors. Phytoestrogens can occur at high levels in milk and infant formula and exhibit significant developmental actions in animal studies. In contrast to other endocrine disruptors, however, phytoestrogens also exhibit an array of beneficial effects that could provide preventative or therapeutic actions in carcinogenesis, heart disease, and osteoporosis. Thus, the phytoestrogens both expand our view of environmental substances with endocrine action and provide a useful tool for investigating the mechanisms by which such compounds produce harmful or beneficial effects.

Phytoestrogens are classically defined as any plant compound that is functionally or structurally similar to estrogen or that produces estrogenic effects.[1] This definition includes compounds that bind to the alpha estrogen receptor, induce estrogen-responsive gene products, stimulate breast cancer cells *in vitro*, induce estrus, and stimulate growth of the female genital tract.[2] The two major classes of phytoestrogens are lignans and isoflavonoids. The latter group is the most intensely studied of the two and is further divided into the isoflavones, isoflavans, and coumestans. Mycoestrogens, or mycotoxins, are a similar group of compounds that can have potent estrogenic effects but are not intrinsic components of plants. They are mold metabolites of the fungal genus *Fusarium*, which frequently infects pasture grasses and legumes including alfalfa and clover. Although they are rarely considered in the discussion of phytoestrogens, they are the compounds that initially generated interest in the topic of naturally occurring estrogens and their effects on health and reproduction. A hierarchy of phytoestrogens is presented in Figure 4.1.

4.2   Dietary Sources of Phytoestrogens

4.2.1   Lignans

Lignans are a minor component of plant cell walls. The plant lignans matairesinol and secoisolariciresinol are converted to the mammalian lignans enterlactone and enterodiol, respectively (see Figure 4.2), by the resident bacterial flora of the gut.[3] Mammalian lignan production has been assessed and quantified by *in vitro* fermentation with human fecal microbiota.[4] The highest concentrations of mammalian lignans are produced from oilseeds, particularly flaxseed, which produces 50-100 times that of nearly every other plant studied. Mammalian lignans are also produced from whole grains, cereal brans, legumes, and vegetables. The *in vitro* production of lignans from some common foods is listed in Table 4.1.

Flavonoids
    Flavanones
        4',7-Dihydroxyflavanone
        Naringenin
    Flavones
        Apigenin
        4',5-Dihydroxyflavone
        4',6-Dihydroxyflavone
    Flavonols
        Kaempferol
    Hydroxychalcones
        Phloretin
        Isoliquiritigenin
        4,4'-Dihydroxychalcone
    Isoflavonoids
        Isoflavones
            Daidzein
            Formononetin
            Genistein
            Biochanin A
        Isoflavanones
            O-Desmethylangolensin
        Isoflavans
            Equol
        Coumestans
            Coumestrol
Lignans
    Enterlactone
    Enterodiol
Mycoestrogens
    Zearalenone
    Zearalenol
    Zearalanol (zeranol)

FIGURE 4.1
Hierarchy and classification of phytoestrogens.

4.2.2 Isoflavonoids

The isoflavonoids are divided into three major classes: isoflavones, isoflavans, and coumestans. The major mammalian isoflavones are genistein and daidzein, which are formed from the plant precursors formononetin and biochanin A, respectively. The most significant isoflavan is equol (see Figure 4.2), a metabolite of daidzein. Coumestrol is the major coumestan. Very little is known about the coumestans compared to the other isoflavonoids. Coumestrol is the most potent phytoestrogen, with a relative potency of .202 compared to estradiol (100).[5]

Phytoestrogenic isoflavonoids are less prevalent than lignans. Legumes contain the most, with the highest concentrations found in soybeans and

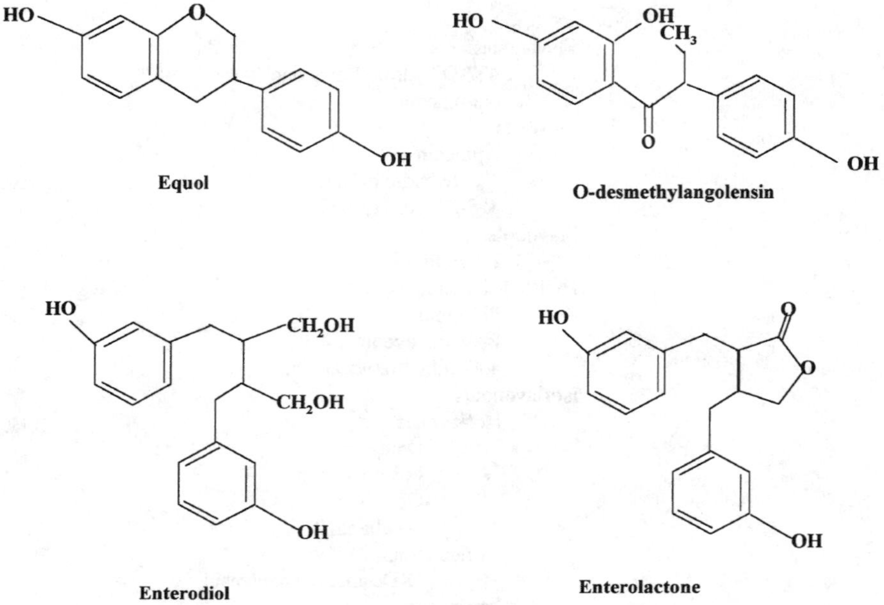

FIGURE 4.2
Mammalian metabolites of isoflavones (equol, o-desmethylangolensis) and lignans (enterodiol, enterolactone).

soybean-based products. These foods contain approximately 0.2-1.6 mg of isoflavones per gram dry weight.[2] Alfalfa produces only small amounts, but clover can contain up to 5% dry weight of estrogenic isoflavones, including genistein, formononetin, and biochanin A.[6] It is this legume that caused sterility in pasture-grazing sheep in the 1940s, hence the name "clover disease" for the affliction. All of the legumes are susceptible to infection by *Fusarium* fungus, which produces high levels of mycoestrogens such as zearalenone. Once infected, many legumes elevate their own phytoestrogen production, further increasing the exogenous estrogen exposure for any animal grazing on infected pasture. Whole grain products, potatoes, fruits, and vegetables also contain detectable levels of isoflavonoids.[7] In nearly all foods, the most prevalent group of isoflavonoids are the isoflavones. The isoflavone content of a variety of soy-based foods is summarized in Table 4.2.

4.3   Metabolism

In plants, phytoestrogens are found most frequently in their glycosidic form. Once ingested, metabolism into the mammalian forms is carried out by the

TABLE 4.1

Human Lignan Production from Various Foods

Food	Enterodiol (μg produced by fecal flora/100 g)	Enterolactone (mg/100 g)
Flaxseed meal	59,024	8,517
Flaxseed flour	40,861	11,818
Soybeans	170	693
Rapeseed	155	975
Oat bran	386	265
Wheat bran	298	269
Barley	74	41
Brown rice	128	169
Garlic	326	81
Asparagus	238	136
Broccoli	65	161
Potatoes	50	33
Pears	69	112
Bananas	14	55

Note: The values in the table are expressed in mg produced by human fecal flora from 100g of nondessicated sample.

Adapted from data presented by Thompson, L. U., Robb, P., Serraine, M., and Cheung, F., *Nutr. Canc.*, 16, 43, 1991. With permission.

resident microflora of the gut. Both the metabolites and a variable amount of the original compounds are absorbed and then undergo enterohepatic circulation. The exact metabolic processes of how each individual compound is converted are not completely characterized and vary between species. In all mammals, gut flora are essential for the initial hydrolysis and metabolism of these compounds. Only after this has occurred can the metabolites be absorbed by the animal, where they may undergo further conjugation and degradation by the liver enzymes. Complete metabolism in most species involves several intermediate compounds, some of which are more estrogenic than the end products.

For example, two of the most commonly studied isoflavones, daidzein and genistein, can be produced through the hydrolysis of their glucoside conjugates or though metabolism of formononetin and biochanin A, respectively. Daidzein is further metabolized into dihydrodaidzein, then equol, and finally O-demethylangolensin (O-DMA) in humans (see Figure 4.2). In sheep, genistein is metabolized into dihydrogenistein before ultimately becoming p-ethylphenol, which has no known estrogenic properties.[2] In humans, the metabolism of genistein more closely parallels that of daidzein and ultimately becomes 6'-hydroxy-O-demethlangolensin (6'-OH-O-DMA), which has unknown effects.[10]

Phytoestrogen absorption proceeds through a series of conjugation and deconjugation steps facilitated by the gut bacterial flora and the liver. In

TABLE 4.2

Isoflavone Content of Various Foods

Food	Daidzein (µg/g)	Genistein (µg/g)	Coumestrol (µg/g)	Method	Ref
Soy beans, dry, whole	700	200	None detected	HPLC	8
Soybean seeds, dry	846.25	1106.75	None detected	HPLC	9[a]
Soybean seeds, roasted	848.1	1105.5	None detected	HPLC	9
Soybean seeds, boiled	68.5	69.4	None detected	HPLC	9
Green soybeans	54.6	72.9	None detected	HPLC	9
Soy flour	523.5	854.1	None detected	HPLC, GC-MS	7-9[b]
Soy protein, textured	523.25	636.25	None detected	HPLC	8[c]
Soy nuts	575	935	None detected	HPLC	8
Soybean sprouts	138	230	7	HPLC	8
Soy hot dogs	49	139	N/A	HPLC	8
Soy cheese	14	20	N/A	HPLC	8
Tempeh	190	320	N/A	HPLC	8
Tofu	76	166	None detected	HPLC	8
Soy sauce	8	5	None detected	HPLC	8
Poppy seeds	17.9	16.7	N/A	GC-MS	7
Green split peas	72.6	None detected	None detected	HPLC	9
Kala chana seeds, dry	None detected	6.4	61.3	HPLC	9
Alfalfa sprouts	None detected	None detected	46.8	HPLC	9
Clover sprouts	None detected	3.5	280.6	HPLC	9
Garlic	2.08	1.45	N/A	GC-MS	7
Carrots	1.6	1.7	N/A	GC-MS	7

[a] Table values are averages of the values from all reported trials in the referenced paper.
[b] Table values are averages of the values reported in all three papers.
[c] Table values are averages of the values listed in the referenced paper.

humans, after absorption from the small intestine, phytoestrogens are conjugated with glucuronic acid and sulfate by hepatic phase II enzymes. In ruminants, the liver contributes very little to the conjugation process, and rumen microorganisms likely account for most of the degradation.[11] Like endogenous estrogens, mammalian lignans and isoflavonoid phytoestrogens are all diphenols structurally similar to endogenous estrogens and found in all bodily fluids, including urine, feces, blood, and bile.[12] They can exist in a wide variety of conjugate forms, which are only beginning to be identified. Once absorbed and conjugated, they undergo enterohepatic circulation and can be deconjugated by the gut flora, only to reenter the same absorption cycle or be further metabolized and degraded in the large intestine.

Human metabolism and excretion of phytoestrogens show substantial variation both between populations and among individuals. Series of studies in several countries have all revealed that vegetarians excrete the highest levels of lignans, while breast cancer patients excrete the lowest. Japanese men and women have among the highest urinary and plasma levels of isoflavones but low values of lignans. These differences have been summarized and reviewed by Adlercreutz et al.[7,13] Most of these differences are due to dietary variation. Asian diets are particularly high in soy, resulting in isoflavone consumption as high as 1 mg/kg body weight, while vegetarian diets are high in whole grains, vegetables, legumes, and other sources of lignans. These dietary exposures result in plasma concentrations as high as 0.4 μM isoflavones and 0.5 μM lignans in vegetarians and 1 μM isoflavones in Japanese subjects, whereas plasma concentrations of both isoflavones and lignans are less than 0.07 μM in omnivores.

Urinary concentrations of phytoestrogenic metabolites also vary widely among individuals within populations, but these differences are only beginning to be elucidated. Several studies have now demonstrated that many individuals apparently lack the ability to metabolize daidzein to equol or can only produce it in negligible quantities.[3,14,15] In one study designed to detect plasma levels of phytoestrogens after a dietary challenge, only four of 12 subjects were able to produce detectable levels of equol.[16] Men have been shown to excrete more enterolactone and less enterodiol than women, suggesting a gender difference in the metabolism of lignans.[17] This phenomenon has not been studied widely and may also apply to isoflavone metabolism.

This variation might be due to individual differences in the quantity and composition of intestinal microflora. Specific gender differences in gut colonization are unknown, as are differences between populations. A portion of this variation can also be attributed to specific dietary intake because the phytoestrogen content of soy and other foods varies widely due to differences in processing and preparation. Soy processing also appears to influence isoflavone bioavailability. In a study reported by Hutchins et al.,[14] urinary recovery of daidzein and genistein in men was higher for subjects consuming tempeh than those consuming unfermented soy, suggesting that the aglycone conjugate of isoflavones, found in fermented food, may be more bioavailable than the glucoside conjugates. The phytoestrogenic content of edible plants also changes from season to season and year to year, depending on the growing conditions.[5] What has not been considered to date when attempting to account for individual variability is the effect of body size and body composition, which may play a critical role in the metabolism of these compounds.

Metabolism of phytoestrogens is also species specific. Cows produce significantly more equol than sheep, and clear it from their systems twice as slowly,[11] while many humans lack the ability to make equol at all.[6] Similarly, in ruminants, many of the isoflavones, including genistein and biochanin A, are broken down to nonestrogenic p-ethyl phenol and organic acids in the rumen. Humans, on the other hand, absorb considerable amounts, and conjugates of the isoflavones are found in all bodily fluids.[10,12] When using animal models to examine the possible biological effects of phytoestrogens in humans, this factor needs to be taken into consideration. To assess accurately the effects of phytoestrogenic compounds on mammalian tissue, their exact metabolic pathways must be characterized on a species-by-species basis. Greater attempts must also be made to characterize and identify the sources of variability in urine and plasma levels between individuals, and particularly between men and women.

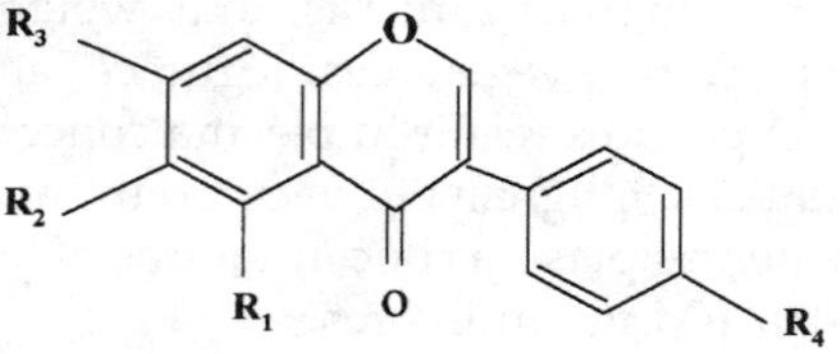

Isoflavone Structures

Isoflavone	R_1	R_2	R_3	R_4
Genistein	OH	H	OH	OH
Daidzein	H	H	OH	OH
Formononetin	H	H	OH	OCH_3
Biochanin A	OH	H	OH	OCH_3
Glycetin	H	OCH_3	OH	OH

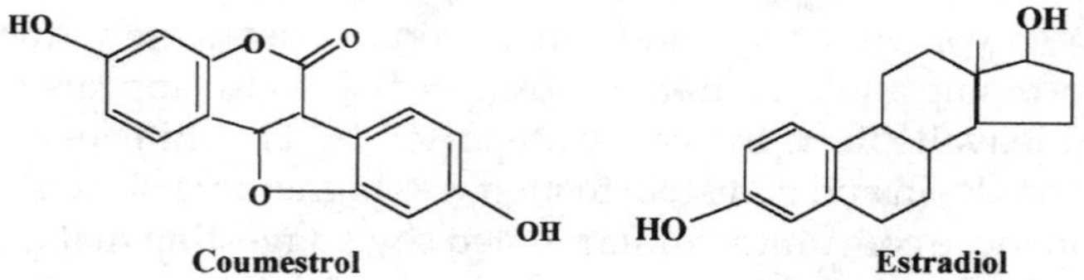

Coumestrol   **Estradiol**

FIGURE 4.3
Structure of isoflavones and coumestans compared to 17β-estradiol.

4.4   Activity

4.4.1   Estrogen Receptor Binding

Phytoestrogens get their name from their ability to mimic the actions of endogenous estrogens. Structurally, the isoflavonoid phytoestrogens and endogenous estrogens are markedly similar, as shown in Figure 4.3. For both groups of compounds, the A-ring is aromatic. There is a hydroxyl group at the C3 position in steroidal estrogens and in the equivalent position in phytoestrogens (7 in ring A and 4′ in ring B). The D ring of natural estrogens is a cyclopentano ring, but the terminal ring is aromatic in the isoflavonoids.[18] The lignans show less structural similarity to natural estrogens. All are diphenols but have a strikingly different conformation.

Because of their structural similarity to endogenous estrogens, isoflavonoid phytoestrogens can bind with the estrogen receptor (ER). Successful binding to the ER occurs through two distinct steps: receptor recognition and stabilization of the receptor-ligand complex.[19] For endogenous estrogens, receptor recognition is achieved by hydrogen bonding between the C3 hydroxyl group on the estrogen and amino acid side chain in the binding domain of the ER. Stabilization is also achieved through hydrogen binding to the D ring but does not require a hydroxyl group.[19,20] Both zearalenol and estrone stabilize the receptor-ligand complex with a ketone. Biological potency of phytoestrogens relative to estradiol appear to be determined by their ability to stabilize this complex.

Once formed, the ligand-receptor complex is taken into the cell and functions as a nuclear transcription factor by binding to an estrogen response element (ERE) and facilitating assembly of a functional transcription complex. Because of their structural similarity to endogenous estrogens, coumestrol and the isoflavones can all bind weakly to the alpha estrogen receptor (ERα). Once bound, they mimic the effects of estrogen, with variable potencies based on the effective ability of the ER-phytoestrogen complex to promote gene transcription. For example, genistein's ability to regulate gene expression through the alpha estrogen receptor is nearly 50-fold less than the mycoestrogen zearalenone, but its affinity is only two- to three-fold less.[18] Thus, even though their ability to bind to the receptor is about the same, zearalenone is a much more potent agonist.

Many attempts have been made to quantify the relative binding affinities, and potencies of phytoestrogens compared to estradiol. Depending on which assay is used, widely different values have been obtained, creating discrepancies about which phytoestrogens are the most estrogenic. There is little doubt that the mycoestrogens are the most potent and have the highest binding affinities with values in the range of 8.7-0.07 depending on the assay used and the fungal mycoestrogen tested.[21,22] Coumestrol is the most potent of the isoflavonoids, with a potency of around 0.67.[22,23] The next most potent are genistein and equol, with potencies in the range of 0.011 to 0.2 depending on the assay used.[22,24] Biochanin A, formononetin, and genistein are less potent, with values ranging from <0.0006 up to 0.0091.[5,22] Although the exact order in which these phytoestrogens should be placed in relation to estrogenic potency is not clear, these studies and others comparing them to each other and to other related compounds reveal that the 4'-hydroxy position on the B ring and its spacial orientation in relation to the 7-position hydroxy group on the A ring are primarily responsible for the estrogenicity of flavonoids.[25] This is illustrated by the reduced potency of biochanin A compared with genistein. Biochanin A has a methyl group in this position but is otherwise structurally identical to genistein and has a much lower potency. This structural difference is depicted in Figure 4.3.

There is some confusion over why many phytoestrogens appear to be both estrogen agonists and antagonists at the same time. All phytoestrogens are estrogen agonists in that they can produce an estrogenic response, although with a much lower potency than any endogenous estrogen. When significant numbers of estrogen receptors are bound to certain phytoestrogens in the presence of estrogen, the estrogenic response is much lower than it would be normally if those receptors could bind to endogenous estrogen. This phenomenon makes phytoestrogens appear to be estrogen antagonists in some situations. At concentrations 100-1000 times that of estradiol, a few phytoestrogens may effectively compete with circulating levels of endogenous estrogens, bind to the ER, and prevent normal levels of estrogen-stimulated DNA transcription.[13] These concentrations may sound high but are not biologically unattainable and have frequently been detected in the plasma of vegetarians and other people consuming a diet with a relatively high phytoestrogen content.[26-28] In cell culture, the most potent phytoestrogens, coumestrol and genistein, do not function as antiestrogens at any concentration, but weaker phytoestrogens, such as biochanin A, exhibit antiestrogenic activity in a dose-dependent fashion.[23]

Lignans have not been shown to bind with any great affinity to the primary binding site on estrogen receptor, which is not remarkable given that they are not as structurally similar to natural estrogens as the isoflavonoids. However, Adlercreutz et al. have also discovered that both the isoflavonoids and some lignans can compete with estradiol for the rat uterine nuclear type II estrogen binding sites.[26] Equol and daidzein bind with the highest affinity, and not all lignans have been shown to have binding ability. There is some preliminary evidence that estrogen-stimulated growth is at least partially regulated by activity at this site, which may indicate that antiestrogenic activity of phytoestrogens may be mediated by this site to some extent.

Recently a second estrogen receptor, designated the beta estrogen receptor (ERβ) was discovered.[29] A comparison of the amino acid sequence of this novel ER and the original ER (ERβ) revealed a high level of conservation in the DNA-binding domain (96%) but only a moderate level of conservation in the ligand-binding domain (58%). Although 17β-estradiol binds with high affinity to ERβ, it binds slightly better to ERβ.[29] This difference in the amino acid sequence of the ligand-binding domain opens up the possibility that phytoestrogens bind with different affinities to ERβ than to ERα. There are early indications that coumestrol binds to ERβ with a higher affinity than any of the endogenous estrogens, and genistein binds to ERβ with a much higher affinity that it does to ERα.[30]

One of the major questions surrounding this newly discovered second ER is whether it has its own specific set of functions or merely acts as a backup to ERα. ERα knockout (ERKO) mice develop with no gross physiological abnormalities but can experience reproductive defects. Although there is early indication that both receptors activate DNA transcription in some of the same DNA regions, it is possible that this newly discovered receptor activates different genes than ERα.

Originally, ERβ was detected in the ovaries and prostate of rats[31] and subsequently in the spleen, thymus, ovaries, testes,[29] vasculature, and aorta[32] of human adults. In rats, this second ER has also been detected in the bladder and different regions of the brain, including the hypothalamus and the paraventricular and arcuate nuclei.[33] A recent study also detected it in a variety of tissues in the midgestational human fetus. ERβ mRNA was expressed at higher levels than ERα mRNA in fetal ovaries, testes, adrenal gland, and placenta, but the reverse was true in the uterus.[34] ERβ was also present at relatively high levels in fetal spleen and at lower levels in the lungs, thymus, kidney, and skin. Both ERs were present in fetal long bone in low amounts. Overall, ERβ appears to have a more uniform distribution than ERα in the midgestational fetus, indicating that it may play a significant role in the growth and development of the fetus. This second estrogen receptor also may play a critical role in adult female reproductive function, particularly in the follicular phase of the menstrual cycle, because its mRNA is expressed in higher amounts than ERα mRNA in the adult ovary. This expression is primarily localized to the granulosa cell layer of small, growing, and preovulatory follicles and declines as the follicle reaches maturity.[35] ERβ downregulates quickly following the preovulatory luteinizing hormone (LH) surge and in the presence of other gonadotropins, including human chorionic gonadotropin.

The discovery of a second estrogen receptor introduces a whole new level of complexity to the actions and activity of phytoestrogens in animals. It appears that some tissues, which contain no alpha receptors, may contain high levels of beta receptors, particularly in development. This could mean that phytoestrogens could influence developmental processes and have a more profound impact through this second receptor than through the alpha receptor. This is an area of phytoestrogen activity that remains, for the most part, unexplored but is particularly interesting given that ERβ mRNA is expressed in such high quantities in the prostate, and genistein, which has been shown to bind to ERβ, and has also been associated with cancer-protective effects in the prostate as well as many other organs.[25,36]

4.4.2 Mechanisms of Action Not Mediated by Estrogen Receptors

Phytoestrogens can also produce their effects in ways not mediated through an ER pathway. Enterolactone, genistein, and daidzein have been shown *in vitro* to stimulate synthesis of hormone-binding globulin (SHBG) in liver cells.[26] By elevating circulating SHBG levels, phytoestrogens can reduce the biological activity of endogenous estrogens and testosterone by reducing their concentrations in circulation.[3] Isoflavones have also been shown *in vivo* to reduce circulating LH and follicle stimulating hormone (FSH) levels in premenopausal women.[37] Isoflavones and lignan phytoestrogens, including equol, genistein, and biochanin A, are also potent inhibitors of the ovarian aromatase enzyme, which produces estrogen from androstenedione and testosterone in humans.[38,39] Phytoestrogens bind to the active site of this enzyme in a different orientation from that in ERα.[40] Coumestrol has been shown *in vitro* to reduce the conversion of [^{3}H]-estrone to [^{3}H]-estradiol by inhibiting the estrogen-specific enzyme 17β-hydroxysteroid oxidoreductase Type 1, in a dose-dependent fashion beginning with concentrations as low as 0.12 μM.[41] Genistein was more weakly inhibitory but demonstrated a similar dose-dependent effect.

Genistein is a unique phytoestrogen with a variable array of physiological effects. In addition to the effects listed above, genistein is a potent inhibitor of tyrosine protein kinases (PTKs).[42,43] PTKs catalyze phosphorylation of their own tyrosine residues and those of other proteins, including growth factors involved in tumor cell proliferation. By inhibiting PTKs, genistein potentially can slow tumorogenesis. Genistein can also inhibit DNA topoisomerases I and II, enzymes essential for DNA replication.[2,44] In addition, recent studies done *in vitro* have revealed a diverse range of cardioprotective effects, including the ability to lower blood cholesterol, reduce platelet aggregation, and inhibit the effects of growth factors on artherosclerotic plaques.[45]

4.5   Physiological Effects

Phytoestrogens were first discovered to have physiological effects early this century when Australian sheep grazing on legume-rich pasture began to develop unusual reproductive abnormalities. Abortion rates were extraordinarily high in several flocks, and many ewes became permanently sterile. In 1946, Bennetts et al. described severe clinical abnormalities in these animals, including prolapse of the uterus, dystocia in ewes, low lambing rates, enlargement of the bulbo-urethral glands, and death.[46] This syndrome, which came to be known as "clover disease," is still a potential problem that must be carefully managed by farmers today.

Permanent infertility in ewes was ultimately discovered to be caused by the failure of the cervix to permit normal transport of spermatozoa after insemination.[6,47] In the ewe, the genes controlling sexual differentiation do not completely deactivate after birth. Exposure to high levels of estrogen for several months can continue the differentiation process, similar to the process that happens to males *in utero*. This differentiation results in the cervix becoming more like the uterus in both histological appearance and function, which then prevents normal sperm transport. The discovery that certain plants could induce reproductive abnormalities, including sterility, prompted an intense investigation aimed at identifying which phytochemicals could produce physiological effects in animals and humans and what exactly those effects were.

Not all of the physiological effects of phytoestrogens are problematic. There is mounting evidence that they can play a significant role in the prevention and treatment of cancer. Their high concentrations in the urine and plasma of vegetarians and Asian women, groups known to be resistant to breast cancer, and their low concentrations in breast cancer patients suggest that consumption of phytoestrogens may help prevent estrogen-dependent carcinomas, including breast and prostate cancer.[13,48] Phytoestrogens may also lower cholesterol, prevent bone mass reduction in postmenopausal women, and reduce the symptoms of menopause, including hot flashes. Lignans have been shown to have antiviral and antifungal effects and may play a significant role in bolstering the immune system.[12]

4.5.1 Hormonal and Reproductive Effects

Phytoestrogens are estrogenic by definition and can act as weak estrogens in mammalian systems, giving them the ability to produce a whole range of hormonal effects in a variety of animals. Heifers grazing on phytoestrogen-rich red clover developed 35% longer teats on average and had an accumulation of fluid in the vagina and uterus. Uterine tone increased, as did uterine size in ovariectomized animals.[49] Although phytoestrogen-induced infertility in cattle is rare, phytoestrogens can also cause cystic ovaries, irregular estrus, and anestrus.[6] A myriad of studies have demonstrated that the isoflavones can stimulate uterine growth in rodents.[50] Of all the biological effects with which phytoestrogens have been affiliated, infertility is the one that causes the most concern.

First seen in sheep, phytoestrogen-related infertility has now been observed in an array of species. A 1976 study confirmed that the breeding success of California quail depends on the phytoestrogen content of forbs growing in their breeding ranges.[51] Genistein and formononetin were present in significantly higher concentrations in forbs growing in dry years than in forbs growing in wet years. Consequently, as a result of consuming a phytoestrogen-rich diet, breeding was generally unsuccessful, and many birds left California as early as June for their winter roosts.

One of the most recent examples of phytoestrogen-related infertility involves captive cheetahs. In the 1980s, high mortality coupled with low fertility threatened to drastically reduce captive cheetah populations in North American zoos. The most prevalent cause of death in these animals was liver disease of unknown etiology, and nearly 60% of all North American cheetahs had venocclusive disease.[52] Additionally, only 9-12% of North American captive female cheetahs were producing live cubs, compared to 60-80% of African captive female cheetahs. The vast majority of these animals were fed primarily a commercially prepared diet made mostly from horse meat. When four cheetahs at the Cincinnati Zoo were fed a chicken diet for 3 months, their liver condition improved significantly, and a few females became pregnant, implying that something in the commercial diet was contributing to the illness and the infertility. This commercial preparation contained between 5 and 13% soy protein, exposing each cheetah to 50 mg/d of phytoestrogens (approximately 1 mg/kg body weight), and the preparation had particularly high levels of genistein and daidzein.[52] Estrogens are known to produce changes in blood coagulation with secondary liver involvement[53] and to have cholestatic effects, which cause bile retention and alterations in the shunting of substances into the vascular compartment.[54] Phytoestrogens, by nature of their estrogenicity, may produce similar effects. The metabolism of daidzein and genistein in cheetahs and other large felines will have to be characterized before any definitive conclusions can be made about the reproductive effects of phytoestrogens in these animals, but their improved reproduction in the absence of an estrogen-rich diet suggests that phytoestrogens have a potentially potent effect on their reproductive ability.

Humans may be facing a very similar situation. Infertility among young couples inexplicably tripled between 1965 and 1982,[55] and several studies have now documented a steady decline in mean sperm density and seminal volume over the past 50 years.[56,57] Exogenous estrogens are hypothesized to be one of the primary causes of declining human fertility[58] and may be particularly detrimental to men. The exact role phytoestrogens play in this emerging problem is unclear, but there are some indications that they can influence human fertility.[59]

Phytoestrogens are a common component of alcoholic beverages and the reproductive toxicity of ethyl alcohol in chronic alcoholics is well documented, but phytoestrogens also may contribute to the reproductive dysfunction seen in chronic alcoholics. Male alcoholics frequently have atrophied seminiferous tubules, and hypoplastic spermatogonia in addition to severe liver abnormalities. Chronic consumption of alcohol ultimately results in hypoandrogenism that usually results in testicular atrophy and impotence.[60] Alcoholic beverages are made from a wide variety of plant sources, including hops, rice, corn, and barley, all of which contain phytoestrogens. Many alcoholic beverages, including beer, bourbon, and red wine, all produce estrogen effects both *in vitro* and *in vivo*.[61]

Phytoestrogens may also alter the menstrual cycle. Women consuming 10 g of flax seed powder in addition to their regular diet for three cycles had increased luteal phases and higher progesterone to estradiol ratios than women consuming only their regular diet. In addition, the study group had no anovulatory cycles, while three women in the control group each had one.[62] Dietary supplements of ISP or soy milk, providing isoflavone intakes of 0.6-3 mg/kg body weight, have both increased and reduced cycle length, with variable effects on serum estradiol and progesterone.[37,63,64] These results indicate that the menstrual cycle can be altered by phytoestrogen intake, but many more studies of longer duration and with a larger subject pool need to be conducted to further characterize this effect. The menstrual cycle is extremely variable, both within one woman, between individuals, and across populations. This variability makes it difficult to attribute cycle alterations specifically to one dietary element.

4.5.2 Developmental Effects

Estrogens and androgens play a critical role in development and influence growth and differentiation in tissues, including the gonads and the brain.

TABLE 4.3

Developmental Effects of Phytoestrogens and Mycoestrogens in Rodents

Tissue	Phytoestrogen	Effect	Reference
Uterus	Coumestrol, zearalenone	Reduced number of glands and ER	68,70
Vagina	Coumestrol, genistein	Cornification, metaplasia, delayed opening	66,71,72
Breast	Genistein	Increased duct development	73
Anogenital	Genistein	Decreased distance in males	66
Prostate	Coumestrol, Daidzein	Increased c-fos, prevention of DES lesions	74
Hypothalamus	Coumestrol	Premature anovulation, abnormal sexual behavior in males	71,75
Pituitary	Coumestrol, genistein, zearalenone	Altered LH response, decreased basal LH	69,76
SDN-POA	Coumestrol, genistein	Enlarged in females	69,76

Because of their ability to produce estrogenic effects, phytoestrogens may influence fetal development and ultimately affect reproductive physiology and behavior in adulthood. As a fetus develops, there are specific, sensitive periods when it is particularly responsive to hormones. In rats, this sensitive period lasts through the final third of gestation and into the first 10 d of life.[65] This period of enhanced sensitivity suggests that timing of exposure may be as or even more important than the level of exposure. When examining the effects of phytoestrogens on fetal development, it is important to consider the stage of development along with the level of phytoestrogen exposure.

The developmental effects of phytoestrogens have been studied mostly in rats and interpreted to have implications for human health. The results of some of these studies are presented in Table 4.3. Genistein exposure at doses of 25,000 µg and 5000 µg on days 16 through 20 of gestation produces a variety of developmental effects, including low birth weight females, shortened anogenital distances in males, and delayed vaginal opening in females.[66] Persistent exposure to coumestrol through lactation after the first 10 post-natal days produces acyclicity in early adulthood and suppresses early growth, resulting in lower than average weight at vaginal opening.[67] Exposure to 10–100 µg of coumestrol immediately after birth also causes a significant increase in uterine weight, accompanied by severely reduced ER levels.[68] By post-natal day (PND) 20, however, uterine weight in exposed animals is significantly lower than the controls and ER levels are still below normal. Neonatal exposure to equol also lowers uterine weight by PND 20 but does not affect ER levels.

A hormone-sensitive period for differentiation of the sexually dimorphic nucleus in the preoptic area of the hypothalamus (SDN-POA) occurs between gestation day 16 and day 5 of life. This nucleus is larger in males and plays a role in male mating activity.[65] Females exposed to diethylstilbestrol (DES), zearalenone, and genistein during the critical period have significantly larger SDN-POA volumes than female controls.[69]

Early exposure to phytoestrogens may influence reproductive physiology and behavior in adulthood. Exposure to coumestrol at doses as low as 0.1 μg on the first 10 d of life significantly reduces pituitary responsiveness to gonadotrophin-releasing hormone (GnRH) and elevates basal LH levels in females when they reach adulthood. Adult males show elevated basal LH levels after neonatal exposure to 1 μg coumestrol but do not have reduced pituitary sensitivity.[65] Females may be affected by lower doses of coumestrol and other phytoestrogens because they are more susceptible to the masculinizing effects of low dose estrogens. Male rats exposed to coumestrol through lactation exhibit a number of deficits in sexual behavior as adults. Exposed males have a lower ejaculation rate, a longer latency to first mount interval, and fewer overall mount attempts than unexposed males.[67] Very few studies have examined the influence of phytoestrogens on sexual behavior, and more research in this area is badly needed.

The impact of phytoestrogens on human fetal development is unclear, but the teratogenic results of diethylstilbestrol (DES) exposure confirmed that estrogen exposure can have profound effects. The parenteral doses required for developmental actions in rodents (0.01–10 mg/kg) are similar to doses reported for developmental actions by estrogenic pesticides. Over the past 30–50 years, the incidences of testicular cancer, cryptorchidism, and hypospadias have markedly increased and are hypothesized to be the result of exposure to exogenous estrogens.[58] It is unclear how phytoestrogens might be involved in these changes, but it is a role that should be explored.

4.6   Phytoestrogens and Lactation

In light of these developmental actions, concern has been raised in the past decade over infant exposure to phytoestrogens. The presence of phytoestrogens in human urine suggests that these chemicals may also be present in breast milk. There is particular concern over the use of infant formulas made from soy, considering the high isoflavone content of soy-based products. The first high-performance liquid chromatography (HPLC) analysis, done in 1987, revealed high levels of isoflavones in infant soy milk products, with genistein and daidzein being present in the highest quantities.[77] Subsequent analyses by Setchell et al. in 1997 have confirmed that soy formula contains significantly more isoflavones than breast milk or bovine-based milk formula.[78]

Setchell's 1997 study is the only study to date that compared plasma isoflavone concentrations of infants consuming different formula types or breast milk. It clearly showed that infants fed a soy milk diet exclusively have significantly higher mean plasma concentrations of isoflavones (particularly daidzein and genistein) than infants fed bovine milk formula or breast milk. This indicates that an infant fed only soy formula consumes approximately

TABLE 4.4

Isoflavone Content of Commercial Soy Infant Formulas

Soy Product (dry)	Daidzein μg/g	Genistein μg/g	Method	Milk Level[a]	Ref.
Prosobee	17.0	22.0	HPLC	21 μM	77
Isomil	19.0	23.0	HPLC	23 μM	77
Isomil	15.0	19.0	GC-MS	18 μM	85
Jevity Isotonic	0.3	3.1	GC-MS	2 μM	7

[a] Based on a reconstitution of 8.7 g formula per 60 ml water.

6–9 mg/kg body weight per d, which is considerably higher than the amounts regularly consumed by adult vegetarians or Asians, who consume approximately 0.3–1.2 mg/kg/d on average.[79] Infants fed soy formula have circulating phytoestrogens at concentrations of approximately 1 μg/ml, 13,000–22,000 times higher than endogenous estrogens, which range from 40–80 pg/ml in infancy.[80] These levels are more than two times higher than the levels required to produce physiological effects such as alteration of cycle length in adult women.

Equol was the only phytoestrogen present in significant concentrations in the plasma of infants fed bovine milk-based formulas. This result is consistent with data showing that cows produce and excrete more equol than any other phytoestrogen.[6] Only four of the seven infants fed soy-based formula had detectable levels of equol in their plasma, suggesting that the ability to produce equol varies in infants as well as adults. Infants, however, do not have full complement of gut flora and acquire this population as they mature. The age of the infant must be considered in metabolic studies before any conclusions can be made about when the ability to synthesize equol arises.

The isoflavone levels in different formulas can vary between brands and lot preparations due to natural variation within the soybean plants themselves and manufacturing conditions, as shown in Table 4.4.[77] Composition of human breast milk is even more variable, not only between different women but also within one woman over the course of a day. After consuming a meal rich in soy and soy proteins, isoflavones reach maximum levels in the milk 10-12 h post-consumption but may not reach baseline values until 2–4 d later (close to zero), depending on the level of soy in the meal.[81] Milk concentrations of isoflavones, including genistein and daidzein conjugates, increase rapidly after consumption, decrease to near basal levels, then increase again before dropping to baseline. This biphasic pattern is most likely due to enterohepatic circulation. Consumption of only 5 g of roasted soybeans produced daidzein and genistein breast milk levels in the range of 10–30 nM within 12 h. Consumption of 25 g of roasted soybeans produced milk levels in the range of 50–70 nM. Although these levels are substantial, they are considerably less than the 2–23 μM concentrations present in soy-based formula.

Ever since soy-based formulas were introduced, there have been health problems associated with them. Soy-induced goiter is a well known phenomenon first discovered in animals in the 1930s.[82] These high-uptake goiters are characterized by a greatly increased iodine requirement after thyroxin depletion through fecal wastage. Thyroxin (T_4) undergoes enterohepatic circulation and must be reabsorbed and recirculated to preserve normal plasma levels. Even a slight impairment in reabsorption could lead to significant fecal wastage. Soy formula is thought to interfere with this resorption, resulting in lower circulating levels of thyroxin.[83]

In the 1960s, the manufacturers switched from a high fiber soy flour preparation to one made from isolated soy protein. This new formula was also supplemented with iodine to further decrease the risk of goiter. This change in formulation has virtually eliminated soy-induced goiter in infants but may have other hidden consequences. Infants fed soy formula may still have lower circulating levels of thyroxine than infants fed milk formula or breast milk.[84] This effect is of particular concern for infants born with congenital hypothyroidism or other problems because soy formula is often recommended for children with "milk allergies." Soy protein also contains more isoflavones than soy flour, exposing infants to higher levels of exogenous estrogens.

The developmental effects of these compounds in infants, as well as their potential cancer protective benefits, are the subject of great debate. Before this question can be approached, the metabolism and relative bioavailability of these compounds must be understood. This process is just beginning to be elucidated in the adult, but limited research in this area has been conducted in infants. Adults and infants are thought to have very different intestinal microflora, and great variation in the composition of gut flora is also suspected between infants fed commercial formulas and infants fed breast milk.[78] Differences in plasma levels give some clues, but further research in this area is badly needed.

4.7 The Cancer Connection

Cancer is the leading cause of death in adults aged 25 through 64 in the United States, and nearly one-third of these deaths are attributable to dietary factors.[86] It is widely accepted that agents that promote terminal differentiation of tumor cells inhibit cancer cell proliferation.[87] Cell proliferation is promoted by enzymes such as protein tyrosine kinases (PTKs) and DNA topoisomerases. Inhibition of these enzymes results in the repression of cancer proliferation and often the promotion of cell differentiation. PTKs are oncogene products that catalyze phosphorylation of their own tyrosine residues as well as those in other proteins, including growth factors. DNA topoisomerases catalyze topologic changes in DNA and are required for

DNA replication.[2] Mammary tumors in rats have over 60 times more topoisomerase II enzymatic activity than healthy mammary tissue. Similarly, mammary tumors also contain more tyrosine phosphopeptides indicating increased protein tyrosine kinase activity.[88]

The first evidence that certain phytoestrogens may have cancer-protective effects came from epidemiological studies of vegetarians, Asian populations, and breast cancer patients. Low risk countries such as Japan and China have breast cancer incidence rates five-fold lower than high risk countries, including the United States and Europe. Vegetarians also have a lower overall cancer risk than groups consuming a more typical Western diet. Similar studies also have revealed analogous risk patterns for prostate, colon and other types of cancer.[89-91] Migrants to high risk countries have risk levels closer to those for the high risk countries, indicating an environmental rather than geographic basis for the variation.[92]

Dietary surveys from as far back as the 1960s indicate that Japanese populations consume 90 times more legumes than individuals in the United States.[25] This high consumption of soy foods is reflected as high isoflavone levels in their blood, urine and feces.[7] Several epidemiological studies have demonstrated that urinary and plasma levels of phytoestrogens correlate negatively with rates of breast and prostate cancer risk.[13,48,93] Men from low risk countries, such as China, also have higher levels of phytoestrogens, particularly the isoflavones, in their prostatic fluid then men from high risk countries. A study comparing prostatic fluid from men in Hong Kong, Portugal, and Manchester, England, revealed that the Chinese men had up to 15 times more daidzein and as much as 17 times more equol in their prostatic fluid than the European men.[94] Interestingly, the concentrations of the phytoestrogens examined were higher in prostatic fluid than in plasma, indicating that the prostate has the ability to concentrate these compounds.

Equivalent studies have examined the relationship between phytoestrogens and breast cancer and produced similar findings. An extensive case control study of 144 breast cancer patients and 144 carefully matched controls in Australia found lower phytoestrogen excretion levels among the cancer patients. Data from premenopausal and postmenopausal women were analyzed separately, and both showed a positive correlation between high phytoestrogen excretion and reduced cancer risk.[48] Nipple aspirate fluid (NAF) from Asian and western women has also been compared and examined for the effects of a soy diet on the quality of cells collected. Chinese and Japanese women have lower NAF volume, lower mean levels of gross cystic disease fluid protein (GCDFP), fewer hyperplasic cells, and fewer atypical epithelial cells in their NAF than American women.[64] To test directly the effects of soy on NAF, 14 premenopausal and 10 postmenopausal women consumed two packets of powdered soy protein, each containing 18.7 mg of genistein, daily for six months in addition to their normal diet. Although a 30% decrease in the mean concentration of GCDFP-15 was found in the premenopausal women, NAF volume increased two- to six-fold, and epithelial hyperplasia was observed in 29% of premenopausal women, suggestive of an estrogenic rather than a protective effect. Estradiol was erratically elevated, suggesting an effect on the hypothalamic-pituitary-gonadal axis. This study illustrates some of the difficulties of predicting outcomes for substances that impact a broad range of tissues and exhibit biphasic actions and highlights the need for careful investigation of potential adverse, along with beneficial, effects.

Phytoestrogens have been shown to be cancer protective for many different types of cancer, including breast cancer, prostate cancer, leukemia, endometrial cancer, liver cancer, and melanoma, among others.[13,95] Cell culture and other *in vitro* studies have helped elucidate the mechanisms behind the anticarcinogenic effects of phytoestrogens. These effects are probably not mediated solely by the estrogen receptor as originally hypothesized but rather by a combination of other effects at multiple levels. Phytoestrogens, like endogenous steroids, have more than just genomic effects. As explained earlier, they influence hormone production and the release of gonadotropins, can bind to numerous enzymes and other proteins and can reduce circulating levels of endogenous estrogens by increasing SHBG production. Multiple whole animal and mammalian cell studies have demonstrated that phytoestrogens have a wide range of biological activities including antioxidant effects, inhibition of the proliferation and development of numerous cell types, promotion of cell differentiation, and inhibition of both topoisomerase and protein kinase enzyme activity.[3] The results of many of these studies have been summarized and reviewed by Adlercreutz et al.[3,13]

4.7.1   The Cancer Specialist — Genistein

Of all the phytoestrogens, genistein appears to be the most significant cancer fighter and has the greatest diversity of effects. It is also the most intensely studied phytoestrogen, with over 1000 papers in publication since 1990 investigating its effects. Genistein is antiproliferative at concentrations above 10 μM in both ER+ and ER− human breast cancer cells grown *in vitro* but is a pure estrogen agonist and thus proliferative at concentrations below 10 μM.[25,96] This biphasic effect indicates that there is a significant dose effect of genistein and possibly other phytoestrogens on cancer proliferation. At low concentrations, the proliferative effects of genistein on breast cancer cells are mediated through the alpha estrogen receptor.[97] At higher concentrations, the chemoprotective effects of genistein are mediated by multiple mechanisms independent of estrogen receptors.

Genistein is the most powerful antioxidant of all the phytoestrogens, with the ability to both increase the activities of antioxidant enzymes as well as directly inhibit hydrogen peroxide production. Female rats fed 250 ppm of genistein daily for 30 d showed a 10-30% increase in the activities of glutathione peroxidase, glutathione reductase, catalase, and superoxide dismutase.[98] Genistein is a potent inhibitor of PTKs, although other phytoestrogens can do this to a much lesser extent.[43] This effect may be one of the most important and significant mechanisms for the cancer protective effects of genistein, along with its ability to inhibit DNA topoisomerase activity. Several studies have now confirmed that genistein can inhibit both topoisomerase I and II.[2,99] Genistein can also suppress angiogenesis through mechanisms to be discussed in a later section. However, because all of these effects require micromolar concentrations, it is not clear whether they are physiologically relevant (see below).

4.7.2 Breast Cancer

A multitude of epidemiological studies have shown that subjects with breast cancer excrete lower amounts of lignans and isoflavonoids than healthy women, and that women living in low risk countries have higher amounts of these compounds in their plasma and urine than women living in high risk countries.[3,28,48,89-92] The mechanism behind this protection may come from reduced exposure to endogenous estrogens. Asian women have much lower levels of circulating estrogens than western women.[100,101] It is unclear if these lower levels are attributable to diet or genetics, a point that needs to be clarified before a diet high in phytoestrogens can be endorsed for western women.

Several *in vitro* studies have elucidated some of the breast cancer-protective mechanisms of phytoestrogens. Lignans and isoflavonoids inhibit three ovarian enzymes, essential for estradiol production: 3β-hydroxysteroid dehydrogenase, aromatase, and 17β-hydroxysteroid oxidoreductase type I.[7] This combination of inhibitory effects could result in the decreased reduction of estradiol production and thus, lower circulating levels. Many phytoestrogens can slow or even completely prevent breast cancer cell proliferation, but only when they are present in sufficient quantities.[25] Doses below about 10 μM can actually stimulate proliferation, rather than suppress it.[97]

Early exposure to genistein may be critical for reducing the risk of breast cancer in adulthood. Female rats injected with 500 mg of genistein per kg body weight on postnatal days 2, 4, and 6 developed fewer dimethylbenz[a]anthracene (DMBA)-adenocarcinomas and had an increased meantime to tumor development compared to control rats. The treated rats, however, had significantly reduced circulating progesterone, earlier vaginal opening, and follicular abnormalities, including atretic antral follicles and fewer corpora lutea.[73] In a second study, female rats injected with 500 mg/kg genistein on postnatal days 16, 18, and 20 also developed nearly half as many DMBA-induced mammary tumors as controls, but showed none of the reproductive side effects documented in the earlier study.[102] In both studies, genistein caused immediate and significant proliferation in the mammary glands, resulting in the creation of more differentiated terminal ductal structures (lobules II). Premenarchal women have many undifferentiated terminal ductal structures that progress to more differentiated lobules during pregnancy. The earlier pregnancy is achieved, the lower the risk of breast cancer, indicating the protective effect of differentiation. Prepubertal administration of genistein by injection in rats causes rapid and prolific differentiation of breast tissue, which may be one mechanism of how genistein could protect against breast cancer.

4.7.3 Precautions and Directions for Future Research

The epidemiological evidence in humans suggesting that a diet high in phytoestrogens can reduce the risk of cancer is compelling, but whole animal and *in vitro* studies have been much more controversial, and many have produced conflicting results. Part of the conflict has arisen because of the different doses used to test for anitproliferative effects of phytoestrogens. Studies that use small concentrations (<1 to 10 µM) have discovered that some phytoestrogens, including genistein, daidzein, biochanin A, enterolactone, and coumestrol, actually stimulate tumor proliferation, while others using higher concentrations of the same compound have found antiproliferative effects.[96,97,103] This biphasic dose response is significant, and the mechanism producing this effect warrants further examination, particularly because human plasma levels are most often in the lower dose range. This would seem to suggest that phytoestrogen consumption would result in an increased cancer risk, but this is in direct conflict with the extensive epidemiological data. This apparent paradox would be resolved if organs such as the breasts and prostate have the ability to concentrate phytoestrogens. One study has already discovered that the prostate has this ability,[94] and the concentration of endogenous estrogens in normal breast ductal fluid is as much as 40-fold higher than that in serum, indicating that the breast may have the ability to concentrate phytoestrogens as well.[25] This paradox makes understanding the effects of phytoestrogens on cancer cell growth at both high and low doses critical and emphasizes the need to pay particular attention to the concentration of phytochemicals in human tissues, not just plasma levels.

There is also some controversy surrounding the doses required *in vivo* to produce effects seen *in vitro* and how to normalize data gathered from different *in vitro* assays. Yeast estrogen screening assays are sensitive enough to produce results at much lower concentrations than those required for mammalian cell cultures,[23] but there are a multitude of them developed by different labs, and not all of them are capable of adequately testing for antiestrogenic effects.[22] Because phytoestrogens can bind to SHBG and other proteins, the concentrations needed to produce biological effects in an animal or human will necessarily be much higher than the concentrations needed in an *in vitro* assay or cell culture.[104] The trick is to determine how those two concentrations correlate with each other and to be able to predict one from the other.

4.7.4 Interactions Between Phytoestrogens and Other Xenoestrogens

New evidence exists that may indicate a synergistic effect of curcumin and genistein on the inhibition of environmental estrogen-stimulated growth in human breast cancer cells *in vitro*.[105] Cells stimulated with synthetic, estrogenic pesticides, including DDT and endosulfane, were tested along with cells stimulated with estradiol. In both cases, the administration of genistein or curcumin alone reduced proliferation, but cells exposed to both curcumin and genistein together stopped proliferating completely. A combination of 5 μM each of endosulfane, chlordane, and DDT has a proliferative potency of 125, as compared to 100 for 17-β estradiol. However, when 25 μM of genistein is added, the proliferative potency drops to 34.5. If 10 μM of curcumin is also added, the proliferative potency drops to zero. This is one of the first studies to show that phytoestrogenic compounds may reduce the estrogenic effects of other exogenous estrogens, and more are certainly needed to conform the results. Environmental estrogens, particularly pesticides, have been suspected of increasing breast cancer risk. If phytoestrogens are proven to reduce the estrogenic effect of these xenoestrogens in addition to all their other cancer protective effects, there would be compelling evidence for the recommendation of increased phytoestrogen intake.

4.8 Cholesterol and Heart Disease

There is a large body of literature indicating that soy products lower total blood cholesterol levels in animals and humans, particularly LDL and VLDL cholesterol.[106,107] Research from as early as 1940 confirmed that animal protein (casein) is more atherogenic than soy protein.[108] More recent studies have made similar conclusions. LDL and VLDL concentrations in male peripubertal rhesus monkeys dropped 30% after the animals were fed a high-fat diet supplemented with soy flour for 24 weeks. Females experienced a 40% drop, along with a 15% increase in HLDC concentrations.[109] Free thyroxine, plasma estradiol, SHBG, and testosterone concentrations were not affected; neither were average testicular weight, prostate weight, or uterine weight. Plasma cholesterol reductions ranging from 8 to 16% have been reported for human patients with moderate to severe type II hypercholesterolemia after consuming soy protein.[107] The question now is not whether soy foods can lower cholesterol, but how and under what conditions.

The exact mechanism of how soy products can lower blood cholesterol is unknown, but there are several theories. The most prominent attributes the cardioprotective effects of soy to their tendency to increase T_4 levels, which then results in lower serum cholesterol levels. Multiple animal studies using rabbits, rats, pigs, and gerbils have all shown elevated T_4 levels in response to soy consumption,[110] and soy-induced goiter was once problematic in infants fed soy formula.[83] Hamsters fed isolated soy protein (ISP) had elevated T_4 levels, but hamsters fed soy protein concentrate (SPC) did not, even though both groups had significantly lower blood cholesterol levels compared to the control animals.[111] SPC is only about 70% protein compared to

ISP, which is nearly 90% protein. Thus, a number of other, potentially biologically active compounds could be present in the SPC that could influence cholesterol reduction and hormonal effects. Most animals studies to date have been conducted using ISP products and thus may only represent a limited range of soy effects. Human studies also have revealed an increase in T_4 levels in mildly hypercholesterolemic men after consuming 20 g of ISP daily. However this elevation was not significant when compared to levels in men who had consumed milk proteins.[112] This hypothesis appears to account at least partially for the effects of soy foods on cholesterol, but other soy products besides ISP need to be considered before any definitive conclusions can be drawn.

Another proposed mechanism for the actions of soy protein on cholesterol is a direct effect on hepatic metabolism of cholesterol. 3-Hydroxy-3methylglutaryl coenzyme A (HMG CoA) reductase activity increased in rats fed soy in addition to their normal diets.[113] This theory has not received as much attention and has only been studied in a limited range of animals. There is good evidence, however, that soy foods increase fecal excretion of bile acids. This depletes the body's store of bile and results in the recruitment of circulating cholesterol for increased bile production. This mechanism for the hypocholesterolemic effect of soy has been well documented in rabbits and rats,[113] but reports in other species, especially humans, are less consistent and thus less conclusive.[114]

The mechanism for the ability of soy products to reduce total serum cholesterol is far from being characterized, and more human and animal studies will be necessary to elucidate the process. Part of the difficulty arises over confusion over which compounds within soy are actually producing the effects. In addition to isoflavones, soy foods also contain high levels of saponins, phytic acid, and trypsin inhibitors, along with a variety of proteins and amino acids. All of these could possibly contribute to the cholesterol-lowering effects of soy foods.

Estrogen is cardioprotective, which is why postmenopausal women have an elevated risk of heart disease compared to premenopausal women. Estrogen replacement therapy has been shown to decrease this risk in both humans and animal studies.[115] Isoflavones are all weak estrogens and can bind to the estrogen receptors, resulting in similar cardioprotective effects. Isoflavones, particularly genistein, could also act through other nongenomic mechanisms that have yet to be elucidated. Ipriflavone, a synthetic isoflavone, is also effective at reducing cholesterol levels in the livers of adult, ovariectomized rats.[116] The amino acids and peptides of soy foods have been studied to a great extent, and it is now widely accepted that amino acid mixtures are not as effective as the intact proteins at lowering blood cholesterol.[117] Animals fed diets high in animal fat have significantly greater concentrations of lysine, arginine, valine, and isoleucine in their serum than animals fed a diet high in soy protein.[110] These amino acids may play a role in elevating serum cholesterol. Saponins can decrease serum cholesterol levels in animals on high animal protein diets but produces no changes in animals on a high soy protein diet because they bind to the soy proteins and form an insoluble complex.[113] Saponins reduce cholesterol by increasing bile excretion. Administration of this compound may help lower cholesterol in animals and humans consuming an animal product-based diet but may not be a significant mechanism for cholesterol reduction in animals and humans already consuming a soy-based diet. Phytic acid and trypsin inhibitors do not appear to play a significant role in the hypocholesterolemic effects of soy.

Artherosclerosis is a common disease in older Americans that results from the formation of plaques on the inner layers of the arteries. The development and proliferation of these plaques is regulated by a long list of cytokines and growth factors. PTKs phosphorylate many of the proteins that regulate cell function, and many growth factors depend on PTK activity to bind properly to their receptor. As discussed earlier, genistein is a potent inhibitor of PTKs. Genistein also has been shown to inhibit vascular permeability factor-induced relaxation in canine coronary arteries, suppress lipopolysaccharide induction of cytokines and NF-κB, and inhibit fibronectin EIIIA mRNA induction in rat aortic rings at levels at or below 37 μM.[45] At higher levels, genistein has been shown to inhibit chemotaxis and smooth muscle growth,[118] alter nitric oxide formation, and inhibit platelet aggregation[119] *in vitro*. A recent study demonstrated that after consuming high doses of isoflavones for 6 months, artherosclerotic female macaques had enhanced arterial dilator response to acetylcholine.[120]

It has long been known that a diet high in soluble fiber helps protect against heart disease. A recent study in middle-aged, Finnish, male smokers found that supplementing a normal diet with only 10 g of fiber reduces the risk of coronary death by 18%.[121] It is unclear whether any of the lignans are responsible for this reduction. Epidemologic studies demonstrate that whole grains are cardioprotective in addition to being cancer-protective. Dietary fiber is only one potenially important component of whole grains. Lignans, undigestable starch, antioxidants, trace minerals, and phenolic compounds are all found in whole grains and could reduce the risk of heart disease.[122]

4.9 Menopause and Osteoporosis

Menopause produces a wide range of hypoestrogenic symptoms in women, including hot flashes, and a reduction in bone density. In the United States, the hot flash is the most common symptom of menopause, and the progressive decrease in bone density can lead to osteoporosis, which increases a woman's risk of fracturing a bone. Asian populations have a much lower incidence of both hot flashes and osteoporosis than American populations,[89] suggesting that phytoestrogens may reduce the incidence of these symptoms.

The hypothesis that diet can play a role in the onset of menopausal symptoms, particularly bone loss, is not a new one, but it has generally been focused on calcium intake. Although postmenopausal women are encouraged to take calcium supplements, studies have only dealt with a narrow range of doses, creating confusion over dosage recommendations. A recent study has shown that a considerable amount of calcium must be ingested, in the 1417-2417 mg range, for any appreciable amount of bone loss to be prevented.[123] Even more disturbing is that population studies have not been able to demonstrate clearly a correlation between calcium intake and bone loss, bone mass, or fracture rates.[124] Estrogen replacement therapy can help prevent bone loss in postmenopausal women, and because of their weak estrogenicity, phytoestrogens may help as well.

Although relatively few studies have been done, both *in vitro* and *in vivo* research indicate that phytoestrogens can prevent bone loss and help protect against osteoporosis. Coumestrol has been shown *in vitro* both to inhibit bone resorption and stimulate bone mineralization.[125] Bone loss was significantly reduced in the spine and femur of oophorectomized rats injected with 1.5 μmol of coumestrol twice weekly for six weeks (~1.5 mg/kg), and overall bone loss was completely prevented.[126] The coumestrol reduced urine calcium excretion and the bone resorption markers pyridinoline and deoxypyridinoline after only 1 week of treatment. Rats fed 131.25 mg of a phytoestrogen mixture weekly (~0.5 mg/kg) did not show any less bone loss than the control animals. This could indicate that the dose given was too low or too infrequent to produce physiological effects or that oral ingestion of phytoestrogens cannot prevent bone loss in rats. These results emphasize the need for dose–response studies of phytoestrogens on bone loss and the importance of evaluating animal studies carefully before making any conclusions about the effects of phytoestrogens on human health.

There is strong evidence that ipriflavone, a synthetic isoflavone derivative, can prevent bone loss in postmenopausal women. Ipriflavone reduces osteoclast recruitment and differentiation, thereby inhibiting bone resorption. This effect may be achieved by the direct inhibition of parathyroid hormone on bone.[127] A recent long-term study in postmenopausal women gives strong *in vivo* support to the positive results obtained *in vitro*. Women given 200 mg of ipriflavone daily (2.5 mg/kg) over a 2-year period along with a 1-g calcium supplement showed significantly lower bone loss then women given a placebo treatment along with the calcium supplement.[128] Women given GnRH agonists to treat a variety of severe estrogen-dependent conditions including endometriosis and uterine fibroids, enter a hypoestrogenic state, which alleviates the symptoms of the condition but produces a variety of menopausal side effects, including hot flashes and the reduction of bone metabolism and bone density. Women given 600 mg of ipriflavone along with 500 mg calcium every day for 6 months showed no bone loss compared to women given the calcium supplements alone. One of the breakdown products of ipriflavone is daidzein.[129] Nearly 10% of all ipriflavone consumed in a day will be metabolized into daidzein, which may indicate that daidzein, taken at higher doses (e.g., >1.8 mg/kg), may produce similar effects.

TABLE 4.5

Phytoestrogen Doses and Effects

Dose/BW	Species	Effect
0.01–10 mg/kg	Rats, mice	Altered reproductive tract and brain development
2–10 mg/kg	Rat	Slowed tumor development
500 mg/kg	Rat	Developmentally induced breast cancer resistance
1.0 mg/kg	Cheetah	Infertility, liver disease
9.0 mg/kg	Rhesus monkey	Reduced LDL, VLDL
1.0 mg/kg	Human	Breast epithelial cell proliferation
0.6–1.0 mg/kg	Human	Increased E_2
3.0 mg/kg	Human	Reduced E_2
2.5–7.5 mg/kg	Human	Reduced postmenopausal bone loss

4.10 Conclusions

Phytoestrogens are a promising group of compounds that may have many ramifications for the improvement of human health. If the epidemiological data is a true indication of their cancer-protective effects, then increased consumption of these compounds could greatly reduce the risk of cancer and provide other benefits as well, including lowering cholesterol and reducing the risk of osteoporosis. However, there is little data available on the most effective or optimal dose range for any of these compounds, and some animal studies have indicated that they can have severe reproductive consequences if consumed at high levels for long periods of time. Like other estrogens, these natural substances appear to have the capacity to produce both beneficial and adverse effects, and Table 4.5 shows that many of these effects can be produced at a similar range of doses across species. The potential reproductive impact for humans is unclear. There are some indications that beneficial effects may require higher doses than adverse effects, but further studies in this area must be completed before any definite dietary recommendations can be made. Once again, the epidemiological data indicate that populations consuming significant quantities of phytoestrogens, including vegetarians and many Asian cultures, suffer no adverse effects and live long, healthy lives. This may be an indication that lignans and soy foods should be part of the western diet.

References

1. Knight, D. C. and Eden, J. A., A review of the clinical effects of phytoestrogens, *Obstet. Gynecol.*, 87, 897, 1996.
2. Kurzer, M. S. and Xia, X., Dietary phytoestrogens, *Annu. Rev. Nutr.*, 17, 353, 1997.

3. Adlercreutz, H., Phtyoestrogens: epidemiology and a possible role in cancer protection, *Environ. Health Perspect.*, 130, 103, 1995.
4. Thompson, L. U., Robb, P., Serraino, M., and Cheung, F., Mammalian lignan production from various foods, *Nutrition and Cancer*, 16, 43, 1991.
5. Markiewicz, L., Garey, J., Adlercreutz, H., and Gurpide, E., *In vitro* bioassays of non-steroidal phytoestrogens, *J. Steroid Biochem. Mol. Biol.*, 45, 399, 1993.
6. Adams, N. R., Detection of the effects of phytoestrogens on sheep and cattle, *J. Anim. Sci.*, 73, 1509, 1995.
7. Adlercreutz, H. and Mazur, W., Phyto-oestrogens and western diseases, *Ann. Med.*, 29, 95, 1997.
8. Reinli, K. and Block, G., Phytoestrogen content of foods — a compendium of literature values, *Nutr. Canc.*, 26, 123, 1996.
9. Franke, A. A., Custer, L. J., Cerna, C. M., and Narala, K., Rapid HPLC analysis of dietary phytoestrogens from legumes and from human urine, *Proc. Soc. Exp. Biol. Med.*, 208, 18, 1995.
10. Joannou, G. E., Kelley, G. E., Reeder, A. Y., Waring, M., and Nelson, C., A urinary profile study of dietary phytoestrogens. The identification and mode of metabolism of new isoflavonoids, *J. Steroid Biochem.*, 54, 167, 1995.
11. Lundh, T., Metabolism of estrogenic isoflavones in domestic animals, *Proc. Soc. Exp. Biol. Med.*, 208, 33, 1995.
12. Adlercreutz, H., van der Wildt, J., Kinzel, J., Attalla, H., Wähälä, K., Mäkelä, T., Hase, T., and Fotsis, T., Lignan and isoflavonoid conjugates in human urine, *J. Steroid Biochem.*, 52, 97, 1995.
13. Adlercreutz, H., Goldin, B. R., Gorbach, S. L., Höckerstedt, K. A. V., Watanabe, S., Hamalainen, E. K., Markkanen, M. H., Mäkela, T. H., and Wähälä, K. T., Soybean phytoestrogen intake and cancer risk, *J. Nutr.*, 125, 757, 1995.
14. Hutchins, A. M., Slavin, J. L., and Lampe, J. W., Urinary isoflavonoid phytoestrogen and lignan excretion after consumption of fermented and unfermented soy products, *J. Am. Diet. Assoc.*, 95, 545, 1995.
15. Kelley, G. E., Joannou, G. E., Reeder, A. Y., Nelson, C., and Waring, M. A., The variable metabolic response to dietary isoflavones in humans, *Proc. Soc. Exp. Biol. Med.*, 208, 40, 1995.
16. Morton, M. S., Wilcox, G., Wahlqvist, M. L., and Griffiths, K., Determination of lignans and isoflavonoids in human female plasma following dietary supplementation., *J. Endocrinol.*, 142, 251, 1994.
17. Kirkman, L. M., Lampe, J. W., Campbell, D. R., Martini, M. C., and Slavin, J. L., Urinary lignan and isoflavonoid excretion in men and women consuming vegetable and soy diets, *Nutr. Canc.*, 24, 1, 1995.
18. Clarke, R., Hilakivi-Clarke, L., Cho, E., James, M. R., and Leonessa, F., Estrogens, phytoestrogens and breast cancer, in *Dietary Phytochemicals in Cancer Prevention and Treatment*, American Institute for Cancer Research, Ed., Plenum Press, New York, 1996, 63.
19. Raynaud, J. P., Ojasco, T., Bouton, M. M., Bignon, E., Pons, M., and Crastes de Paulet, A., Structure-activity relationships of steroid estrogens, in *Estrogens in the Environment*, McLachlan, J. A., Ed., Elsevier Science Publ. Co., New York, 1985, 24.
20. Anstead, G. M. and Kym, P. R., Benz(a)anthracene diols: predicted carcinogenicity and structure-estrogen receptor binding affinity relationships, *Steroids*, 60, 383, 1995.

21. Miksicek, R. J., Interaction of naturally occurring nonsteroidal estrogens with expressed recombinant human estrogen receptor, *J. Steroid Biochem. Mol. Biol.*, 47, 39, 1994.
22. Coldham, N. G., Dave, M., Sivapathasundaram, S., McDonnell, D. P., Connor, C., and Sauer, M. J., Evaluation of a recombinant yeast cell estrogen screening assay, *Environ. Health Perspect.*, 105, 734, 1997.
23. Collins, B. M., McLachlan, J. A., and Arnold, S. F., The estrogenic and antiestrogenic activities of phytochemicals with the human estrogen receptor expressed in yeast, *Steroids*, 62, 365, 1997.
24. Arts, C. J. M. and Van Den Berg, H., Multi-residue screening of bovine urine on xenobiotic oestrogens with an oestrogen radioreceptor assay, *J. Chromatogr.*, 489, 225, 1989.
25. Zava, D. T. and Duwe, G., Estrogenic and antiproliferative properties of genistein and other flavonoids in human breast cancer cells *in vitro*, *Nutr. Canc.*, 27, 31, 1997.
26. Adlercreutz, H., Mousavi, Y., Clark, J., Höckersted, K., Hämäläinen, E. K., Wähälä, K., Mäkelä, T., and Hase, T., Dietary phytoestrogens and cancer: *in vitro* and *in vivo* studies, *J. Steroid Biochem. Mol. Biol.*, 41, 331, 1992.
27. Whitten, P. L. and Naftolin, F., Dietary estrogens: a biologically active background for estrogen action, in *New Biology of Steroid Hormones*, 74, Hochberg, R. B. and Naftolin, F., Eds., Raven Press, New York, 1991, 155.
28. Adlercreutz, H., Fotsis, T., Lampe, J., Wähälä, K., Mäkelä, T., Brunow, G., and Hase, T., Quantitative determination of lignans and isoflavonoids in plasma of omnivorous and vegetarian women by isotope dilution gas chromatography-mass spectrometry, *Scand. J. Clin. Lab. Invest.*, 53, 5, 1993.
29. Mosselman, S., Polman, J., and Dijkema, R., ERβ: identification and characterization of a novel human estrogen receptor, *FEBS Lett.*, 392, 49, 1996.
30. Kuiper, G. G. J. M., Carlsson, B., Grandien, K., Enmark, E., Häggblad, J., Hilsson, S., and Gustafsson, J.-A., Comparison of the ligand binding specificity and transcript tissue distribution of estrogen receptors α and β, *Endocrinology*, 138, 863, 1997.
31. Kuiper, G. G. J. M., Enmark, E., Pelto-Huikko, M., Nilsson, S., and Gustafsson, J.-A., Cloning of a novel estrogen receptor expressed in rat prostate and ovary, *Proc. Natl. Acad. Sci. U.S.A.*, 93, 5925, 1996.
32. Iafrati, M. D., Karas, R. H., Aronovitz, M., Kim, S., Sullivan, T. R. J., Lubahn, D. B., O'Donnell, T. F. J., Korach, K. S., and Mendelsohn, M. E., Estrogen inhibits the vascular injury response in estrogen receptor α-deficient mice, *Nat. Med.*, 3, 545, 1997.
33. Shughrue, P. J., Komm, B., and Merchenthaler, I., The distribution of estrogen receptor-β mRNA in the rat hypothalamus, *Steroids*, 61, 678, 1996.
34. Brandenberger, A. W., Tee, M. K., Lee, J. Y., Chao, V., and Jaffe, R. B., Tissue distribution of estrogen receptors and alpha (ER-α) and beta (ER-β) in the midgestational human fetus, *J. Clin. Endocrinol. Metab.*, 82, 3509, 1997.
35. Byers, M., Kuiper, G. G. J. M., Gustafsson, J.-A., Park-Sarge, O.-K., Estrogen receptor-β mRNA expression in rat ovary: down-regulation by gonadotropins, *Mol. Endocrinol.*, 11, 172, 1997.
36. Naik, H. R., Lehr, J. E., and Pienta, K. J., An *in vitro* and *in vivo* study of antitumor effects of genistein on hormone refractory prostate cancer, *Anticanc. Res.*, 14, 2617, 1994.

37. Cassidy, A., Bingham, S., and Setchell, K. D. R., Biological effects of a diet of soy protein rich in isoflavones on the menstrual cycle of premenopausal women, *Am. J. Clin. Nutr.*, 60, 333, 1994.

38. Wang, C., Makela, T., Hase, T. A., Adlercreutz, C. H. T., and Kurzer, M. S., Lignans and isoflavonoids inhibit aromatase enzyme in human preadipocytes, *J. Steroid Biochem. Mol. Biol.*, 50, 205, 1994.

39. Pelissero, C., Lenczowski, M., Chinzi, D., Davail-Cuisset, B., Sumpter, J., and Fostier, A., Effects of flavonoids on aromatase activity, an *in vitro* study, *J. Steroid Biochem. Mol. Biol.*, 57, 215, 1996.

40. Chen, S., Kao, Y., and Laughton, C., Binding characteristics of aromatase inhibitors and phytoestrogens to human aromatase, *J. Steroid Biochem. Mol. Biol.*, 61, 107, 1997.

41. Franke, A. A. and Custer, L. J., High-performance liquid chromatographic assay of isoflavonoids and coumestrol from human urine, *J. Chromatogr. B: Biomed. Appl.*, 662, 47, 1994.

42. Piontek, M., Hangels, K. J., Porschen, R., and Strohmeyer, G., Anti-proliferative effect of tyrosine kinase inhibitors in epidermal growth factor-stimulated growth of human gastric cancer cells, *Anticanc. Res.*, 13, 2119, 1993.

43. Boutin, J. A., Minireview — tyrosine protein kinase inhibition and cancer, *Int. J. Biochem.*, 26, 1203, 1994.

44. Okura, A., Arakawa, H., Oka, H., Yoshinari, T., and Monden, Y., Effect of genistein on topoisomerase activity and on the growth of [Val 12] Ha-ras-transformed NIH 3T3 cells, *Biochem. Biophys. Res. Commun.*, 157, 183, 1988.

45. Raines, E. W. and Ross, R., Biology of atherosclerotic plaque formation: possible role of growth factors in lesion development and the potential impact of soy, *J. Nutr.*, 125, 624, 1995.

46. Bennetts, H. W., Underwood, E. J., and Shier, F. L., A specific breeding problem of sheep on subterranean clover pastures in Western Australia, *Aust. Vet. J.*, 22, 2, 1946.

47. Adams, N. R., Organizational and activational effects of phytoestrogens on the reproductive tract of the ewe, *Proc. Soc. Exp. Biol. Med.*, 208, 87, 1995.

48. Ingram, D., Sanders, K., Kolybaba, M., and Lopez, D., Case-control study of phyto-oestrogens and breast cancer, *Lancet*, 350, 990, 1997.

49. Nwannenna, A. I., Madej, A., Lundh, T. J.-O., and Fredriksson, G., Effects of oestrogenic silage on some clinical and endocrinological parameters in ovariectomized heifers, *Acta Vet. Scand.*, 35, 173, 1994.

50. Whitten, P. L., Russell, E., and Naftolin, F., Effects of a normal human-concentration phytoestrogen diet on rat uterine growth, *Steroids*, 57, 98, 1992.

51. Leopold, A., Erwin, M., Oh, J., and Browning, B., Phytoestrogens: adverse effects on reproduction in California quail, *Science*, 191, 98, 1976.

52. Setchell, K. D. R., Gosselin, S. J., Welsh, M. B., Johnston, J. O., Balistreri, W. F., Kramer, L. W., Dresser, B. L., and Tarr, M. J., Dietary estrogens — a probable cause of infertility and liver disease in captive cheetahs, *Gastroenterology*, 93, 225, 1987.

53. Almen, T., Hartel, M., Nylander, G., and Olivercrona, H., The effect of estrogen on the vascular endothelium and its possible relation to thrombosis, *Surg. Gynecol. Obstet.*, 140, 938, 1975.

54. Adlercreutz, H. and Tenhunen, R., Some aspects of the interaction between natural and synthetic female hormones and the liver, *Am. J. Med.*, 49, 630, 1970.

55. Mosher, W. D. and Pratt, R. F., Fecundity and infertility in the United States, 1965-1982, in Advance Data from Vital and Health Statistics, 104, Public Health Service, New York, 1985.

56. Carlsen, E., Giwercman, A., Keiding, N., and Skakkebaek, F., Evidence for decreasing quality of semen during the past 50 years, *Br. Med. J.*, 305, 609, 1992.

57. Feichtinger, W., Environmental factors and fertility, *Hum. Reprod.*, 6, 1170, 1991.

58. Sharpe, R. M. and Skakkebaek, N. E., Are oestrogens involved in falling sperm counts and disorders of the male reproductive tract? *Lancet*, 341, 1392, 1993.

59. Dobrzynska, A. D. and Basaran, N., Effect of various genotoxins and reproductive toxins in human lymphocytes and sperm in the Comet assay, *Teratogen. Carcinogen. Mutagen.*, 17, 29, 1997.

60. Lester, R. and Van Thiel, D. H., Gonadal function in chronic alcoholic men, *Adv. Exp. Med. Biol.*, 85a, 399, 1977.

61. Gavaler, J. S., Rosenblum, E. R., Deal, S. R., and Bowie, B. T., The phytoestrogen congeners of alcoholic beverages: current status, *Proc. Soc. Exp. Biol. Med.*, 208, 98, 1995.

62. Phipps, W. R., Martini, M. C., Lampe, J. W., Slavin, J. L., and Kurzer, M. S., Effect of flax seed ingestion on the menstrual cycle, *J. Clin. Endocrinol. Metab.*, 77, 1215, 1993.

63. Lu, L.-J. W., Anderson, K. E., Grady, J. J., and Nagamani, M., Effects of soya consumption for one month on steroid hormones in premenopausal women: implications for breast cancer risk reduction, *Canc. Epidemiol. Biomarkers Prev.*, 5, 63, 1996.

64. Petrakis, N. L., Barnes, S., King, E. B., Lowenstein, J., Wiencke, J., Lee, M. M., Miike, R., Kirk, M., and Coward, L., Stimulatory influence of soy protein isolate on breast secretion in pre- and postmenopausal women, *Canc. Epidemiol. Biomarkers Prev.*, 5, 785, 1996.

65. Preslock, J. P. and McCann, S., Lesions of the sexually dimorphic nucleus of the preoptic area: effects upon LH, FSH, and prolactin in rats, *Brain Res. Bull.*, 18, 127, 1987.

66. Levy, J. R., Faber, K. A., Ayyash, L., and Hughes, C. L., Jr., The effect of prenatal exposure to the phytoestrogen genistein on sexual differentiation in rats, *Proc. Soc. Exp. Biol. Med.*, 208, 60, 1995.

67. Whitten, P. L., Lewis, C., Russell, E., and Naftolin, F., Phytoestrogen influences on the development of behavior and gonadotropin function, *Proc. Soc. Exp. Biol. Med.*, 208, 82, 1995.

68. Medlock, K. L., Branham, W. S., and Sheehan, D. M., Effects of coumestrol and equol on the developing reproductive tract of the rat, *Proc. Soc. Exp. Biol. Med.*, 208, 67, 1995.

69. Faber, K. A. and Hughes, C. L. J., The effect of neonatal exposure to diethylstilbestrol, genistein, and zearalenone on pituitary responsiveness and sexually dimorphic nucleus volume in the castrated adult rat, *Biol. Reprod.*, 45, 649, 1991.

70. Sheehan, D. M., Branham, W. S., Medlock, K. L., and Shamugasundaram, E. R. B., Estrogenic activity of zearalenone and zearalanol in the neonatal rat uterus, *Teratology*, 29, 383, 1984.

71. Whitten, P. L., Lewis, C., and Naftolin, F., A phytoestrogen diet induces the premature anovulatory syndorme in lactationally exposed female rats, *Biol. Reprod.*, 49, 1117, 1993.

72. Burroughs, C. D., Long-term reproductive tract alterations in female mice treated neotanally with coumestrol, *Proc. Soc. Exp. Biol. Med.*, 208, 78, 1995.

73. Lamartiniere, C. A., Moore, J. B., Brown, N. M., Thompson, R., Hardin, M. J., and Barnes, S., Genistein suppresses mammary cancer in rats, *Carcinogenesis*, 16, 2833, 1995.

74. Mäkelä, S., Chemoprevention of prostate cancer. Role of plant estrogens in normal and estrogen-related growth of rodent prostate, *Turun Yliopiston Julkaisuja Ann. Univ. Turkuensis*, Ser. D, 170, 1995.

75. Leavitt, W. W. and Meismer, D. M., Sexual development altered by neonatal oestrogens, *Nature*, 218, 181, 1968.

76. Register, B., Bethel, M. A., Thompson, N., Walmer, D., Blohm, P., Ayyash, L., and Hughes, C., Jr., The effect of neonatal exposure to diethylstilbestrol, coumestrol, and β-sitosterol on pituitary responsiveness and sexually dimorphic nucleus volume in the castrated adult rat, *Proc. Soc. Exp. Biol. Med.*, 208, 72, 1995.

77. Setchell, K. D. R. and Welsh, M. B., High-performance liquid chromatographic analysis of phytoestrogens in soy protein preparations with ultraviolet, electrochemical and thermospray mass spectrometric detection, *J. Chromatogr.*, 386, 315, 1987.

78. Setchell, K. D. R., Zimmer-Nechemias, L., Cai, J., and Heubi, J. E., Exposure of infants to phyto-oestrogens from soy-based infant formula, *Lancet*, 350, 23, 1997.

79. Barnes, S., Effect of genistein on *in vitro* and *in vivo* models of cancer, *J. Nutr.*, 125, S777, 1995.

80. Winter, J. S. D., Hughes, I. A., Reyes, F. I., and Faiman, C., Pituitary-gonadal relations in infancy: patterns of serum gonadal steroid concentrations in man from birth to two years of age, *J. Clin. Endocrinol. Metab.*, 42, 679, 1976.

81. Franke, A. A. and Custer, L. J., Daidzein and genistein concentrations in human milk after soy consumption, *Clin. Chem.*, 42, 955, 1996.

82. McCarrison, R., The goitrogenic action of soya-bean and ground-nut, *Ind. J. Med. Res.*, 21, 179, 1933.

83. Jabbar, M. A., Larrea, J., and Shaw, R. A., Abnormal thyroid function tests in infants with congenital hypothyroidism: the influence of soy-based formula, *J. Am. Coll. Nutr.*, 16, 280, 1997.

84. Chorazy, P. A., Himelhoch, S., Hopwood, N. J., Greger, N. G., and Postellon, D. C., Persistent hypothyroidism in an infant receiving a soy formula: case report and review of the literature, *Pediatrics*, 96, 148, 1995.

85. Lu, L. J. W., Broemeling, L. D., Marshall, M. V., and Ramanujam, V. M. S., A simplified method to quantify isoflavones in commercial soybean diets and human urine after legume consumption, *Canc. Epidemiol. Biomarkers Prev.*, 4, 497, 1995.

86. Yang, C. S., Pence, B. C., Wargovich, M. J., and Landau, J. M., Diet, nutrition, and cancer prevention: research opportunities, approaches, and pitfalls, in *Dietary Phytochemicals in Cancer Prevention and Treatment*, 401, American Institute for Cancer Research, Ed., Plenum Press, New York, 1996, 231.

87. Sartorelli, A. C., Malignant cell differentiation as a potential therapeutic approach, *Br. J. Canc.*, 52, 293, 1985.

88. Constantinou, A. I., Mehta, R. G., and Vaughan, A., Inhibition of N-methyl-N-nitrosourea-induced mammary tumors in rats by the soybean isoflavones, *Anticanc. Res.*, 16, 3293, 1996.

89. Tang, G., The climacteric of Chinese factory workers, *Maturitas*, 19, 177, 1994.

90. Rose, D. P., Boyar, A. P., and Wynder, E. L., International comparison of mortality rates for cancer of the breast, ovary, prostate, and colon, and per capita food consumption, *Cancer*, 58, 2363, 1986.

91. Armstrong, B. E. and Doll, R., Environmental factors and cancer incidence and mortality in different countries with special reference to dietary practices, *Int. J. Canc.*, 15, 617, 1975.

92. Stanford, J. L., Herrinton, L. J., Schwartz, S. M., and Weiss, N. S., Breast cancer incidence in Asian migrants to the United States and their descendants, *Epidemiology*, 6, 181, 1995.

93. Carter, B. S., Cater, H. B., and Isaacs, J. T., Epidemiologic evidence regarding predisposing factors to prostate cancer, *The Prostate*, 16, 187, 1996.

94. Morton, M. S., Chan, P. S. F., Cheng, C., Blacklock, N., Matos-Ferreira, A., Abranches-Monteiro, L., Correia, R., Lloyd, S., and Griffiths, K., Lignans and isoflavonoids in plasma and prostatic fluid in men: samples from Portugal, Hong Kong, and the United States, *The Prostate*, 32, 122, 1997.

95. Goodman, M. T., Wilkens, L. R., Hankin, J. H., Lyu, L.-C., Wu, A. H., and Kolonel, L. N., Association of soy and fiber consumption with the risk of endometrial cancer, *Am. J. Epidemiol.*, 146, 294, 1997.

96. Wang, C. and Kurzer, M. S., Phytoestrogen concentration determines effects on DNA synthesis in human breast cancer cells, *Nutr. Canc.*, 28, 236, 1997.

97. Dees, C., Foster, J. S., Ahamed, S., and Wimalasena, J., Dietary estrogens stimulate human breast cancer cells to enter the cell cycle, *Environ. Health Perspect.*, 105, 633, 1997.

98. Wei, H., Bowen, R., Cai, Q., Barnes, S., and Wang, Y., Antioxidant and antipromotional effects of the soybean isoflavone genistein, *Proc. Soc. Exp. Biol. Med.*, 208, 124, 1995.

99. Constantinou, A., Kiguchi, K., and Huberman, E., Induction of differentiation and DNA strand breakage in human HL-60 and D-562 leukemia cells by genistein, *Canc. Res.*, 50, 2618, 1990.

100. Shimizu, H., Ross, R. K., Pike, M. C., and Henderson, B. E., Serum oestrogen levels in postmenopausal women: comparison of American whites and Japanese in Japan, *Br. J. Canc.*, 62, 451, 1990.

101. Bernstein, L., Ross, R. K., Pike, M. C., Brown, J. B., and Henderson, B. E., Hormone levels in older women: a study of postmenopausal breast cancer and healthy population controls, *Br. J. Canc.*, 61, 298, 1990.

102. Murrill, W. B., Brown, N. M., Zhang, J., Manzolillo, P. A., Barnes, S., and Lamartiniere, C. A., Prepubertal genistein exposure suppresses mammary cancer and enhances gland differentiation in rats, *Carcinogenesis*, 17, 1451, 1997.

103. Mousavi, Y. and Adlercreutz, H., Enterolactone and estradiol inhibit each other's proliferative effect on MCF-7 breast cancer cells in culture, *J. Steroid Biochem. Mol. Biol.*, 14, 615, 1992.

104. Arnold, S. F., Collins, B. M., Robinson, M. K., Guillette, L. J., Jr., and McLachlan, J. A., Differential interaction of natural and synthetic estrogens with extracellular binding proteins in a yeast estrogen screen, *Steroids*, 61, 642, 1996.

105. Verma, S. P., Salamone, E., and Goldin, B., Curcumin and genistein, plant natural products, show synergistic inhibitory effects on the growth of human breast cancer MCF-7 cells induced by estrogenic pesticides, *Biochem. Biophys. Res. Commun.*, 233, 692, 1997.

106. Carrol, K. K. and Kurowska, E. M., Soy consumption and cholesterol reduction: review of animal and human studies, *J. Nutr.,* 125, 594, 1995.
107. Sirtori, C. R., Lovati, M. R., Manzoni, C., Monetti, M., Pazzucconi, F., and Gatti, E., Soy and cholesterol reduction: clinical experience, *J. Nutr.,* 125, 598, 1995.
108. Kritchevsky, D., Dietary protein, cholesterol and artherosclerosis: a review of the early history, *J. Nutr.,* 125, 589, 1995.
109. Anthony, M. S., Clarkson, T. B., Hughes, C. L., Jr., Morgan, T. M., and Burke, G. L., Soybean isoflavones improve cardiovascular risk factors without affecting the reproductive system of peripubertal rhesus monkeys, *J. Nutr.,* 126, 43, 1996.
110. Forsythe, W. A., III, Soy protein, thyroid regulation and cholesterol metabolism, *J. Nutr.,* 125, 619, 1995.
111. Potter, S. M., Pertile, J., and Berber-Jimenez, M. D., Soy protein concentrate and isolated soy protein similarly lower blood serum cholesterol but differently affect thyroid hormones in hamsters, *J. Nutr.,* 126, 2007, 1996.
112. Ham, J. O., Chapman, K. M., Esses-Sorlie, D., Bakhit, R. M., Prabhudesai, M., Winter, L., Erdman, J. W., and Potter, S. M., Endocrinological response to soy protein and fiber in mildly hypercholesterolemic men, *Nutr. Res.,* 13, 873, 1993.
113. Potter, S. M., Overview of proposed mechanisms for the hypocholesterolemic effect of soy, *J. Nutr.,* 125, 606, 1995.
114. Fumagalli, R., Soleri, L., Farini, R., Musanti, R., Mantero, O., Noseda, G., Gatti, E., and Sirtori, C. R., Fecal cholesterol excretion studies in type II hypercholesterolemic patients treated with soybean protein diet, *Atherosclerosis,* 43, 341, 1982.
115. Wagner, J. D., Cefalu, W. T., Anthony, M. S., Litwak, K. N., Zhang, L., and Clarkson, T. B., Dietary soy protein and estrogen replacement therapy improve cardiovascular risk factors and decrease aortic cholesterol ester content in ovariectomized cynomolgus monkeys, *Metabolism,* 46, 698, 1997.
116. Arjmandi, B. H., Kahn, D. A., Juma, S. S., and Svanborg, A., The ovarian hormone deficiency-induced hypercholesterolemia is reversed by soy protein and the synthetic isoflavone, ipriflavone, *Nutr. Res.,* 17, 885, 1997.
117. Nagata, Y., Tanaka, K., and Sugano, M., Studies on the mechanism of the antihypercholesterolemia action of soy protein and soy protein-type amino acid mixtures in relation to their casein counterparts in rats, *J. Nutr.,* 112, 16147, 1982.
118. Shimokado, K., Umezawa, K., and Ogata, J., Tyrosine kinase inhibitors inhibit multiple steps of the cell cycle of vascular smooth muscle cells, *Exp. Cell Res.,* 220, 266, 1995.
119. Gaudette, D. C. and Holub, B. J., Effect of genistein, a tyrosine kinase inhibitor, on U46619-induced phosphoinositide phosphorylation in human platelets, *Biochem. Biophys. Res. Commun.,* 170, 238, 1990.
120. Honore, E. K., Williams, J. K., Anthony, M. S., and Clarkson, T. B., Soy isoflavones enhance coronary vascular reactivity in atherosclerotic female macaques, *Fertil. Steril.,* 67, 148, 1997.
121. Pietinen, P., Rimm, E., and Korhonen, P., Intake of dietary fiber and risk of coronary heart disease in a cohort of Finnish men: the ATBC study, *Circulation,* 94, 2720, 1996.
122. Slavin, J., Jacobs, D., and Marquart, L., Whole-grain consumption and chronic disease: protective mechanisms, *Nutr. Canc.,* 27, 14, 1997.

123. Michaelsson, K., Bergstrom, R., Holmberg, L., Mallmin, H., Wolk, A., and Ljunghall, S., A high density calcium intake is needed for a positive effect on bone density in Swedish postmenopausal women, *Osteoporosis Int.*, 7, 155, 1997.

124. Kanis, J. A. and Passmore, R., Calcium supplementation of the diet: not justified by present evidence, *Br. Med. J.*, 298, 205, 1989.

125. Tustsumi, N., Effect of coumestrol on bone metabolism in organ culture, *Biol. Pharmaceut. Bull.*, 18, 1012, 1995.

126. Draper, C. R., Edel, M. J., Dick, I. M., Randall, A. G., Martin, G. G., and Prince, R. L., Phytoestrogens reduce bone loss and bone resorption in oophorectomized rats, *J. Nutr.*, 127, 1795, 1997.

127. Valente, M., Bufalino, L., Castiglione, G., D'Angelo, R., Mancuso, A., Galoppi, P., and Zichella, L., Effects of 1-year treatment with ipriflavone on bone in postmenopausal women with low bone mass, *Calcified Tissue Int.*, 54, 377, 1994.

128. Adami, S., Bufalino, L., Cervetti, R., Di Marco, C., Di Munno, O., Fantasia, L., Isaia, G., Serni, U., Vecchiet, L., and Passeri, M., Ipriflavone prevents radial bone loss in postmenopausal women with low bone mass over 2 years, *Osteoporosis Int.*, 7, 119, 1997.

129. Gambacciani, M., Spinetti, A., Piaggesi, L., Cappagli, B., Taponeco, F., Manetti, P., Weiss, C., Teti, G. C., Commare, P. I., and Facchini, V., Ipriflavone prevents the bone mass reduction in premenopausal women treated with gonadotropin hormone-releasing hormone agonists, *Bone Miner.*, 26, 19, 1994.

5

Estrogens, Xenoestrogens, and the Development of Neoplasms

Ana M. Soto and Carlos Sonnenschein

CONTENTS

5.1 Introduction

Sharpe and Skakkebaek postulated that environmental, hormone-like chemicals may be the underlying cause of the increases in testicular cancer, undescended testis, and malformations of the male genital tract during the last half of this century.[1] Davis extended this correlation to the increase in breast cancer incidence during the same time interval.[2] Epidemiological studies and experimental carcinogenesis in animal models that reveal a strong link between hormonal exposure and neoplasia are the bases for both hypotheses.

Endogenous estrogens are considered the main risk factor in the development of breast cancer. Also, estrogen replacement therapy has been shown to increase the incidence of endometrial cancer. Exposure to diethylstilbestrol (DES) *in utero* resulted in the development of clear cell carcinoma of the vagina that appeared after exposed females reached puberty. The recent discovery of hormonally active compounds in the environment, as well as in materials such as food packaging, food additives, cosmetics, and toiletries, suggested that in addition to exposure to exogenous hormones for medical purposes, humans are exposed to many synthetic chemicals that have hormonal activity.

While the role of natural estrogens in carcinogenesis is well documented, the role of other sex steroids, such as androgens, is less compelling. Androgens are a main factor in the development of prostate cancer; however, there is no evidence at present of environmental contaminants that act as androgen mimics. Some environmental contaminants do, however, possess antiandrogenic properties. Although these compounds may disrupt the development of the male genital tract, it is not yet known whether they play a role in carcinogenesis.

5.2 Xenoestrogens

Xenobiotics of widely diverse chemical structures have estrogenic properties.[3-5] This diversity makes it difficult to predict the estrogenicity of chemicals solely on a structural basis. Hence, their identification as estrogens has relied on bioassays using diverse end points on which estrogens play a direct or indirect role (cell proliferation, uterine growth, induction of specific genes). Hertz argued convincingly that the proliferative effect of natural estrogens on the female genital tract is the hallmark of estrogen action; thus, this property was selected to determine whether or not a chemical is an estrogen in animals or in cell culture models.[6] This requires measuring increases of proliferative activity in tissues of the female genital tract after estrogen administration. An equally reliable, easy, and rapid-to-perform method was developed, using estrogen-target, serum-sensitive breast cancer MCF7 cells, that measures cell proliferation as a specific marker of estrogenicity (E-SCREEN assay).[7,8] Other *in vitro* assays rely on the induction of endogenous genes, such as PS2 and PgR, or transfected reporter genes.[9,10]

5.2.1 Cumulative Effect of Xenoestrogens

Humans and wildlife are exposed to a variety of chemicals simultaneously.[11,12] Residues of diverse estrogenic xenobiotics coexist in the fat and body fluids of exposed individuals;[12] hence, it is likely that they may become bioavailable, such as during fasting or nursing. At such a time, they may act cumulatively; that is, when present at individual levels lower than those needed to express overt estrogenicity, their activity may add up to a level sufficient to trigger a full estrogenic response.[13-15] We explored this concept and found that xenoestrogens indeed act cumulatively in the E-SCREEN assay.[13,14] In fact, the effect of some mixtures is more than additive by three- to five-fold. Hence, measuring the total estrogenic burden due to environmental contaminants present in plasma/tissue samples may be more meaningful than measuring the levels of each of the known xenoestrogens individually. This has significant implications for the study of human conditions suspected to be caused by xenoestrogens, such as undescended testis (cryptorchidism), testicular and breast cancer, and the decrease of sperm counts and quality during the last 50 years.[1,16,17]

5.2.2 Novel Xenoestrogens

Novel xenoestrogens were found among antioxidants (alkylphenols, butylhydroxyanisole), plasticizers (bisphenol-A [BPA], dibutylphthalate, butylbenzylphthalate), PCB congeners, disinfectants (o-phenylphenol), and pesticides (toxaphene, dieldrin, endosulfan and lindane) (Table 5.1).[18,19] The

TABLE 5.1

Xenobiotics Tested by the E-SCREEN Assay

Estrogenic Xenobiotics	Nonestrogenic Xenobiotics	

I. Herbicides

None	2,4 D	2,4 DB
	Alochlor	Atrazine
	Butylate	Cyanazine
	Dacthal	Dinoseb
	Hexazinone	Picloram
	Propazine	Simazine
	Trifluralin	

II. Insecticides

pp' DDT	Bendiocarb	Carbofuran
op' DDT	Chlordane	Chlordimeform
op' DDE	Diazinon	Chlorpyrifos
op' DDT	Heptachlor	Dicamba
DDT*	Kelthane	Metoalchlor
Dieldrin	Malathion	Mirex
Chlordecone (kepone)	Methoprene	Pyrethrum
Endosulfan[a]	Parathion	Rotenone
alpha Endosulfan		
beta Endosulfan		
Lindane		
Methoxychlor		
Toxaphene		

III. Fungicides

None	Chlorothalonil	Thiram
	Maneb	Zineb
	Metiram	Ziram

IV. Industrial Chemicals

2,3,4 TCB	Butylated Hydroxytoluene	2 CB
2,2',4,5 TCB	2,5 DCB	4 CB
2,3,4,5 TCB	2,6 DCB	2,3,6 TCB
2,4,4',6 TCB	3,5 DCB	2,3,5,6 TCB
2,2',3,3',6,6' HCB	2,3',5 TCB	2,3,3'4,5' PCB
2 OH-2',5' DCB	2,3,4,4' TCB	2,2',3,3',5,5' HCB
3 OH-2',5' DCB	2,3,4,5,6 PCB	2 OH-3,5 DCB
4 OH-2',5' DCB	2 OH-2',3',4',5,5' PCB	DecaCB
4 OH-2,2',5 TCB	3 OH-3,5 DCB	Dimethyl Isophthalate
4 OH-2',4',6' TCB	4 OH-3,5 DCB	Dimethyl Terephthalate
3 OH-2',3',4',5' TCB	1,2-Dichloroethylene	Dinonyl Phthalate
4 OH-2',3',4',5' TCB	Hexachlorobenzene	

TABLE 5.1 (continued)

Xenobiotics Tested by the E-SCREEN Assay

Estrogenic Xenobiotics	Nonestrogenic Xenobiotics	
4 OH-alkyl-phenols	Irganox 1640	Octachlorostyrene
Bisphenol-A (BPA)	2,3,7,8 TCDD[b]	Styrene
BPA dimethacrylate	Tetrachloroethylene	
OH-biphenyls		
t-Butylhydroxyanisole		
Benzylbutylphthalate		
Dibutylphthalate		

[a] Denotes a technical grade isomer mixture.
[b] This compound inhibits estrogen action.

newly identified estrogens not only induce cell proliferation but also increase the expression of pS2 and progesterone receptor (PgR). These xenoestrogens compete with estradiol for binding to the estrogen receptor. Their relative binding affinities to the estrogen receptor correlate well with their potency to induce cell proliferation and with the induction of marker gene products such as pS2 and PgR.[19]

No qualitative differences could be found when comparing animal assays and MCF7-based assays; that is, the estrogenic properties of compounds characterized using animal bioassays were also ascertained by measuring cell proliferation or gene induction. From a pharmacokinetic perspective, the *in vitro* assays measure estrogenicity at the target cell level under conditions where estrogen levels are mostly constant, much like the ones achieved when animals are treated with estrogen-filled silastic implants. This approach is more relevant to chronic environmental exposure than that of measuring acute effects after a single dose. Estrogen target cells in culture have a limited metabolic repertory. For example, nonylphenol diethoxylate was estrogenic for MCF7 cells; since it does not compete for estradiol binding to the estrogen receptor, it is likely that the estrogenic activity results from nonylphenol diethoxylate metabolism to the free phenol.[20] Methoxychlor was also believed to be inactive until metabolized to free phenols, presumably in the liver; again, methoxychlor tested positive when assayed by the E-SCREEN test. Therefore, even though the putative proestrogens tested so far were estrogenic when assayed by the E-SCREEN test, an added step in the quest for identifying all xenoestrogens may include their metabolic activation by liver microsome extracts prior to their testing by the E-SCREEN assay.

Regarding quantitative effects, while kepone is 100,000 to 1,000,000 times less potent than estradiol according to the E-SCREEN assay, an increase of the rat uterine wet weight comparable to that of estradiol occurred with a 1000- to 5000-fold higher dose of kepone than of estradiol.[3] This discrepancy may be due to rapid metabolism of estradiol and persistence and bioaccumulation of kepone in animals. BPA, the only novel xenoestrogen tested so far for endocrine disruption, upon exposure *in utero* was found to produce effects at doses lower than expected from its potency measured in adult animals and *in vitro*.[21,22] Moreover, when BPA was given to adult animals, it was found also to be more potent than what was expected from *in vitro* data.[23,24]

5.3 Neoplasia

One of the most vexing biological problems is finding an accurate definition for cancer. No single, comprehensive definition of cancer addresses all aspects of this disease, which indicates a tacit acceptance of a lack of knowledge on its pathogenesis. Cancer is both a biological problem and a medical one. Historically, its study interested physicians, who were concerned with curing patients with "tumors" (etymologically, lumps). Physicians described the disease and divided "tumors" into two categories, benign and malignant, according to their clinical behavior. "Neoplasia" (new growth) denotes an accumulation of cells in a tissue. However, each one of the properties of neoplasias could also be expressed in normal cells (i.e., invasiveness, ability to proliferate, etc.). From an evolutionary perspective, neoplasias appear with the advent of multicellular organisms; their purview spans several hierarchical levels of organization, from the cellular to the organismal. The process by which neoplasias are generated is called carcinogenesis. In epithelia, these precursor lesions are called hyperplasia (increased cell proliferation), metaplasia (the ectopic appearance of otherwise normal epithelium), dysplasia (the epithelium shows altered organization and signs of increased proliferative activity), and carcinoma *in situ* (the epithelium resembles a neoplasia that has not yet invaded normal adjacent tissue).

Definitions of neoplasias and even of their precursor lesions are fraught with unwarranted assumptions about the carcinogenetic process.[25] They are usually circular, and in addition, they are contradicted by either the behavior of a particular neoplasm or by that of a normal cell type. For example, the widely used definition proposed by Willis states that "a tumor is an abnormal mass of tissue, the growth of which exceeds and is uncoordinated with that of the normal tissues, and persists in the same excessive manner after cessation of the stimuli which evoked the change."[26] This definition (1) fails to distinguish a simple hyperplasia from a neoplasia, (2) does not establish in which regard this "abnormal mass of tissue" differs from other anomalies that are not neoplastic, (3) invokes stimuli that are presently unknown, and (4) does not take into consideration the phenomenon of regression that may occur during carcinogenesis or even neoplasia. True and complete spontaneous regression of early stage melanomas[27] and some neuroblastomas[28] is a well documented phenomenon. Regression often occurs in hormonal carcinogenesis after hormone withdrawal. Another drawback of Willis's definition is that it does not take into consideration the tissular organization defects that allow the diagnosis of neoplasia at the histological level. For all these reasons, we will leave neoplasia undefined, and we will paraphrase the pronouncement of the judges of the U.S. Supreme Court about pornography: while it is difficult to define, we recognize it when we see it.

Neoplasias are viewed in three contexts: (a) as an aberration of development, (b) as a problem of tissular organization, and (c) as an aberration of the control of cell proliferation.

5.4 Theories on the Mechanisms of Carcinogenesis

5.4.1 Genetic Origin and the Somatic Mutation Theory of Carcinogenesis

The major reason to invoke a genetic origin for certain cancers is the existence of familial cancers inherited through the germinal line. However, this fact by itself does not provide an explanation of how carcinogenesis takes place. The lethal (2) giant larvae mutant [l(2)gl] in *Drosophila* is the best-studied model. Homozygosity of this mutant gene results in the appearance of neuroblastomas in the third instar larvae.[29] The normal gene codes for an intracellular, cytoskeleton-associated protein, which is expressed in the early embryo, long before the morphogenesis of the nervous system takes place. Replacement of the mutated sequence in early homozygous embryos with the wild allele results in normal flies, indicating that expression of this gene at this embryonal stage, not later, is required for the development of normal neuroblasts.[30] The difficulty remains in trying to understand how the affected gene resulted in a neoplasia, since this protein does not appear to have a direct role in the control of the proliferation of neuroblasts.

The somatic mutation theory of cancer has survived practically unchallenged as dogma for almost a century. Since first articulated by Boveri in 1914, it has been updated from time to time to accommodate new findings; however, it has never predicted outcomes that would validate or falsify it. In other words, a theory that can accommodate all outcomes is not useful. In its latest incarnation it postulates that cancer arises through mutations in putative oncogenes (positive mediators) and in tumor-suppressor genes (negative mediators), which have been proposed to regulate cell proliferation.[31]

Research on chemical carcinogenesis is based on the premise that, in addition to its intoxicating effects, these chemicals generate somatic mutations. This research led to the two-stage model, whereby an "initiating" agent causes permanent DNA damage and a "promoting" agent that is unspecific induces proliferation of the genetically altered cells.[32] Although this view is somewhat consistent with some experiments on skin carcinogenesis, there is a substantial body of experimental evidence that contradicts this simplistic interpretation of the data.[33,34] Despite the many reports favoring the somatic mutation theory, the unequivocal identification of the candidate mutated genes responsible for tumor formation has been elusive. This much has been formally acknowledged by Varmus[35] and by Bishop,[36] the original proponents of a crucial role for oncogenes in carcinogenesis.

5.4.2   Epigenetic Origin: Development and Neoplasia

The epigenetic origin is invoked on the basis of two experimental phenomena that rule out DNA mutation as the ultimate cause of carcinogenesis. The first is the development of embryonal carcinomas when blastocysts are implanted in the testes of mice. When a few of these tumor cells were injected into normal blastocysts, they contributed to normal progeny in different tissues of the "mosaic" mice, including oocytes and spermatozoa, that in turn, generated normal individuals.[37] The second experimental phenomenon is the development of normal tadpoles when nuclei of tetraploid frog renal carcinoma cells were transplanted into enucleated diploid eggs.[38] In addition, certain tumors, arising during development from fetal tissue, appear in association with developmental anomalies (nephroblastoma with horseshoe kidney, hypospadias, and cryptorchidism), suggesting that neoplasias may develop when normal development is affected.[39] The frequent regression of neuroblastomas in infants suggests that cancer cells may revert to normalcy when placed in a permissive environment. Thus, the dictum "once a cancer cell, always a cancer cell" is unsupported by data.[40]

The major obstacle preventing research in epigenetic causation has been the absence of a paradigm to study how the developmental program is materialized. It is hoped that the recent advances in the study of pattern formation, histogenesis, and organogenesis will lead to the underlying mechanisms involving cell-to-cell and tissue-to-tissue communication. In contrast, the somatic mutation hypothesis points to research at the genetic level, an endeavor in which powerful technologies are being used to study mutational phenomena. The problem with the mutational approach is that, in the long run, if the identified gene is not directly responsible for the neoplasm, as in the case of the lethal (2) giant larvae mutant, once again the question of where and when the ultimate cause acts remains unanswered. Neither the somatic mutation theory nor the epigenetic theory has produced a compelling explanation for the events that lead to carcinogenesis. This difficulty may arise from the fact that phenomena at the whole-organism level cannot be reconstructed from the properties of its components; probably, this is because when hierarchical levels of complexity are crossed, emergent properties arise or disappear.[41,42]

5.4.3 Control of Cell Proliferation and Neoplasia

A significant shortcoming in establishing a successful research program in carcinogenesis is the lack of resolution of the fundamental controversy regarding the default proliferative state of cells in metazoa.

Self-replication is the sine qua non of life. It is accepted that proliferation is a built-in property of the cells of unicellular organisms and metaphyta. Unicellular organisms and metaphyta cells dissociated from tissues and placed in culture proliferate maximally as long as they are exposed to nutrients. The state of proliferative quiescence appeared with the advent of multicellularity. There are only two choices to be made: the first proposes that the default of cells in metazoa is quiescence; the other posits that proliferation is the default state of these cells. Researchers studying metazoa assume that the quiescent state observed *in situ* is the default state. This means that cells will not proliferate unless stimulated. However, evolutionarily speaking, this argument is not compelling, since multicellular organisms evolved from unicellular ones.

The prevailing idea that quiescence appeared as a new default state in metazoans has never been adequately supported by either argument or data. Multicellular organisms have quiescent cells. However, there is no reason to believe that the quiescent state is a newly acquired default state rather than the consequence of a regulatory event imposed by the organism on specific cell types. How can organisms relinquish the fundamental property of self-replication? Every organism starts as a single cell. It is impossible for that single cell to forgo the property of self-replication. The finding that there is almost complete homology between the machinery to replicate yeast cells and human cells suggests that the machinery for cell replication has remained constant through evolution. If one considers quiescence as a newly acquired default state, a number of incompatibilities become obvious. For instance, if one proposes that the somatic cells lost this property, one must explain how this may be the case when well-known facts suggest the opposite: (1) the genome is similar in all cells of the organism, and in experimental conditions, somatic cell nuclei may generate whole individuals when placed in enucleated oocytes, and (2) the segregated germ cells, like their somatic counterparts, undergo control of cell proliferation, as shown by the "dormancy" of oogenesis and spermatogenesis at certain developmental stages. If the built-in capacity to proliferate within these cells were not curtailed by organismal control, their exponential proliferation would destroy the soma.

The choice made by cancer researchers about the default state in metazoan cells subsequently shapes their research program. Those accepting quiescence as the default state search for growth factors and other possible stimulators of cell proliferation, while those accepting proliferation as the default state search for inhibitory factors.

5.4.3.1   Control of Cell Proliferation by Sex Steroids

Sex hormones (androgens and estrogens) regulate the proliferative activity of their target cells. Studies in animal models have shown that estrogens and androgens control epithelial cell numbers in their target organs by (1) inhibiting cell death,[43] (2) inducing cell proliferation (Step-1), and later (3) inhibiting cell proliferation (proliferative shutoff effect, Step-2).[44,45] These three effects may be segregated in different experimental models, suggesting that they are controlled by discrete, separate mechanisms.

5.4.3.2   Control of Initiation of Cell Proliferation
by Estrogens (Step-1)

Three hypotheses aim at explaining the role of estrogens on the induction of cell proliferation: The direct positive hypothesis proposes that estrogens trigger per se the proliferation of their target cells.[46] The indirect positive hypothesis proposes that estrogens induce the synthesis of growth factors that, in turn, cause proliferation of estrogen-sensitive cells via stroma-epithelium, paracrine,[47] or autocrine[48] interactions. And the indirect negative hypothesis posits that estrogens cancel the effect of plasma-borne inhibitory molecules (estrocolyone-I).[49-51] The first two hypotheses are based on the premise that proliferation is an inducible function (that is, the default state of cells is quiescence). On the contrary, the third hypothesis assumes that proliferation is a constitutive property of cells. Either a "falsification" or a synthesis of one of the two premises has yet to emerge. This implies that important evidence needed to fully understand estrogen control of cell proliferation is either still missing or remains unacknowledged. A brief reference to data collected using a variety of models follows, and a resolution of the controversy will be proposed.

5.4.3.2.1   Whole Animal Models

After estradiol administration to ovariectomized or immature rodents, the expression of cellular oncogenes,[52] growth factors,[53] and their receptors[54] are augmented in a temporal pattern consistent with their involvement in the proliferative process. In support of this notion, it was proposed that estrogens act by inducing epidermal growth factor (EGF) receptors and EGF synthesis in uterine epithelium *in situ*.[53] EGF implants induced both cell proliferation and estrogen-regulated genes in uterine and vaginal epithelia in mice.[55] However, EGF does not induce uterotropic effects in estrogen receptor-knockout mice.[56] These contradictory results leave unresolved the identity of the ultimate causal agent responsible for entry into the cell cycle.

5.4.3.2.2 Primary Culture Experiments

Rodent uterine epithelial cells are fully responsive to estrogens for the induction of specific genes; however, estradiol does not increase their proliferative rate.[57,58] In fact, these cells proliferate both in estrogenless and serumless defined medium, suggesting that estrogens may act indirectly in order to induce cell proliferation.[58-60] However, lack of a proliferative effect by estrogens in primary cultures is inconsistent with the autocrine hypothesis. Moreover, proliferation occurs even in the absence of growth factors.[59] Also, mice mammary luminal epithelial cells are estrogen-sensitive for gene expression but not for cell proliferation.[61] Inferred paracrine mechanisms involving stromal cells are inconsistent with data obtained using vaginal explants from ovariectomized mice.[62] Epithelial cells in these explants undergo rapid proliferation in basal medium devoid of growth factors, regardless of the presence of estrogens. This suggests that the intact stroma, present in the explant, fails to mediate estrogen-induced epithelial cell proliferation, and that these cells are released from inhibitory signals operating in the animal.[62]

5.4.3.2.3 Established Estrogen-Target Cell Lines

Estrogen-mediated proliferation in culture conditions occurs only when the medium contains serum made estrogenless by charcoal-dextran stripping (CD). Contradictory data were reported on the proliferative effect of estrogens in serumless medium; it varied from a much reduced[63] to a null effect.[64-66] These discrepancies may be due to (1) the presence of a proliferation inhibitor in serum,[50,51,65,66] (2) a permissive effect of serum growth factors,[67] or (3) a synergism between these growth factors and estrogens.[68] Human breast MCF7 cells become quiescent in culture when growth medium is supplemented with CD serum, and estrogens release them from this proliferative quiescence specifically.[49] A subline of MCF7 cells (MCF7-SF9) has been propagated in defined medium without growth factors for several thousand generations.[69] These cells proliferate at comparable rates in defined medium regardless of the presence of estrogens. Still, CD serum inhibits their proliferation, while estrogens cancel the CD serum-mediated inhibition. The very existence of these cell lines challenges the notion of synergism between growth factors and estrogen and strongly supports the existence of a negative control mechanism involving a serum-borne inhibitor, estrocolyone-I.[49-51] Remarkably, these human cells form tumors only in estrogen-treated athymic mice.[70]

5.4.3.2.4 The Role of Serum Inhibitors

Serum fractionation protocols resulted in the coelution of the inhibitory activity with serum albumin. Removal of human albumin (HA) from charcoal-dextran-stripped serum resulted in a preparation lacking the inhibitory effect. HA inhibition was cell type- and protein-specific. Only estrogens cancelled HA inhibition; recombinant growth factors and other hormones were ineffective. Recombinant HA and a truncated peptide spanning Domains I and II inhibited cell proliferation; Domain I was also inhibitory, albeit less potent that HA.[51] Domain III lacked inhibitory activity. These results suggest that (1) albumin or a portion of it (most likely within Domains I and II) is the specific inhibitory signal for the proliferation of human estrogen-target, serum-sensitive cells, (2) estrogens specifically cancel this inhibition, (3) inhibitory signals prevail over putative growth factors, and (4) the default state in these cells is proliferation.

5.4.3.2.5   Role of Estrogen Receptors (ER) on Induction of Cell Proliferation by Estrogens

Stable expression of transfected αER gene constructs in previously αER-negative cells renders these cells able to evoke an estrogen-induced proliferative shutoff (Step-2); however, no induction of estrogen-sensitive cell proliferation has been observed.[71] This suggests that αER expression is necessary but not sufficient for conferring estrogen-sensitivity for induction of cell proliferation. In contrast, βER is not present in serum-sensitive, estrogen target cells, and most likely, it does not play a role on the control of the proliferation of these cells.

5.4.3.3   Control of the Expression of the Proliferative Shutoff by Estrogens (Step-2) in Normalcy, Carcinogenesis, and Tumor Regression

Stormshak et al. found that estrogens not only induced the proliferation of their target cells in rats but that their chronic administration resulted in a proliferative shutoff.[44] Later, Gorski's and Stancel's groups demonstrated that this inhibitory effect is a physiological response to estrogens,[72,73] while Bruchovsky et al. showed a parallel behavior of rat prostate cells to androgens.[74] Mukku et al. found that a second injection of estradiol, given 18 h after the first one, reduces the peak of mitosis normally observed in the endometrium 24 h after a single hormone dose.[73] Wilklund et al. explored the difference in responses of the anterior pituitary in Holtzman and Fischer rats; estrogen implants induced a proliferative response which lasted only 5-6 d in female Holtzman rats, while it continued in Fisher rats; eventually, rats of this strain went on to develop pituitary tumors. Wiklund et al. concluded that "…the quantitative relationships of estrogen doses to 'refractoriness' suggest to us that estrogens induce the accumulation of some product that limits the ability of the cells to respond to additional estrogen."[75]

High doses of estrogens induce regression of clinical breast cancer at rates similar to those obtained with antiestrogens. In fact, the usefulness of tamoxifen was tested in comparison with DES; both were equally effective, but tamoxifen was adopted because of its less severe side effects.[76] As mentioned above, transfection of ER into mammary breast cells, fibroblasts, HeLa cells, etc., resulted in a phenotype expressing Step-2 only. In dimethylbenz[a]-anthracene

(DMBA)-induced tumors, high doses of estrogen inhibited the development of mammary tumors.[77] The development of variants of the MCF7 cell line that exclusively express either Step-1 and Step-2, both, or neither suggests that these two effects are controlled through independent pathways.[78,79] The existence of an estrogen-induced shutoff effect indicates that the proliferative effect does not follow a linear dose-response curve.[79,80] We have postulated that Step-2 is mediated by estrogen-induced intracellular effectors (estrocolyone-II). A comparable pattern was described in the human prostate cancer cell line LNCaP.[81,82]

5.4.4 Epigenetic Origin: Tissue Maintenance and Neoplasia

We postulate that the process of carcinogenesis in adulthood takes place at the hierarchical level of tissue organization. We posit that there are discrete units of tissue maintenance and/or organization in normal, adult, multicellular organisms. They comprise the parenchyma and the stroma of an organ. The proposed name tissulon abbreviates this concept. Like the morphogenetic fields that act during embryogenesis to instruct the formation of tissues and organs, tissulons operating during postnatal life are tridimensional and carry positional information. They maintain the normal architecture of all organs and guide tissue turnover, remodeling, and healing through a dynamic process. During embryogenesis, the stroma exerts instructive and permissive influences on the overlying epithelium, dictating its phenotypic characteristics. According to data collected by J.W. Orr and his colleagues almost half a century ago, these properties are maintained by the stroma during adulthood;[83] carcinogen-exposed stroma was able to evoke a neoplastic phenotype in adjacently grafted epithelia never exposed to the carcinogen. In our view, tissulons, present within all organs, are the ultimate targets of carcinogenic agents. There are likely to be tissulons that are more susceptible to carcinogenesis than others (breast, prostate, colon, uterus, etc.).

Developmental biology is now tackling the problems of pattern formation and morphogenesis, and thus providing the basis for the study of interactions among cells and tissues. It is hoped that the application of these principles in the context of the tissulon theory will shed light on the study of carcinogenesis.

5.5 Hormonal Carcinogenesis

It is difficult to establish without ambiguity the role played by hormones in the development of neoplasias. Within the somatic mutation theory, two roles have been postulated for hormones, namely, that they induce mutations and that they act as promoters. For proponents of the epigenetic perspective, extemporaneous exposure to hormones is considered teratogenic. Hence, neoplasia is the result of altered development. Finally, some think that the genetic and epigenetic options are not mutually exclusive. In this case, sex hormones would contribute to the development of neoplasia by acting at these three end points (mutation, control of cell proliferation, and organo-genesis-tissue maintenance).

5.5.1   Hormones as Mutagens

Supporters of the genetic causation hypothesis (two-step model of carcino-genesis) propose that certain estrogens are able to form DNA adducts; this would lead to mutations in yet-to-be-identified genes that, in turn, through yet-to-be-defined pathways would result in neoplasms. These inferential pathways involve entities such as "oncogenes" and suppressor genes.

The main research program in this endeavor has been to elucidate meta-bolic pathways leading to the formation of estrogen metabolites that form DNA adducts in estrogen-target tissues. These DNA adducts, when misre-paired, would originate mutations. One prediction of the mutagenic hypoth-esis is that not all estrogenic compounds are carcinogenic, which means that only those that are mutagenic are expected to induce tumor formation. For example, 2-fluoroestradiol, a compound with an estrogenic potency similar to estradiol, does not induce tumorigenesis in the Syrian hamster model, while estradiol does. This is explained by the ability of estradiol to be metab-olized to 2-hydroxy metabolites, while 2-fluoroestradiol is not metabolized.[84] From a similar perspective, DES is metabolized to an unstable semiquinone that can react with DNA;[85,86] others have postulated that DES may interact with spindle formation causing aneuploidy.[87] Bradlow et al. suggested that estradiol is metabolized through two mutually exclusive pathways, resulting in a 2-OH estrone and 16α-estrone; they propose that their genotoxic activity is entirely due to 16α-estrone.[88,89] From this perspective, carcinogenesis may be induced by chemicals that affect the metabolism of natural estrogens enhancing the formation of 16α-estrone. Estrogens have also been implicated in the development of prostate cancer in rats:[90] mutational mechanisms were invoked.[91] These hypotheses are based on circumstantial evidence, and a firm demonstration of causality is still missing.

5.5.1.1   *Xenoestrogens and the Mutational Hypothesis*

Xenoestrogen exposure appears to be a risk factor for neoplasms of the female genital tract, breast, and prostate. If mutations are the first step in carcinogenesis, how are xenoestrogens expected to act? Accumulation in a target cell would be proportional to the binding affinity for the xenoestrogens by estrogen receptors. Therefore, a linear dose-response curve may be assumed when associating exposure to effects. However, once xenoestrogens are accumulated in the target tissue, the rate of conversion to the metabolites able to produce DNA adducts must be dependent on their affinity for the enzymes involved in this pathway. If xenoestrogens act by altering the metabolism of endogenous estrogens, the mutagenic activity would be disassociated from the estrogenic activity and linked, instead, with the ability of these xenoestrogens to induce or activate enzymes that regulate the metabolism of endogenous estrogens. Therefore, a linear dose-response curve would be expected. However, mutagenic potency may not be directly related to estrogenic potency. In conclusion, while the estrogenic potency of xenoestrogens may be important, it does not seem to be the main determinant for their potential mutagenicity.

5.5.2 Hormones as Promoters

Animal models and observational data in humans indicate that tumors in estrogen and androgen target organs are rare in individuals that had been gonadectomized before or during early adulthood. It is postulated that the role of sex steroids in this context is to sustain cell proliferation in genetically susceptible individuals (i.e., only certain strains develop tumors upon sustained hormone exposure).

In normal sex hormone-target tissues, a tight regulation of cell number operates, whereby sex steroids both induce cell proliferation (Step-1) and later inhibit it (Step-2). The "initiated" cells must overcome the restraining mechanisms of Step-2 in order to proliferate selectively and become a hyperplasia and, later on, a tumor. Once the tumor develops, it may or may not require hormones to propagate further (hormone-sensitive or insensitive, respectively). In this view, a cell "mutated" in its ability to proliferate would acquire a selective advantage to multiply over those impervious to the carcinogen-mutagen. This is a rarely analyzed paradox. The paradox could be reconciled if those mutations are shown to be only in suppressor genes or colyogenes. Proponents of oncogenes state that cancer cells have lost the ability to respond to organismal signals that inhibit cell proliferation.[92] However, none of these hypotheses take into consideration that the precursor lesions that appear during carcinogenesis show altered tissue organization.

Hormones are not only necessary during the process of carcinogenesis but may also play a role in the propagation of these tumors. Thus, breast and prostate cancers in humans regress after estrogens or androgens, respectively, are withdrawn or suppressed. In animal models, regression may "cure" the tumor, whereas in humans, clinical regressions are temporary due to the selection of "hormone-insensitive" phenotypes. This process is called tumor progression; this recurrence has been attributed to genetic (further mutations) and/or epigenetic (adaptive) mechanisms due to short-lived therapeutic regimes.[79,82,93,94]

5.5.2.1   Xenoestrogens and the Promotional Hypothesis

As explained above, the issue regarding how estrogen levels may affect proliferation and carcinogenesis remains unsolved. To assess whether or not xenoestrogens significantly increase normal adult women's exposure to estrogen, one first has to ask how ovarian estrogen levels affect proliferation in their target organs. For example, ductal cell proliferation in the breast is maximal from the late follicular phase and throughout the luteal phase (i.e., when endogenous estrogen levels are high).[95] Further increases in the estrogen levels may not affect cell proliferation, since the endogenous levels of estrogen at this point are already triggering a full proliferative response followed by a proliferative shutoff. The ubiquitous presence of xenoestrogens in foods, their persistence in the environment, lack of binding to the plasma carrier protein sex hormone binding globulin, and cumulative action[13,14,19,96,97] may increase the "basal" levels of estrogens during the early follicular phase of the menstrual cycle. This may result in an early onset of proliferative activity of the organs of the female genital tract and breast, consequently prolonging the period of proliferative activity during each cycle, leading to a higher incidence of breast tumors in later years. Hence, the assumption of a linear dose-response curve is not appropriate when evaluating the role of xenoestrogens as promoters.

5.5.3   Hormones as Teratogens

Developmental biologists assign the role of extemporaneous hormonal activity as being essentially teratogenic. These untimely exposures would favor the persistence of cell populations past the point at which they should disappear during normal development.[98-100]

5.5.3.1   The DES Model

Genital tract organogenesis occurs in humans during the first trimester of gestation and at gestational days 9-16 in mice. The role of estrogenic hormones in the normal development of the mammalian reproductive tract is not completely understood, although it is clear that ER must be present for estradiol to mediate biological activity.[101] Exposure to exogenous estrogens during early development results in several anomalies of the genital tract, including neoplasia. Some of these effects entail the persistence of tissues that regress or express different cellular markers during development. For example, Müllerian ducts (structures that give rise to organs of the female genital tract) regress during development in males, but they persist in those exposed to estrogens during development. Women exposed to DES *in utero* manifested a series of anomalies of the genital tract (adenosis, ectropion, and anomalies of the cervix) and an increased incidence of clear cell adenocarcinoma of the vagina (risk from birth to 34 years of age is 1:1000).[102] Exposure to DES occurred before the 13th week of pregnancy in women that developed clear cell adenocarcinoma. The fact that 90% of the cases were diagnosed between ages 15 and 27 suggests that in addition to *in utero* exposure the hormonal environment present at puberty is also required for the development of this lesion. Interestingly, in the mouse model, a main effect of DES exposure was that animals developed adenocarcinomas of the uterus after 4 months of age.[103] Before this time point in development, exposed mice had exhibited hypoplastic uteri with few or no glands.[104] This suggests that the primary effect may neither be a proliferative one nor a mutational one. Instead, the primary effect may be developmental (epigenetic?) in the sense that cell populations that should have disappeared did not.

DES-exposed women are just now entering the fifth decade of life. Therefore, it is not yet known whether *in utero* exposure to DES also increases the risk of hormone-related neoplasms (endometrium, breast) at the age in which these neoplasms appear in the unexposed population. Bern[105,106] and Newbold and McLachlan[103] studied the effect of prenatal and early postnatal exposure to DES on the genital tract of mice and found that the most important feature of this syndrome is that some of the morphological alterations are not readily recognizable at birth, but they manifest themselves during puberty and adult life. In the uterus, cystic endometrial hyperplasia, leiomyomas, adenocarcinomas, and stromal cell sarcomas were observed. In the vagina, the proliferative lesions reported were basal cell hyperplasia combined with hyperkeratinization, epidermoid tumors, and adenocarcinomas. It should be noted that vaginal adenocarcinomas appeared when mice were exposed to relatively low doses (2.5 µg/kg/d), while uterine adenocarcinomas appeared at higher exposure levels (100 µg/kg/d) on days 9 to 16 of gestation.[107] Ovariectomy before puberty prevented the development of these neoplasias. Prolactinomas were observed in mice exposed on days 16–17 of prenatal development.[108] Another interesting consequence of neonatal exposure to DES in mice infected with murine mammary tumor viruses is a shortened latency period and an increased incidence of mammary tumors. In the CD-1 strain of mice, which has high incidence of spontaneous mammary tumors, offspring of females exposed *in utero* had a significantly higher incidence of ovarian and mammary tumors than offspring of females exposed to vehicle.[109] DES induced vaginal adenocarcinomas and squamous cell carcinomas in Wistar rats treated on days 18 to 20 of gestation.[110] More recently, it was reported that male mice exposed *in utero* to DES can transmit a carcinogenic effect to their offspring.[111] Walker and Kurth showed that female mice exposed *in utero* can transmit a carcinogenic effect to their offspring.[112] Using blastocyst transfers, it was shown that offspring of normal blastocysts, which had been transferred to mice exposed prenatally to DES, developed uterine adenocarcinomas (7%). Offspring from blastocysts from female mice exposed to DES *in utero*, transferred to mice exposed to vehicle, also developed endometrial adenocarcinomas (16%). Hence, the neoplastic effects of intrauterine exposure may be due to "germ cell modification" (mutation or gene imprinting), as well as to alteration of the maternal environment.

5.5.3.2   *Xenoestrogens and the Developmental Hypothesis*

Time of exposure appears to be crucial for eliciting developmental mishaps. In addition, some of the developmental alterations mediated by estrogens occurs at significantly lower doses than those necessary for causing estrogenic effects in adults. For example, Burroughs et al. have found that hypoplasia of uterine glands occur after neonatal exposure to extremely low doses of coumestrol, a phytoestrogen.[113,114] In addition, vom Saal observed significant increases in the size of the prostate in adult animals exposed *in utero* to higher levels of estrogen due to a positional effect (a male between two females versus a male between two males).[115,116] Moreover, *in utero* exposure to low doses of BPA also resulted in increased prostate size in the adult.[22] It should be noted that in vom Saal's experiments, the dose-response curve looks like an inverted U. This means that the highest doses were less effective in inducing these effects than the lower ones.[21,22] In summary, there are stages of particular vulnerability during development, and the developing organism seems to be far more sensitive to minute variations of hormone levels than the adult organism.

5.5.4   Hormones as Agents of Tissue Maintenance and Remodeling

During postnatal life, the mammary gland and the endometrium undergo massive architectural changes, comparable to those usually associated with organogenesis. These changes occur in response to various physiological hormonal environments, such as those of puberty and pregnancy. For example, the mammary gland ducts grow by invading the adjacent connective tissue. A similar process takes place in the prostate gland during development and maturation. Moreover, these changes can be induced repeatedly in experiments by endocrine manipulation. These organizational changes occur through interactions between the stroma and the epithelium.[117,118]

5.6   Animal Models for Hormonal Carcinogenesis

5.6.1   "Spontaneous" Neoplasia of Estrogen-Target Organs in Animal Models

Neoplasias of endocrine and reproductive organs seldom occur in wildlife and laboratory animals subjected to a restricted diet. Long-term studies in laboratory animals revealed that mammary tumors occur spontaneously in some laboratory rat and mouse strains. For example, Sprague-Dawley and ACI aging virgin females develop mammary tumors spontaneously. Ovariectomy and multiple pregnancies during early adulthood significantly decreased the incidence of these tumors. Endometrial tumors also develop in Han:Wistar, BDII/Han, and Donryu strains.[119] Ovariectomy inhibits the development of these neoplasias.[120] Spontaneous prolactinomas develop in certain rat (Sprague-Dawley) and mouse strains (C57BL/6).[121] Adenoma and adenocarcinoma of the magnum of the oviduct and leiomyoma of the ventral ligament of the oviduct are the most frequent spontaneous neoplasias in the reproductive tract of hens,[122] which correlate with high plasma estrogen levels.[123]

5.6.2 Experimental Neoplasia as a Result of Hormonal Manipulation in Animal Models

Studies of hormonal carcinogenesis started as a result of experiments to study the role of endocrine organs by means of organ ablation-hormone replacement experiments.[39] Ovarian hormones were found to play a role in tumor development of the mammary gland. Pituitary tumors could be obtained by estrogen treatment (rat) and were also induced by thyroidectomy in mice. Thyroid tumors in mice were induced by goitrogens, through an increase in TSH plasma levels. Ovarian tumors were induced by transplanting the ovary into the spleen in ovariectomized rats and mice (presumably gonadotropin-induced). Gonadectomy induced adrenocortical tumors in guinea pigs, rats, mice and hamsters.

5.6.3 Ovarian Hormones and Neoplasia

The search for a role for ovarian hormones in breast neoplasia can be traced to the end of the nineteenth century, when Beatson reported that ovariectomy resulted in clinical regression of advanced breast cancer.[124] This result may be interpreted today as evidence for the trophic role of estrogens in tumor growth and cell survival; ovariectomy drastically reduced the incidence of breast cancer. Endometrial cancer in humans is also related to estrogen exposure. Vaginal clear cell carcinoma in young women appears as a consequence of *in utero* exposure to DES. Understandably, experimentation in humans is restricted by ethical concerns. On the other hand, animal models provide valuable insights, although not always are they directly applicable to humans. Estrogens were found to induce pituitary neoplasia (rat, mouse, European hamster), mammary cancer (rat and mouse), and kidney tumors in male Syrian and European hamsters. These kidney tumors are estrogen-sensitive. Although they do not seem to have an equivalent in human pathology, they are currently used to explore the role of estrogens as mutagens.

5.6.3.1 *Endometrial Tumors*

Endometrial tumors occur at a relatively high incidence in certain strains of rats. DES exposure throughout adult life results in a 1.7% incidence of uterine adenocarcinoma in mice, while neonatal (day 1-5) administration results in 90% incidence. Tumors did not develop in animals ovariectomized before puberty.[107] These tumors required estrogens for continuous growth when transplanted. Adenocarcinomas of the uterus may also be developed by administration of the carcinogen n-nitroso-n-methylurea (NMU) to intact adult mice;[125] progestagens inhibited the development of tumors in estrogen-treated animals.[126]

In humans, endometrial adenocarcinoma rates increased in women taking estrogen-replacement therapy.[127] Simultaneous administration of estrogens and progestagens (hormone-replacement therapy) results in a much lower incidence of this type of cancer (almost similar to those of untreated women).[128,129] Recently, it has been suggested that the xenoestrogen hypothesis should be tested by focusing on endometrial rather than breast cancer.[130] This is predicated by the rapid increase in the incidence of endometrial cancer in postmenopausal women treated with unopposed estrogens and the low incidence of this malignancy when compared with that of breast cancer. However, it is likely that xenoestrogen exposure would not increase the risk of endometrial cancer in mature, cycling women since their ovaries produce progesterone. Regarding postmenopausal women, many are taking hormone-replacement therapy to avoid osteoporosis and heart disease. Only those post-menopausal women not taking progesterone may be at risk of developing endometrial tumors.

5.6.3.2 *Mammary Gland Tumors*

In 1928, Murray demonstrated that mammary cancer could be induced to appear in male mice of a strain in which almost 100% of the females developed mammary cancer when ovaries were transplanted into males.[131] Lacassagne reproduced these results by treating male mice with ovarian extracts ("folliculin").[132] While it is possible to obtain a high tumor yield by prolonged treatment of susceptible rats with estrogens, this only happens in mice infected with mouse mammary tumor viruses.

Mammary tumors can be induced in the Sprague-Dawley and other rat strains by prolonged treatment with estrogens. Estrogens shorten the latency period and increase the incidence of tumors that otherwise would appear if those animals were observed for their entire life span. For example, the spontaneous incidence of mammary adenocarcinomas in female ACI rats was reported to be 7%, whereas treatment with 5-mg pellets of DES at 80 d of age increased the incidence to 52% after 200 d of observation.[133] Regardless of whether or not the resulting neoplasia behaves as a hormone-sensitive tumor, it develops only in intact, nonovariectomized animals.[134]

Experimental estrogen-induced mammary tumors required prolonged treatment with hormones; the latency periods were extremely long, and the incidence was usually low. The discovery that chemical carcinogens such as methylcholanthrene and 7,12-DMBA induced mammary carcinomas in some rat strains greatly facilitated the study of these tumors, since the latency period was shortened and the percent incidence was higher than that of estrogen-induced tumors. Interestingly, the tumors obtained with DMBA or nitroso-methylurea (NMU) were histologically similar to human breast tumors. Several factors play a role in the induction of mammary carcinomas by these agents: genetic background, estrogen exposure, pituitary hormone exposure, and age.[135]

Tumors only develop in certain strains. Over 80% of these carcinogen-treated rats present tumors after 90 d of observation when they belong to the Fisher, Wistar/Furth, Sprague/Dawley, and other inbred and outbred strains; this incidence is significantly lowered or nonexistent when other strains, like Copenhagen, are used.

In nulliparous Sprague/Dawley rats, mammary cancer develops spontaneously. Similarly, estrogens are necessary for the development of DMBA- and NMU-induced mammary cancer in rats. Ovariectomy prior to carcinogen treatment inhibits tumor formation; estrogen treatment of ovariectomized animals results in comparable tumor incidence rates and latency periods as those observed in intact animals. Paradoxically, high doses of estrogen increase the latency period, decrease the size of tumors, and result in a lower tumor yield per animal.[77] Hence, estrogens also have a biphasic effect on the induction of mammary carcinoma.

Hypophysectomy prevents the development of DMBA-induced tumors. Prolactin appears to stimulate the growth of DMBA-induced mammary carcinomas in ovariectomized, adrenalectomized, and hypophysectomized rats.[136] However, estrogens seem to be essential for the prolonged growth of these tumors.[137,138] This contradicts the hypothesis that estrogens act by inducing the secretion of prolactin.

In DMBA-induced mammary cancer in rats, a "window of vulnerability" was identified between the 45th and 55th day of life;[139] carcinogen administration during this period significantly increases the incidence of carcinomas and decreases the latency period. Multiparity further decreases the incidence of carcinomas. These effects are explained by the intense proliferative activity of structures called terminal end buds, from which new gland ducts are originated during this "window of vulnerability" period.[135] Further development of the gland produces structures that become "carcinogen-resistant."[139]

In humans, only a small percentage (5–10%) of breast cancer is attributed to genetic inheritance; otherwise, risk factors are mostly related to cumulative lifetime exposure to endogenous ovarian hormones,[140] from early menarche and late menopause. Pregnancy also plays a role; nulliparous women have a higher risk than those that undergo full-term pregnancies in their early twenties; first pregnancy in the late 30s and 40s increases the risk of breast cancer.[140] There is also some evidence that the level of estrogen exposure during development *in utero* may influence the risk of breast cancer.[141] Exposure to radiation during adolescence and early adulthood is also a risk factor. Epidemiological studies have, for the most part, examined exposure to estrogens from the viewpoint that they act as promoters. For example, a study by Toniolo et al. showed a significant correlation between free (unbound to sex steroid binding globulin) estrogen levels in postmenopausal women and their incidence of breast cancer a few years later.[142]

5.6.3.3   Pituitary Tumors

Chronic estrogen treatment in Fischer, ACI, or Wistar-Furth rats results in the development of pituitary adenomas and transplantable neoplasms that grow as estrogen-sensitive tumors. The proliferative response to estrogens ceased after a few days, in spite of the continuous presence of estrogens in strains that did not develop adenomas (proliferative shutoff).[72,143] Rat strains in which the proliferative response was maintained as long as estrogens were administered developed neoplasms. Hence, tumors developed in animals that lost the ability to express the estrogen-induced proliferative shutoff.

5.6.3.4   Testicular Neoplasias

There are no animal models that closely parallel the human disease. Hence, we will discuss current thoughts about the genesis of this disease in humans. Germ cell tumors develop from carcinoma *in situ*.[144] The age-specific pattern of tumor incidence in males shows a small peak from birth to 4 years of age, and a second increase after puberty reaches another peak between 20–30 years of age for malignant teratoma and 30-40 years for seminoma.[145] While incidence has increased recently in young men, there is no clear evidence of an increase in boys.[146] Although histological examination of testicular parenchyma adjacent to tumors in adult men revealed the presence of carcinoma *in situ*, this association was not found in tissue from boys;[147] this suggests separate etiologies. The age distribution for incidence of testicular cancer suggests that exposure to risk factors occurs early in life, and progression from carcinoma *in situ* to clinical cancer is influenced by androgens and/or pituitary hormones. The risk of testicular cancer is increased in men with a history of testicular maldescent, gonadal dysgenesis, androgen insensitivity, intersex states, and infertility. Maldescent is associated with a five- to ten-fold relative risk increase. When undescent is unilateral, testicular cancer may arise in the contralateral testicle, or in both.[148] In addition, orchidopexy may not prevent testicular cancer.[149] This suggests that an inherent germinal defect present in germinal epithelium may be responsible for the two pathologies.[150] Testicular dysgenesis is an etiologic factor in cryptorchidism.[151] Also, dysgeneic tissue is frequently found in undescended testis.[152] In addition, approximately 20% of the cases of testicular cancer have a history of maldescent. A two-fold increase in incidence of undescended testis has been reported from 1950 to 1970;[153] similar increases in hypospadias have been reported.[154-156] The hypothesis that high estrogen exposure *in utero* may be a risk factor for testicular cancer is supported by the increased incidence of this pathology in dizygotic twins (a condition that results in increased estrogen exposure).[157]

Mouse strains where testicular cancer arises spontaneously have been described.[145] Mice exposed *in utero* to DES offer a model for testicular maldescent;[104] this pathology is correlated strongly with testicular cancer of germinal cell origin in humans. However, the testicular cancer associated with DES exposure in mice originates in the rete testis (nongerminal origin). For the most part, hormone-induced testicular cancers in laboratory rodents are Leydig cell adenomas; DES treatment induces these tumors in European hamsters.[158]

5.6.3.5 Prostate Cancer

The etiology of human prostate cancer is unknown. However, like other cancers of the genital tract, its incidence is practically nonexistent in men who were castrated before 40 years of age.[159] In addition, most cases of clinical prostate cancer regress after castration. Several models for prostate cancer have been developed in animal systems. Most pathologists believe that rat ventral prostate tumors are not representative of the human disease, while those of the dorsolateral prostate are good models for human carcinoma.[160]

5.6.3.5.1 *Spontaneous Cancer*

Cribriform carcinoma of the ventral prostate develops frequently in the aging ACI rat[160] and the AXC rat.[161] Adenocarcinoma of the dorsolateral prostate develops in the Lobund-Wistar rat.[160] One interesting feature of the ACI tumors is that their incidence rate increases in animals exposed to a high-fat diet.[162] This is consistent with correlations derived from human studies.

5.6.3.5.2 *Hormone-Induced Cancer*

Prostate cancer may be induced in rats by treatment with chemical carcinogens, androgens, carcinogens plus androgens, and androgens plus estrogens. Treatment with chemical carcinogens in otherwise normal males resulted in ventral prostate tumors in the F344 and MRC rat.[160] Lobund-Wistar rats developed spontaneous prostate cancer. Prolonged treatment with testosterone increased the tumor yield, and the latency period decreased.[163] Interestingly, increasing the fat content in the diet resulted in further shortening of the latency period. Combinations of chemical carcinogens and testosterone in various protocols increased the tumor incidence over that obtained with carcinogen alone. Moreover, carcinomas also appeared in the seminal vesicles and coagulating glands. However, the most striking results are those obtained with a combination of estradiol or ethynyl-estradiol and testosterone. Noble originally found that estradiol plus testosterone was more effective than testosterone alone.[164] These hormones induce epithelial dysplasia and, subsequently, adenocarcinoma in the dorsolateral prostate of NBL rats[164] and F344 rats treated with the carcinogen 3,2'-dimethyl-4 aminobiphenyl (DMAB).[165] An interesting feature of the DMAB model is that testosterone alone, as well as testosterone plus ethynyl-estradiol, significantly decreases the incidence of ventral prostate carcinoma below that obtained with DMAB alone, while increasing carcinoma incidence of the lateral, dorsal, and anterior prostates. Testosterone and estrogen levels increased two- to three-fold during this treatment. The role of estrogens in this process is unknown. However, several studies found a cooperative effect of estrogens given together with androgens in normal prostate growth.[166,167] Others have suggested that the role of estrogens is to produce DNA damage.[91] Most interestingly, 5α-dihydrotestosterone, which is not metabolized into estrogens, failed to induce prostate cancer in Lobund-Wistar rats[168] and in the DMAB model.[165]

5.7 Endocrine Disruptors and Neoplasia in Animal Models

5.7.1 DDT and Estrogen-Sensitive Tumor Growth

Estrogen-sensitive mammary MT2 cells grow as a tumor when inoculated into ovariectomized syngeneic hosts treated with estradiol. The full estrogen agonist o,p'DDT sustained tumor growth at the same rate achieved with estradiol pellets. The congener p,p'DDD, which is a partial agonist less potent than p,p'DDT, did not increase the tumor size over that found in ovariectomized controls.[169]

5.7.2 Neoplasias in Animals Treated with Estrogenic Pesticides

As reviewed above, natural estrogens induce neoplasias in reproductive and endocrine organs. There is no consensus regarding whether they do so through nonhormonal mechanisms (as mutagens) or through their hormonal activity (promotional, developmental, and tissue organization effects). In addition, carcinogens devoid of hormonal activity, such as NMU, induce mammary neoplasias that behave as estrogen-sensitive tumors. Carcinogenicity studies done by long-term exposure to maximal tolerable doses of a chemical are unsuitable to address the question of whether or not their carcinogenicity is mediated by their hormonal activity. The results of the few studies reported in the literature are summarized below. It should be noticed that, for the most part, interpretation of these long-term studies is obfuscated by high mortality due to general toxicity, sample loss, or insufficient sampling.[170,171]

Mammary Gland Neoplasias — Methoxychlor treatment resulted in a doubling of the mammary tumor incidence in Osborne-Mendel female rats.[170] In this strain endosulfan induced fibroadenomas and carcinomas.[171]

Neoplasias of the Female Genital Tract — Endosulfan increased the incidence of benign endometrial polyps, stromal cell sarcoma, and endometrial adenocarcinoma.[171]

Pituitary Neoplasias — Methoxychlor increased the percentage of pituitary adenomas and carcinomas in Osborne-Mendel female rats.[170] Lindane increased the incidence of adenomas and carcinomas both in female and male Osborne-Mendel rats.[172]

Ovary Neoplasias — DDT, methoxychlor, and lindane induced carcinomas in Osborne-Mendel rats; these tumors were not seen in the vehicle-treated controls.[170,172-174]

Testicular Neoplasias — Methoxychlor induced interstitial cell carcinomas in Balb/c mice; these tumors were also induced by estrogens in the Balb/c strain.[170]

Adrenal Gland Neoplasias — Methoxychlor doubled the incidence of adenomas and carcinomas in female Osborne-Mendel rats.[170] Lindane also increased the number of these tumors in females and males.[172]

Thyroid Neoplasias — Lindane exposure resulted in an increased incidence of adenomas and adenocarcinomas in both male and female Osborne-Mendel rats.[172]

5.8 Pesticides and Breast Cancer

Among the estrogenic xenobiotics, PCBs and DDT were considered suitable markers of exposure for breast cancer because they were released massively into the environment beginning approximately 50 years ago, and they are persistent; their presence in serum may represent cumulative exposure during a lifetime. Early studies that showed no correlation between breast cancer incidence and xenoestrogen levels were comprised of a small number of cases and controls that were not matched for other risk factors. However, three recent studies do show a correlation between the occurrence of breast cancer and the levels of xenoestrogens. Wolff et al. found that serum DDE levels correlated with breast cancer incidence in a study of 58 breast cancer patients and 171 controls that were well matched for risk factors and age.[17] Another study documented that estrogen-receptor positive breast cancer correlated with higher concentrations of DDE in their tissues.[175] Krieger et al. studied 150 women with breast cancer and 150 controls; each set comprised 50 African-American, 50 Caucasian, and 50 Asian-American women. When the data from all ethnic groups were pooled, no significant correlation was observed between plasma levels of DDE and breast cancer.[176] However, when the cases and matching controls were evaluated separately, according to their ethnic group, high serum DDE levels were correlated to breast cancer incidence in Caucasian and African-American women, but that there was no significant correlation in Asian-American women. Evidence of a link between exposure to PCBs and breast cancer incidence is equivocal.[177] However, these studies correlated exposure to total PCBs, rather than to the levels of specific congeners. In order to clarify the relevance of these findings, epidemiological studies are being conducted involving larger sample sizes. However, testing only for the presence of DDT metabolites and total PCBs will not clarify whether or not xenoestrogens play a role in breast cancer incidence, because (1) not all the PCB congeners are estrogenic and (2) many other environmental estrogens may also play a role. The newly identified estrogens may be less persistent than PCBs and DDT metabolites. However, these new xenoestrogens are widely used. Hence, it may be inferred that exposure occurs steadily due to their presence in foods.[19] Methods to measure the new xenoestrogens in blood plasma are yet to be developed. Nevertheless, the crux of the problem is whether or not the combined exposure to xenoestrogens correlates with breast cancer incidence. Methodology developed to measure the total xenoestrogen burden[14,178] is being used to assess this hypothesis.[179]

5.9   Discussion and Conclusions

The development of neoplasias has been a topic of intense research during the current century. However, little is known about mechanisms underlying this phenomenon. For the most part, in the last four decades, research has focused on the somatic mutation theory, probably due primarily to the technological advances that allow for the study of DNA. In spite of this extensive effort, the somatic mutation theory has not provided a clear understanding of carcinogenesis.

As pointed out at the beginning of this review, most of the data on carcinogenesis have been collected under the premise that the default state of cells in metazoa is quiescence. Instead, we have argued that the default state of all living cells is proliferation.[180] In the context of carcinogenesis, in the first instance, putative carcinogens would play the role of direct or indirect stimulators of cell proliferation. In the alternative paradigm, carcinogens become disruptors of inhibitory processes, by affecting genetic or epigenetic pathways of homeostasis. Their ultimate effects allow cells to ignore inhibitory signals and exercise their built-in capacity to proliferate. The adoption of proliferation as the default state and, consequently, the search for genuine negative signals, may be more productive in harnessing the constitutive ability of cells to proliferate than strategies used so far to learn how cells proliferate and what the role of elusive stimulators of cell proliferation may be.

In contrast to the somatic mutation hypothesis, the epigenetic causation hypothesis has not generated a comparable research program because it has not singled out mechanisms that may result in neoplasia. In addition, epigenetic phenomena may act at several hierarchical levels, which means that they cannot be explored easily using the tools of linear thought and molecular biology, which are the traditional equipment of the genetic hypothesis.

This may soon change, since the theoretical grounds have been articulated (the tissulon theory), and recent advances in developmental biology make it possible now to explore the interactions between tissues and cells that operate in morphogenesis and tissue maintenance.

Endogenous sex steroids are a major causal agent in the development of neoplasias in their target organs; gonadectomy prevents this neoplastic development. The genetic background of animals plays a permissive role in the induction of neoplasms by sex steroids; however, the underlying mechanisms of resistance and susceptibility presently are unknown.

Experimental carcinogenesis studies in animal models and observational studies in humans have produced data consistent with the notion that sex steroids are causal agents because they control the development of their target organs and the proliferation of their target cells. In addition, estrogens induce the formation of DNA adducts, which may result in DNA mutations.

Models for hormone-induced carcinogenesis were developed to obtain high tumor yields with short latency periods. This was done by administering supraphysiological levels of hormones alone or in combination with chemical carcinogens. This contrasts with the normal plasma levels of hormones implicated in carcinogenesis found in susceptible strains that developed hormone-target tumors. The easiest action to take is to blame the genome of these susceptible strains, which indeed plays a role. However, these genetic factors are not a sufficient cause. Estrogens are still required for the development of a neoplasia.

The apparently normal levels of hormones represent a static measure of a time point, which falls within normal ranges. For females, "normal ranges" comprise the wide fluctuations of the estrual and menstrual cycles. Minute increases in estrogen concentration at the beginning of the cycle, when the estrogen level is at its minimum, may be sufficient to produce an effect that does not occur at lower doses. In contrast, an increase in the concentration of estrogens at the point of the cycle where they naturally peak may not produce further effects. In addition, hormones are released in pulses, and this pulsatile pattern of hormone secretion has been shown to be important in determining qualitative aspects of the response. These considerations point to areas of research that have not been explored in relation to carcinogenesis.

The incidence of hormone-induced tumors may be enhanced in animals fed high-fat diets without apparent changes in the plasma levels of hormones. Epidemiological studies also suggest that diet plays an important role in the development of these neoplasias in humans.

It has been observed that extemporaneous administration of sex hormones during development leads to permanent lesions in the genital tract. In turn, this teratogenic effect results in tissues predisposed to neoplasia. Remarkably, developmental effects occur at doses lower than those needed to trigger responses in adult animals. On the other hand, neoplasias of the genital tract in animals exposed *in utero* or neonatally to DES occurred at pharmacological doses. However, recent experiments indicate that females exposed to DES *in utero* transmit a neoplastic phenotype to blastocysts from normal animals.

These data indicate that alterations of the maternal environment may lead to neoplasia.

Whether or not environmental hormonally active agents have a causal role in the development of malignancies of estrogen- and androgen-target organs has not been explored exhaustively. Consequently, it is premature to draw definitive conclusions regarding their contribution to the increase of breast, testicular, and prostate cancer incidence. The plausibility of this hypothesis is based on evidence that exposure to natural estrogens is a main risk factor for endometrial and breast cancers, exposure to androgens is a risk factor for prostate cancer, and estrogenic pesticides induce endocrine and reproductive tumors in some rodent strains. As explained above, our understanding of mechanisms of carcinogenesis in general, and of the role of hormones in this process, is still rudimentary.

The main criticism raised against the xenoestrogen hypothesis is that these chemicals are, in general, less potent than natural estrogens, and that current exposure levels supposedly are insignificant when compared to the levels of endogenous hormones. This criticism is based on a slanted reading of biological phenomena. The few epidemiological studies addressing this problem dealt mostly with exposure to DDT metabolites and organochlorines that are not estrogenic. DDT is just one of the many xenoestrogens to which humans are exposed; evidence of exposure to newly identified xenoestrogens has yet to be gathered. The relatively low potency of xenoestrogens, when compared to ovarian estrogens, is magnified in binding assays and studies done in tissue culture, because these studies do not address metabolic rates and bioavailability. These assays may underestimate the potency of xenoestrogens in whole organisms. A second criticism is based on the assumption of linearity in dose-responses for these chemicals. In this regard, there is evidence that the dose-response to estrogens is not linear but biphasic; it induces cell proliferation at low doses and inhibits it at high doses. From this perspective, the pattern of exposure may be relevant, since estrogen levels are low in the early follicular phase of the menstrual cycle. Steady exposure to xenoestrogens may result in significant increases of the estrogen levels early in the menstrual cycle and, consequently, result in the early onset of proliferative activity in the breast. In contrast, xenoestrogen levels may not affect cell proliferation in the luteal phase, since the endogenous levels of estrogens are already triggering a full proliferative response. Additionally, developmental effects seem to occur at lower doses than those effective in adult animals. The scant dose-response data on developmental effects show an inverted U shape. Moreover, xenoestrogens act cumulatively, and until data on exposure to all known xenoestrogens becomes available, the possibility that their cumulative level is relevant in carcinogenesis cannot be ruled out. The relevance of cumulative effects is heightened by recent evidence indicating that xenoestrogens may act synergistically.[14,15]

Finally, given the many uncertainties about basic mechanisms in the control of cell proliferation and carcinogenesis, the shape of the dose-response curve, levels of xenoestrogen exposure, and timing of exposure, what should be done from the perspective of public and environmental health? Exploring these basic questions will take years, even decades of intense research. Should we wait for the basic science to be done, or should we adopt a preventive approach, diminishing exposures to endocrine disruptors now? The answer is that the enactment of an aggressive preventive approach is not incompatible with a meticulous reappraisal of the implicit premises in this field.

Acknowledgments

This work was partially supported by grants from the NIH-ES08314, NIH-AG13807, NIH-CA13410, and NSF-DCB-9105594. The assistance of The Center for Reproductive Research at Tufts University (P30 HD 28897) is gratefully acknowledged.

References

1. Sharpe, R. M. and Skakkebaek, N. E., Are oestrogens involved in falling sperm count and disorders of the male reproductive tract? *Lancet*, 341, 1392, 1993.
2. Davis, D., Medical hypothesis: xenoestrogens as preventable causes of breast cancer, *Environ. Health Perspect.*, 101, 372, 1993.
3. Hammond, B., Katzenellenbogen, B. S., Kranthammer, N., and McConnell, J., Estrogenic activity of the insecticide chlordecone (kepone) and interaction with uterine estrogen receptors, *Proc. Natl. Acad. Sci. U.S.A.*, 76, 6641, 1979.
4. Meyers, C. Y., Matthews, W. S., Ho, L. L., Kolb, V. M., and Parady, T. E., Carboxylic acid formation from kepone, in *Catalysis in Organic Synthesis*, Smith, G. W., Ed., Academic Press, New York, 1977, 213.
5. Soto, A. M., Michaelson, C. L., Prechtl, N. V., Weill, B. C., Sonnenschein, C., Olea-Serrano, F., and Olea, N., Assay to measure estrogen and androgen agonists and antagonists, in *In Vitro Germ Cell Developmental Toxicology: From Science to Social and Industrial Demand*, del Mazo, J., Ed., Plenum Press, New York, 1998, in press.
6. Hertz, R., The estrogen problem — retrospect and prospect, in *Estrogens in the Environment II — Influences on Development*, McLachlan, J. A., Ed., Elsevier, New York, 1985, 1.
7. Soto, A. M., Justicia, H., Wray, J. W., and Sonnenschein, C., p-Nonyl-phenol: an estrogenic xenobiotic released from "modified" polystyrene, *Environ. Health Perspect.*, 92, 167, 1991.
8. Soto, A. M., Lin, T-M., Justicia, H., Silvia, R. M., and Sonnenschein, C., An "in culture" bioassay to assess the estrogenicity of xenobiotics, in *Chemically-Induced Alterations in Sexual Development: the Wildlife/Human Connection*, Colborn, T. and Clement, C., Eds., Princeton Scientific Publishing, Princeton, NJ, 1992, 295.

9. Routledge, E. J. and Sumpter, J. P., Structural features of alkylphenolic chemicals associated with estrogenic activity, *J. Biol. Chem.*, 272, 3280, 1997.
10. Collins, B. M., McLachlan, J. A., and Arnold, S. F., The estrogenic and antiestrogenic activities of phytochemicals with the human estrogen receptor expressed in yeast, *Steroids*, 62, 365, 1997.
11. Fox, G. A., Epidemiological and pathobiological evidence of contaminant-induced alterations in sexual development in free-living wildlife, in *Chemically-Induced Alterations in Sexual and Functional Development: the Wildlife/Human Connection*, Colborn, T. and Clement, C., Eds., Princeton Scientific Publishing, Princeton, NJ, 1992, 147.
12. Thomas, K. B. and Colborn, T., Organochlorine endocrine dispruptors in human tissue, in *Chemically-Induced Alterations in Sexual Development: The Wildlife/Human Connection*, Colborn, T. and Clement, C., Eds., Princeton Scientific Publishing, Princeton, NJ, 1992, 365.
13. Soto, A. M., Chung, K. L., and Sonnenschein, C., The pesticides endosulfan, toxaphene, and dieldrin have estrogenic effects on human estrogen sensitive cells, *Environ. Health Perspect.*, 102, 380, 1994.
14. Soto, A. M., Fernandez, M. F., Luizzi, M. F., Oles Karasko, A. S., and Sonnenschein, C., Developing a marker of exposure to xenoestrogen mixtures in human serum, *Environ. Health Perspect.*, 105, 647, 1997.
15. Arnold, S. F., Bergeron, J. M., Tran, D. Q., Collins, B. M., Vonier, P. M., Crews, D., Jr., and McLachlan, J. A., Synergistic responses of steroidal estrogens *in vitro* (yeast) and *in vivo* (turtles), *Biochem. Biophys. Res. Commun.*, 235, 336, 1997.
16. Giwercman, A., Carlsen, E., Keiding, N., and Skakkebaek, N. E., Evidence for increasing incidence of abnormalities of the human testis: a review, *Environ. Health Perspect.*, 101, 65, 1993.
17. Wolff, M. S., Toniolo, P. G., Lee, E. W., Rivera, M., and Dubin, N., Blood levels of organochlorine residues and risk of breast cancer, *J. Natl. Canc. Inst.*, 85, 648, 1993.
18. Soto, A. M. and Sonnenschein, C., Environmental sex hormone agonists and antagonists, *Comments Toxicol.*, 5, 329, 1996.
19. Soto, A. M., Sonnenschein, C., Chung, K. L., Fernandez, M. F., Olea, N., and Olea-Serrano, M. F., The E-SCREEN assay as a tool to identify estrogens: an update on estrogenic environmental pollutants, *Environ. Health Perspect.*, 103, 113, 1995.
20. White, R., Jobling, S., Hoare, S. A., Sumpter, J. P., and Parker, M. G., Environmentally persistent alkylphenolic compounds, *Endocrinology*, 135, 175, 1994.
21. vom Saal, F. S., Timms, B. G., Montano, M. M., Palanza, P., Thayer, K. A., Nagel, S. C., Ganjam, V. K., Parmigiani, S., and Welshons, W. V., Prostate enlargement in mice due to fetal exposure to low doses of estradiol or diethylstilbestrol and opposite effects at high doses, *Proc. Natl. Acad. Sci. U.S.A.*, 94, 2056, 1997.
22. Nagel, S. C., vom Saal, F. S., Thayer, K. A., Dhar, M. G., Boechler, M., and Welshons, W. V., Relative binding affinity-serum modified access (RBA-SMA) assay predicts the relative *in vivo* bioactivity of the xenoestrogens bisphenol A and octylphenol, *Environ. Health Perspect.*, 105, 70, 1997.
23. Steinmetz, R., Brown, N. G., Allen, D. L., Bigsby, R. M., and Ben-Jonathan, N., The environmental estrogen bisphenol A stimulates prolactin release *in vitro* and *in vivo*, *Endocrinology*, 138, 1780, 1997.
24. Colerangle, J. B. and Roy, D., Profound effects of the weak environmental estrogen-like chemical bisphenol A on the growth of the mammary gland of Noble rats, *J. Steroid Biochem. Mol. Biol.*, 60, 153, 1997.

25. Peng, A. and Ackerman, A. B., Neoplasm? *Dermatopathology*, 4, 41, 1998.
26. Willis, R. A., *Pathology of Tumors*, Butterworths, London, 1967.
27. Clark, W. H., Tumour progression and the nature of cancer, *Br. J. Canc.*, 64, 631, 1991.
28. Turkel, S. B. and Itabashi, H. H., The natural history of neuroblastic cells in the fetal adrenal gland, *Am. J. Pathol.*, 76(2), 225, 1974.
29. Gateff, E. and Schneiderman, H. A., Neoplasms in mutant and cultured wild-type of Drosophila, *Natl. Canc. Inst. Monogr.*, 31, 365, 1969.
30. Mechler, B. M., Strand, D., Kalmes, A., Merz, R., Schmidt, M., and Torok, I., Drosophila as a model system for molecular analysis of tumorogenesis, *Environ. Health Perspect.*, 93, 63, 1991.
31. Varmus, H. E. and Weinberg, R. A. *Genes and the Biology of Cancer*, Scientific American Library, New York, 1992, 123.
32. Berenblum, I. and Shubik, P., A new quantative approach to the study of the stages of chemical carcinogenesis in the mouse's skin, *Br. J. Cancer*, 1346, 383, 1947.
33. Iversen, O. H., The reverse experiment in two-stage skin carcinogenesis, *AP-MIS*, 101, 1, 1993.
34. Rubin, H., Epigenetic nature of neoplastic transformation, in *Developmental Biology and Cancer*, Hodges, G. M. and Rowlatt, C., Eds., CRC Press, Boca Raton, FL, 1993, 61.
35. Varmus, H. E., The molecular genetics of cellular oncogenes, *Annu. Rev. Genet.*, 18, 553, 1984.
36. Bishop, J. M., Cellular oncogenes and retroviruses, *Annu. Rev. Biochem.*, 52, 301, 1983.
37. Mintz, B. and Ilmensee, K., Normal genetically mosaic mice produce from malignant teratocarcinoma cells, *Proc. Natl. Acad. Sci. U.S.A.*, 72, 3585, 1975.
38. McKinnel, R. G., Deggins, B. A., and Labbat, D. D., Transplantation of pluripotent nuclei from triploid frog tumors, *Science*, 165, 394, 1969.
39. Foulds, L., *Neoplastic Development*, Academic Press, New York, 1969.
40. Pierce, G. B. and Cox, W. F., Jr., Neoplasms as tissue caricatures of tissue renewal, in *Cell Differentiation and Neoplasia*, Saunders, G. F., Ed., Raven Press, New York, 1978, 57.
41. Soto, A. M. and Sonnenschein, C., Regulation of cell proliferation: is the ultimate control positive or negative? in *New Frontiers in Cancer Causation*, Iversen, O. H., Ed.,Taylor & Francis, Washington, D.C., 1993, 109.
42. Rubin, H., Cancer development: the rise of epigenetics, *Eur. J. Canc.*, 28, 1, 1992.
43. Martin, L., Estrogens, antiestrogens and the regulation of cell proliferation in the female reproductive tract *in vivo*, in *Estrogens in the Environment*, McLachlan, J. A., Ed., Elsevier/North-Holland, New York, 1980, 103.
44. Stormshak, F., Leake, R., Wertz, N., and Gorski, J., Stimulatory and inhibitory effects of estrogen on uterine DNA synthesis, *Endocrinology*, 99, 1501, 1976.
45. Mukku, V. R., Kirkland, J. L., Hardy, M., and Stancel, G. M., Hormonal control of uterine growth: temporal relationships between estrogen administration and deoxyribonucleic acid synthesis, *Endocrinology*, 111, 480, 1982.
46. Stack, G. and Gorski, J., Direct mitogenic effect of estrogen on the prepubetal rat uterus: studies on isolated nuclei, *Endocrinology*, 115, 1141, 1984.
47. Cooke, P. S., Uchima, F. D. A., Fujii, D. K., Bern, H. A., and Cunha, G. R., Restoration of normal morphology & estrogen responsiveness in cultured vaginal & uterine epithelia transplanted with stroma, *Proc. Natl. Acad. Sci. U.S.A.*, 83, 2109, 1986.

48. Dickson, R., McManaway, M. E., and Lippman, M. E., Estrogen-induced factors of breast cancer cells partially replace estrogen to promote tumor growth, *Science*, 232, 1540, 1986.

49. Soto, A. M. and Sonnenschein, C., The role of estrogens on the proliferation of human breast tumor cells (MCF-7), *J. Steroid Biochem.*, 23, 87, 1985.

50. Soto, A. M., Silvia, R. M., and Sonnenschein, C., A plasma-borne specific inhibitor of the proliferation of human estrogen-sensitive breast tumor cells (estrocolyone-I), *J. Steroid Biochem. Mol. Biol.*, 43, 703, 1992.

51. Sonnenschein, C., Soto, A. M., and Michaelson, C. L., Human serum albumin shares the properties of estrocolyone-I, the inhibitor of the proliferation of estrogen-target cells, *J. Steroid Biochem. Mol. Biol.*, 59, 147, 1996.

52. Chiappetta, C., Kirkland, J. L., Loose-Mitchell, D. S., Murthy, L., and Stancel, G. M., Estrogen regulates expression of the jun family of protooncogenes in the uterus, *J. Steroid Biochem. Mol. Biol.*, 41, 113, 1992.

53. Huet-Hudson, Y. M., Chakraborty, C., De, S. K., Suzuki, Y., Andrews, G. K., and Dey, S. K., Estrogen regulates the synthesis of epidermal growth factor in mouse uterine epithelial cells, *Mol. Endocrinol.*, 4, 510, 1990.

54. Stancel, G. M., Chiappetta, C., Gardner, R. M., Kirkland, J. L., Lin, T. H., Lingham, R. B., Loose-Mitchell, D. S., Mukku, V. R., and Orengo, C. A., Regulation of the uterine epidermal growth factor receptor by estrogen, *Prog. Clin. Biol. Res.*, 322, 213, 1990.

55. Nelson, K. G., Takahashi, T., Bossert, N. L., Walmer, D. K., and McLachlan, J. A., Epidermal growth factor replaces estrogen in the stimulation of female genital-tract growth and differentiation, *Proc. Natl. Acad. Sci. U.S.A.*, 88, 21, 1991.

56. Curtis, S. W., Washburn, T., Sewall, C., Diaugustine, R., Lindzey, J., Couse, J. F., and Korach, K. S., Physiological coupling of growth factor and steroid receptor signaling pathways: estrogen receptor knockout mice lack estrogen-like response to epidermal growth factor, *Proc. Natl. Acad. Sci. U.S.A.*, 93, 12626, 1996.

57. Uchima, F. D. A., Edery, M., Iguchi, T., Larson, L., and Bern, H. A., Growth of mouse vaginal epithelial cells in culture: functional integrity of the estrogen receptor system and failure of estrogen to induce proliferation, *Canc. Lett.*, 35, 227, 1987.

58. Uchima, F. D. A., Edery, M., Iguchi, T., and Bern, H. A., Growth of mouse endometrial luminal epithelia cells *in vitro*: functional integrity of the oestrogen receptor system & failure of oestrogen to induce proliferation, *J. Endocrinol.*, 128, 115, 1991.

59. Fukamachi, H. and McLachlan, J. A., Proliferation and differentiation of mouse uterine epithelial cells in primary serum-free culture: estradiol-17B suppresses uterine epithelial proliferation cultured on a basement membrane-like substratum, *In Vitro Cell Dev. Biol.*, 27A, 907, 1991.

60. Julian, J., Carson, D. D., and Glasser, S. R., Polarized rat uterine epithelium *in vitro*: constitutive expression of estrogen "induced" proteins, *Endocrinology*, 130, 79, 1992.

61. Yang, J., Richards, J., Guzman, R., Imagawa, W., and Nandi, S., Sustained growth in primary culture of normal mammary epithelial cells embedded in collagen gels, *Proc. Natl. Acad. Sci. U.S.A.*, 77(4), 2088, 1980.

62. Tsai, P. S. and Bern, H. A., Estrogen-independent growth of mouse vaginal epithelium in organ culture, *J. Exp. Zool.*, 259(2), 238, 1991.

63. Darbre, P. D., Curtis, S., and King, R. J., Effects of estradiol and tamoxifen on human breast cancer cells in serum-free culture, *Canc. Res.*, 44, 2790, 1984.

64. Butler, W., Kirkland, W. L., Gargala, T., Goran, N., Kelsey, W. H., and Berlinski, P., Steroid stimulation of plasminogen activator production in a human breast cancer cell line (MCF-7), *Canc. Res.*, 43, 1637, 1983.

65. Soto, A. M. and Sonnenschein, C., Mechanism of estrogen action on cellular proliferation: evidence for indirect and negative control on cloned breast tumor cells, *Biochem. Biophys. Res. Comm.*, 122, 1097, 1984.

66. Lykkesfeldt, A. E. and Briand, P., Indirect mechanism of oestradiol stimulation of cell proliferation of human breast cancer cell lines, *Br. J. Canc.*, 53, 29, 1986.

67. van der Burg, B., Rutteman, G. R., Blankenstein, M. A., De Laat, S. W., and van Zoelen, E. J., Mitogenic stimulation of human breast cancer cells in a growth factor-defined medium: synergistic action of insulin and estrogen, *J. Cell Physiol.*, 134, 101, 1988.

68. van der Burg, B., De Groot, R. P., Isbrucker, L., Kruijer, W., and De Laat, S. W., Direct stimulation by estrogen of growth factor signal transduction pathways in human breast cancer cells, *J. Steroid Biochem. Mol. Biol.*, 43, 111, 1992.

69. Briand, P. and Lykkesfeldt, A. E., Long-term cultivation of a human breast cancer cell line, MCF7, in chemically defined medium, *Anticanc. Res.*, 6, 85, 1986.

70. Soule, H. D. and McGrath, C. M., Estrogen responsive proliferation of clonal human breast carcinoma cells in athymic mice, *Canc. Lett.*, 10, 177, 1980.

71. Jiang, S-Y. and Jordan, V. C., Growth regulation of estrogen-receptor negative breast cancer cells transfected with cDNAs for estrogen receptor, *J. Natl. Canc. Inst.*, 84, 580, 1992.

72. Wiklund, J., Rutledge, J., and Gorski, J., A genetic model for the inheritance of pituitary tumor susceptibility in F344 rats, *Endocrinology*, 109, 1708, 1981.

73. Mukku, V. R., Kirkland, J. L., Hardy, M., and Stancel, G. M., Stimulatory and inhibitory effects of estrogen and antiestrogen on uterine cell division, *Endocrinology*, 109, 1005, 1981.

74. Bruchovsky, N. and Lesser, B., Control of proliferative growth in androgen responsive organs and neoplasms, *Adv. Sex Horm. Res.*, 2, 1, 1976.

75. Wiklund, J. A. and Gorski, J., Genetic differences in estrogen-induced deoxyribonucleic acid synthesis in the rat pituitary: correlations with pituitary tumor susceptibility, *Endocrinology*, 111, 1140, 1982.

76. Ingle, J. N., Ahman, D. L., and Green, S. J., Randomized clinical trial of DES versus tamoxifen in post-menopausal women with advanced breast cancer, *N. Engl. J. Med.*, 304, 16, 1981.

77. Meites, J., The relation of estrogen and prolactin to mammary tumorigenesis in the rat, in *Estrogen Target Tissues and Neoplasia*, Dao, T. L., Ed., Univ. of Chicago Press, Chicago, 1972, 275.

78. Soto, A. M. and Sonnenschein, C., Cell proliferation of estrogen-sensitive cells: the case for negative control, *Endocrinol. Rev.*, 8, 44, 1987.

79. Sonnenschein, C., Szelei, J., Nye, T. L., and Soto, A. M., Control of cell proliferation of human breast MCF7 cells; serum and estrogen resistant variants, *Oncol. Res.*, 6, 373, 1994.

80. Amara, J. F. and Dannies, P. S., 17 beta-Estradiol has a biphasic effect on gh cell growth, *Endocrinology*, 112, 1141, 1983.

81. Sonnenschein, C., Olea, N., Pasanen, M. E., and Soto, A. M., Negative controls of cell proliferation: human prostate cancer cells and androgens, *Canc. Res.*, 49, 3474, 1989.

82. Soto, A. M., Lin, T. M., Sakabe, K., Olea, N., Damassa, D. A., and Sonnenschein, C., Variants of the human prostate LNCaP cell line as a tool to study discrete components of the androgen-mediated proliferative response, *Oncol. Res.*, 7, 545, 1995.

83. Orr, J. W., The mechanism of chemical carcinogensis, *Br. Med. Bull.*, 14, 99, 1958.

84. Liehr, J. G., Stancel, G. M., Chorich, L. P., Bousfield, G. R., and Ulubelen, A. A., Hormonal carcinogenesis; separation of estrogenicity from carcinogenicity, *Chem. Biol. Interact.*, 59, 173, 1986.

85. Bhat, H. K., Han, X., Gladek, A., and Liehr, J. G., Regulation of the formation of the major diethylstilbestrol-DNA adduct and some evidence of its structure, *Carcinogenesis*, 15, 2137, 1994.

86. Roy, D., Bernhardt, A., Strobel, H. W., and Liehr, J. G., Catalysis of the oxidation of steroid and stilbene estrogens to estrogen quinone metabolites by the beta-naphthoflavone-inducible cytochrome P450 IA family, *Arch. Biochem. Biophys.*, 296, 450, 1992.

87. Barrett, J. C., Wong, A., and McLachlan, J. A., Diethylstilbestrol induces neoplastic transformation of cells in culture without measurable somatic mutation at two loci, *Science*, 212, 1402, 1981.

88. Bradlow, H. L., Davis, D. L., Lin, G., Sepkovic, D., and Tiwari, R., Effects of pesticides on the ratio of 16 alpha/2-hydroxyestrone: a biologic marker of breast cancer risk, *Environ. Health Perspect.*, 103 (Suppl 7), 147, 1995.

89. Davis, D. L., Bradlow, H. L., Wolff, M., Woodruff, T., Hoel, D. G., and Anton-Culver, H., Medical hypothesis: xenoestrogens as preventable causes of breast cancer, *Environ. Health Perspect.*, 101, 372, 1993.

90. Noble, R. L., The development of prostatic adenocarcinoma in Nb rats following prolonged sex hormone administration, *Canc. Res.*, 37, 1929, 1977.

91. Han, X., Liehr, J. G., and Bosland, M. C., Induction of a DNA adduct detectable by 32P-postlabeling in the dorsolateral prostate of NBL/Cr rats treated with estradiol-17 beta and testosterone, *Carcinogenesis*, 16, 951, 1995.

92. Alberts, B., Bray, D., Lewis, J., Raff, M., Roberts, K., and Watson, J. D., *Molecular Biology of the Cell*, Garland Publishing Inc., New York, 1994.

93. Szelei, J., Jimenez, J., Soto, A. M., Luizzi, M. F., and Sonnenschein, C., Androgen-induced inhibition of proliferation in human breast cancer MCF7 cells transfected with androgen receptor, *Endocrinology*, 138, 1406, 1997.

94. Sonnenschein, C. and Soto, A. M., Cell proliferation in metazoans: negative control mechanisms, in *Regulatory Mechanisms in Breast Cancer*, Lippman, M. E. and Dickson, R. B., Eds., Kluwer, Boston, 1991, 171.

95. Meyer, J. S., Cell proliferation in normal human breast ducts, fibroadenomas, and other ductal hyperplasias measured by nuclear labeling with tritiated thymidine, *Hum. Pathol.*, 8, 67, 1977.

96. Brotons, J. A., Olea-Serrano, M. F., Villalobos, M., and Olea, N., Xenoestrogens released from lacquer coating in food cans, *Environ. Health Perspect.*, 103(6), 608, 1994.

97. Olea, N., Pulgar, R., Perez, P., Olea-Serrano, F., Rivas, A., Novillo-Fertrell, A., Pedraza, V., Soto, A. M., and Sonnenschein, C., Estrogenicity of resin-based composites and sealants used in dentistry, *Environ. Health Perspect.*, 104(3), 298, 1996.

98. Takasugi, N., Cytological basis for permanent vaginal changes on mice treated neonatally with steroid hormones, *Int. Rev. Cytol.*, 44, 193, 1976.

99. Ozawa, S., Iguchi, T., Sawada, K., Ohta, Y., Takasugi, N., and Bern, H. A., Postnatal vaginal nodules induced by prenatal diethylstilbestrol treatment correlate with later development of ovary-independent vaginal and uterine changes in mice, *Canc. Lett.*, 58, 167, 1991.

100. Bern, H. A. *Diethylstilbestrol Syndrome: Present Status of Animal and Human Studies in Hormonal Carcinogenesis*, Springer Verlag, New York, 1992.

101. Lubahn, D. B., Moyer, J. S., Golding, T. S., Couse, J. F., Korach, K. S., and Smithies, O., Alteration of reproductive function but not prenatal sexual development after insertional disruption of the mouse estrogen receptor gene, *Proc. Natl. Acad. Sci. U.S.A.*, 90, 11162, 1993.

102. Mittendorf, R., Teratogen update: carcinogenesis and teratogenesis associated with exposure to diethylstilbestrol (DES) *in utero, Teratology*, 51, 435, 1995.

103. Newbold, R. R. and McLachlan, J. A., Diethylstilbestrol associated defects in murine genital tract development, in *Estrogens in the Environment II: Influences on Development*, McLachlan, J. A., Ed., Elsevier Science Publ. Co., New York, 1985, 288.

104. Newbold, R., Cellular and molecular effects of developmental exposure to diethylstilbestrol: implications for other environmental estrogens, *Environ. Health Perspect.*, (Suppl. 7), 83, 1995.

105. Bern, H. A., The fragile fetus, in *Chemically-Induced Alterations in Sexual and Functional Development: The Wildlife/Human Connection*, Colburn, T. and Clement, C., Eds., Princeton Scientific Publishing, Princeton, NJ, 1992, 9.

106. Bern, H. A., Jones, L. A., and Mills, K. T., Use of the neonatal mouse in studying long-term effects of early exposure to hormones and other agents, *J. Toxicol. Environ. Health — Suppl.*, 1, 103, 1976.

107. Newbold, R. R., Bullock, B. C., and McLachlan, J. A., Uterine adenocarcinoma in mice following developmental treatment with estrogens: a model for hormonal carcinogenesis, *Canc. Res.*, 50, 7677, 1990.

108. Walker, B. E. and Kurth, L. A., Pituitary tumors in mice exposed prenatally to diethylstilbestrol, *Canc. Res.*, 53, 1546, 1993.

109. Walker, B. E., Tumors in female offspring of control and diethylstilbestrol-exposed mice fed high-fat diets, *J. Natl. Canc. Inst.*, 82, 50, 1990.

110. Baggs, R. B., Miller, R. K., and Odoroff, C. L., Carcinogenicity of diethylstilbestrol in the Wistar rat: effect of postnatal oral contraceptive steroids, *Canc. Res.*, 51, 3311, 1991.

111. Turusov, V. S., Trukhanova, L. S., Parfenov, Y. D., and Tomatis, L., Occurrence of tumours on the descendants of CBA male mice prenatally treated with diethylstilbestrol, *Int. J. Canc.*, 50, 131, 1992.

112. Walker, B. E. and Kurth, L. A., Multi-generational carcinogenesis from diethylstilbestrol investigated by blastocyst transfers in mice, *Int. J. Canc.*, 61, 249, 1995.

113. Burroughs, C. D., Bern, H. A., and Stokstad, E. L., Prolonged vaginal cornification and other changes in mice treated neonatally with coumestrol, a plant estrogen, *J. Toxicol. Environ. Health*, 15, 51, 1985.

114. Burroughs, C. D., Mills, K. T., and Bern, H. A., Long-term genital tract changes in female mice treated neonatally with coumestrol, *Reprod. Toxicol.*, 4, 127, 1990.

115. vom Saal, F. S., Montano, M. M., and Wang, M. H., Sexual differentiation in mammals, in *Chemically-Induced Alterations in Sexual and Functional Development: The Wildlife/Human Connection*, Colburn, T. and Clement, C., Eds., Princeton Scientific Publishing, Princeton, NJ, 1992, 17.

116. Nonneman, D. J., Ganjam, V. K., Welshons, W. V., and vom Saal, F. S., Intrauterine position effects on steroid metabolism and steroid receptors of reproductive organs in male mice, *Biol. Reprod.*, 47, 723, 1992.

117. Cunha, G. R., Bigsby, R. M., Cooke, P. S., and Sugimura, Y., Stromal-epithelial interactions in adult organs, *Cell Differentiation*, 17, 137, 1985.

118. Hayward, S. W., Rosen, M. A., and Cunha, G. R., Stromal-epithelial interactions in the normal and neoplastic prostate, *Br. J. Urol.*, 79 (Suppl. 2), 18, 1997.

119. Nagaoka, T., Onodera, H., Matsushima, Y., Todate, A., Shibutani, M., Ogasawara, H., and Maekawa, A., Spontaneous uterine adenocarcinomas in aged rats and their relation to endocrine imbalance, *J. Canc. Res. Clin. Oncol.*, 116, 623, 1990.

120. Deerberg, F. and Kaspareit, J., Endometrical carcinoma in BD II/Han rats: model of a spontaneous hormone-dependent tumor, *J. Natl. Canc. Inst.*, 78, 1245, 1987.

121. Greenman, D. L., Highman, B., Chen, J., Sheldon, W., and Gass, G., Estrogen-induced thyroid follicular cell adenomas in C57BL/6 mice, *J. Toxicol. Environ. Health*, 29, 269, 1990.

122. Anjum, A. D. and Payne, L. N., Spontaneous occurrence and experimental induction of leiomyoma of the ventral ligament of the oviduct of the hen, *Res. Vet. Sci.*, 45, 341, 1988.

123. Anjum, A. D. and Payne, L. N., Concentration of steroid sex hormones in the plasma of hens in relation to oviduct tumours, *Br. Poultry Sci.*, 29, 729, 1988.

124. Beatson, G. T., On the treatment of inoperable cases of carcinoma of the mamma: suggestions for a new method of treatment with illustrative cases, *Lancet*, 2, 104, 1896.

125. Niwa, K., Murase, T., Furui, T., Morishita, S., Mori, H., and Tanaka, T., Enhancing effects of estrogens on endometrial carcinogenesis initiated by N-methyl-N-nitrosourea in ICR mice, *Jpn. J. Canc. Res.*, 84, 951, 1993.

126. Niwa, K., Morishita, S., Murase, T., Itoh, N., Tanaka, T., Mori, H., and Tamaya, T., Inhibitory effects of medroxyprogesterone acetate on mouse endometrial carcinogenesis, *Jpn. J. Canc. Res.*, 86, 724, 1995.

127. Ziel, H. K., Estrogen's role in endometrial cancer, *Obstet. Gynecol.*, 60, 509, 1982.

128. Brinton, L. A. and Schairer, C., Estrogen replacement therapy and breast cancer risk, *Epidemiol. Rev.*, 15, 66, 1993.

129. Hulka, B. S., Kaufman, D. G., Fowler, W. C., Jr., Grimson, R. C., and Greenberg, B. G., Predominance of early endometrial cancers after long-term estrogen use, *JAMA*, 244, 2419, 1980.

130. Adami, H. O., Lipworth, L., Titus-Ernstoff, L., Hsieh, C. C., Hanberg, A., Ahlborg, U., Baron, J., and Trichopoulos, D., Organochlorine compounds and estrogen-related cancers in women, *Canc. Causes Control*, 6, 551, 1995.

131. Murray, W. S., Ovarian secretion and tumor incidence, *J. Canc. Res.*, 12, 18, 1928.

132. Lacasagne, A., Aparition de cancers de la mammelle chez la souris male, soumise a des injections de folliculine, *C. R. Hebd. Seanc. Acad. Sci.*, 195, 630, 1932.

133. Shellabarger, C. J., Stone, J. P., and Holtzman, S., Rat differences in mammary tumor induction with estrogen and neutron radiation, *J. Natl. Canc. Inst.*, 61, 1505, 1978.

134. Nandi, S., Guzman, R., and Yang, J., Hormones and mammary carcinogenesis in mice, rats, and humans: a unifying hypothesis, *Proc. Natl. Acad. Sci. U.S.A.*, 92, 3650, 1995.

135. Russo, J. and Russo, I. H., Biological and molecular bases of mammary carcinogenesis, *Lab. Invest.*, 57, 112, 1987.
136. Talwalker, P. K. and Meites, J., Mammary lobulo-alveolar growth induced by anterior pituitary hormones in adreno-ovariectomized and adreno-ovariectomized-hypophysectomized rats, *Proc. Soc. Exp. Biol. Med.*, 107, 880, 1961.
137. Leung, B. S. and Sasaki, G. H., On the mechanism of prolactin and estrogen action in 7,12-dimethylbenzanthracene-induced mammary carcinoma in the rat. II. *In vivo* tumor responses and estrogen receptor, *Endocrinology*, 97, 564, 1975.
138. Welsch, C. W., Host factors affecting the growth of carcinogen-induced rat mammary carcinomas: a review and tribute to Charles Brenton Huggins, *Canc. Res.*, 45, 3415, 1985.
139. Russo, J. and Russo, I. H., DNA labeling index and structure of the rat mammary gland as determinants of its susceptibility to carcinogenesis, *J. Natl. Canc. Inst.*, 61, 1451, 1978.
140. Hulka, B. S. and Stark, A. T., Breast cancer: cause and prevention, *Lancet*, 346, 883, 1995.
141. Ekbom, A., Trichopoulos, D., Adami, H. O., Hsieh, C. C., and Lan, S. J., Evidence of prenatal influences on breast cancer risk, *Lancet*, 340, 1015, 1992.
142. Toniolo, P. G., Levitz, M., Zeleniuch-Jacquotte, A., Banerjee, S., Koenig, K. L., Shore, R. E., Strax, P., and Pasternack, B. S., A prospective study of endogenous estrogens and breast cancer in postmenopausal women, *J. Natl. Canc. Inst.*, 87, 190, 1995.
143. Wiklund, J. A., Wertz, N., and Gorski, J., A comparison of estrogen effects on uterine and pituitary growth and prolactin synthesis in F344 and Holtzman rats, *Endocrinology*, 109, 1700, 1981.
144. Skakkebaek, N. E., Bethelsen, J. G., Giwercman, A., and Muller, J., Carcinoma *in situ* of the testis: possible origin from gonocytes and precursor of all types of germ cell tumors except spermatocytoma, *Int. J. Androl.*, 10, 19, 1987.
145. Horwich, A., Mason, M. D., and Hendry, W. F., Urological cancer, in *Oxford Textbook of Oncology*, Peckham, M., Pinedo, H., and Veronesi, U., Eds., Oxford University Press, New York, 1995, 1407.
146. Moller, H., Jorgensen, N., and Forman, D., Trends in incidence of testicular cancer in boys and adolescent men, *Int. J. Canc.*, 61, 761, 1995.
147. Jorgensen, N., Muller, J., Giwercman, A., Visfeldt, J., Moller, H., and Skakkebaek, N. E., DNA content and expression of tumour markers in germ cells adjacent to germ cell tumours in childhood: probably a different origin for infantile and adolescent germ cell tumours, *J. Pathol.*, 176, 269, 1995.
148. Johnson, D. E., Woodhead, D. M., Pohl, D. R., and Robison, J. R., Cryptorchidism and testicular tumorigenesis, *Surgery*, 63, 919, 1968.
149. Senturia, Y. D., The epidemiology of testicular cancer, *Br. J. Urol.*, 60, 285, 1987.
150. Sohval, A. R., Testicular dysgenesis in relation to neoplasm of the testicle, *J. Urol.*, 75, 285, 1956.
151. Sohval, A. R., Testicular dysgenesis as an etiologic factor in cryptorchidism, *J. Urol.*, 72, 693, 1953.
152. Paulson, D. F., Einhorn, L. H., Peckham, M. J., and Williams, S. D., Cancer of the testis, in *Cancer Principles & Practice of Oncology*, DeVita, V. T., Hellman, S., and Rosenberg, S. A., Eds., J. B. Lippincott Co., Philadelphia, 1982, 786.
153. Chilivers, C., Pike, M. C., Forman, D., Fogelman, K., and Wadsworth, M. E. J., Apparent doubling of frequency of undescended testis in England and Wales in 1962-81, *Lancet*, 330, 1984.

154. Kallen, B., Case control study of hypospadias, based on registry information, *Teratology,* 38, 45, 1988.
155. Kallen, B., Castilla, E. E., Robert, E., Lancaster, P. A., Kringelbach, M., Martinez-Frias, M. L., and Mastroiacovo, P., An international case-control study on hypospadias. The problem with variability and the beauty of diversity, *Eur. J. Epidemiol.,* 8, 256, 1992.
156. Paulozzi, L. J., Erickson, J. D., and Jackson, R. J., Hypospadias trends in two US surveillance systems, *Pediatrics,* 100, 831, 1997.
157. Braun, M. M., Ahlbom, A., Floderus, B., Brinton, L. A., and Hoover, R. N., Effect of twinship on incidence of cancer of the testis, breast, and other sites (Sweden), *Canc. Causes Control,* 6, 519, 1995.
158. Reznik-Schuller, H., Carcinogenic effects of diethylstilbestrol in male Syrian golden hamsters and European hamsters, *J. Natl. Canc. Inst.,* 62, 1083, 1979.
159. Moore, R. A., Benign hypertrophy and carcinoma of the prostate, *Surgery,* 16, 152, 1944.
160. Bosland, M. C., Animal models for the study of prostate carcinogenesis, *J. Cell. Biochem. — Suppl.,* 16H, 89, 1992.
161. Shain, S. A., McCullough, B., Nitchuk, M., and Boesel, R. W., Prostate carcinogenesis in the AXC rat, *Oncology,* 34, 114, 1977.
162. Iizumi, T., Yazaki, T., Kanoh, S., Kondo, I., and Koiso, K., Establishment of a new prostatic carcinoma cell line (TSU-Pr1), *J. Urol.,* 137, 1304, 1987.
163. Pollard, M. and Luckert, P. H., Tumorigenic effects of direct- and indirect-acting chemical carcinogens in rats on a restricted diet, *J. Natl. Canc. Inst.,* 74, 1347, 1985.
164. Noble, R. L., Prostate carcinoma of the Nb rat in relation to hormones, *Int. Rev. Exp. Pathol.,* 23, 113, 1982.
165. Shirai, T., Imaida, K., Masui, T., Iwasaki, S., Mori, T., Kato, T., and Ito, N., Effects of testosterone, dihydrotestosterone and estrogen on 3, 2'-dimethyl-4-aminobiphenyl-induced rat prostate carcinogenesis, *Int. J. Canc.,* 57, 224, 1994.
166. Walsh, P. C. and Wilson, J. D., The induction of prostatic hypertrophy in the dog with androstanediol, *J. Clin. Invest.,* 57, 1093, 1976.
167. Ofner, P., Bosland, M. C., and Vena, R. L., Differential effects of diethylstilbestrol and estradiol-17 beta in combination with testosterone on rat prostate lobes, *Toxicol. Appl. Pharmacol.,* 112, 300, 1992.
168. Pollard, M., Snyder, D. L., and Luckert, P. H., Dihydrotestosterone does not induce prostate adenocarcinoma in L-W rats, *Prostate,* 10, 325, 1987.
169. Robison, A. K., Sirbasku, D. A., and Stancel, G. M., DDT supports the growth of an estrogen-responsive tumor, *Toxicol. Lett.,* 27, 109, 1985.
170. Reuber, M. D., Carcinogenicity and toxicity of methoxychlor, *Environ. Health Perspect.,* 36, 205, 1980.
171. Reuber, M. D., The role of toxicity in the carcinogenicity of endosulfan, *Sci. Tot. Environ.,* 20, 23, 1981.
172. Reuber, M. D., Carcinogenicity of lindane, *Environ. Res.,* 19, 460, 1979.
173. Reuber, M. D., Carcinomas of the liver in Osborne-Mendel rats ingesting DDT, *Tumori,* 64(6), 571, 1978.
174. Reuber, M. D., Carcinomas of the liver in Osborne-Mendel rats ingesting methoxychlor, *Life Sci.,* 24, 1367, 1979.
175. Dewailly, E., Dodin, S., Verreault, R., Ayotte, P., Sauve, L., Morin, J., and Brisson, J., High organochlorine body burden in women with estrogen receptor positive breast cancer, *J. Natl. Canc. Inst.,* 86, 232, 1994.

176. Krieger, N., Wolff, M. S., Hiatt, R. A., Rivera, M., Vogelman, J., and Orentreich, N., Breast cancer and serum organochlorines: a prospective study among white, black, and Asian women, *J. Natl. Canc. Inst.*, 86, 589, 1994.

177. Wolff, M. S. and Toniolo, P. G., Environmental organochlorine exposure as a potential etiologic factor in breast cancer, *Environ. Health Perspect.*, 103, 141, 1995.

178. Sonnenschein, C., Soto, A. M., Fernandez, M. F., Olea, N., Olea-Serrano, M. F., and Ruiz-Lopez, M. D., Development of a marker of estrogenic exposure in human serum, *Clin. Chem.*, 41, 1888, 1995.

179. Pazos, P., Perez, P., Rivas, A., Nieto, R., Botella, B., Crespo, S., Olea-Serrano, F., Fernandez, M. F., Esposito, J., Olea, N., and Pedraza, V., Development of a marker of estrogen exposure in breast cancer patients, in *In Vitro Germ Cell Developmental Toxicology: From Science to Social and Industrial Demand*, del Mazo, J., Ed., Plenum Press, New York, 1998, in press.

180. Soto, A. M. and Sonnenschein, C., Regulation of cell proliferation: the negative control perspective, *Ann. N.Y. Acad. Sci.*, 628, 412, 1991.

6

Differential Regulation of Gene Expression by Estrogenic Ligands: A Potential Basis for the Toxicity of Environmental Estrogens

Salman M. Hyder, John L. Kirkland, David S. Loose-Mitchell, Sari Mäkelä, and George M. Stancel

CONTENTS

6.1   Introduction and Perspective

Chemicals present in the environment can mimic or antagonize the actions of endogenous estrogenic hormones by direct actions at estrogen receptor (ER) sites. In addition, chemicals can affect the biological actions of endogenous hormones secondarily by a variety of mechanisms, e.g., competition for plasma protein binding, influences on the biosynthesis of hormones, or alterations in the elimination of endogenous estrogens. In this chapter we will focus primarily on the potential effects of agents that interact with hormone binding sites on the estrogen receptor, i.e., direct-acting environmental estrogens, since we are interested primarily in the regulation of gene expression by estrogens as the basis for their proliferative actions. For background information, interested readers are referred to a number of important references that trace the development of this field[1-3] and several recent reviews[4-6] for an entré to the current literature.

At the outset we wish to emphasize several critical points. First, it is unequivocally established in the laboratory that the environmental estrogens discussed in this chapter can bind to the ER, affect transcription of estrogen target genes, and cause proliferation of hormone-responsive cells *in vivo* and *in vitro*. These observations raise genuine concerns about the reproductive tract toxicity of these chemicals in humans and wildlife. However, the affinities of most environmental estrogens for the ER are quite low, and there are other reasons to suspect that some environmental estrogens, such as the phytoestrogens present in certain foods, may actually have beneficial effects on human health.[4,5] Thus, it is not clear at present if the levels or disposition of these chemicals in the environment have significant effects, either detrimental[1-3,7] or beneficial,[5,8,9] on human or animal health.

6.2   Major Classes of Environmental Estrogens

There are three major types of environmental estrogens that are produced and enter the biosphere from different sources. Phytoestrogens are compounds produced by plants, mycoestrogens are agents produced by fungi, and xenoestrogens are manmade chemicals synthesized for commercial use or formed as byproducts of manufacturing processes, combustion of wastes, or other processes. Humans and animals may thus come in contact with these agents via the diet, air, water, or occupational exposures. There are three major classes of phytoestrogens: isoflavones, coumestans, and lignans. Isoflavones and coumestans bind directly to estrogen receptors, although they also have other activities (e.g., the isoflavone genistein inhibits protein tyrosine kinases)[10] that could account for some of their biological actions. It is not established unequivocally that lignans produce their effects directly via the ER. All known mycoestrogens are β-resorcylic acid derivatives, and these compounds exhibit some of the highest affinities for estrogen receptors of all known environmental estrogens. Xenoestrogens do not fall neatly into chemical classes based upon their structures, but rather a bewildering array of manmade chemicals seem to have estrogenic or antiestrogenic actions in biological systems. The major classes of xenoestrogens include a number of pesticides and agricultural chemicals, phenolic compounds used in synthesis of plastics and other formulated products, and halogenated aromatic hydro-carbons used as insulating materials and for other commercial purposes. Figure 6.1 illustrates the structures of some of these environmental estrogens, along with the structures of estradiol and the synthetic estrogen diethylstil-bestrol (DES). We have included this figure to emphasize the great structural diversity of environmental estrogens and to suggest at the outset that these varied chemical structures raise the possibility that these compounds may produce conformational changes in the estrogen receptor that are distinct from those produced by endogenous estrogens such as estradiol. As discussed throughout this chapter, we believe this has several important implications when considering potential mechanisms of toxicity of these compounds.

Quite recently pthalates, such as butylbenzylphthalate and dibutylphthalate, have also been reported to exhibit estrogenic activity,[11-13] but since little is known about the mechanism of action of these chemicals, they will not be discussed further in this chapter.

Environmental estrogens were initially identified because they produced biological effects (e.g., vaginal cornification, uterine growth, proliferation of hormone responsive tumor cells, etc.) very similar to endogenous estrogens such as estradiol and synthetic estrogens such as DES, which have been used therapeutically in the past. Thus, it was predictable that once environmental estrogens were discovered, there was great concern that they might produce toxicities similar to those produced by endogenous hormones or synthetic estrogens used therapeutically. Since it has been recognized for many years that many cancers of the breast and female reproductive tract are estrogen responsive, there has always been the concern that environmental estrogens would contribute to these and other proliferative diseases in the human population. These fears were further heightened with the discoveries in the 1970s that *in utero* exposure to DES led to an increase in the incidence of a rare type of vaginal cancer and other abnormalities[14] and in the 1980s that unopposed estrogen replacement therapy led to an increase in endometrial cancer in postmenopausal women.[15] For these reasons, we have devoted much of this chapter to a discussion of how environmental estrogens might affect cell proliferation and the expression of genes thought to be involved in regulating the growth of hormone-responsive tumors and normal target tissues such as the uterus.[16-18] Readers interested specifically in the regulation of human breast cancer cell proliferation by these compounds are referred

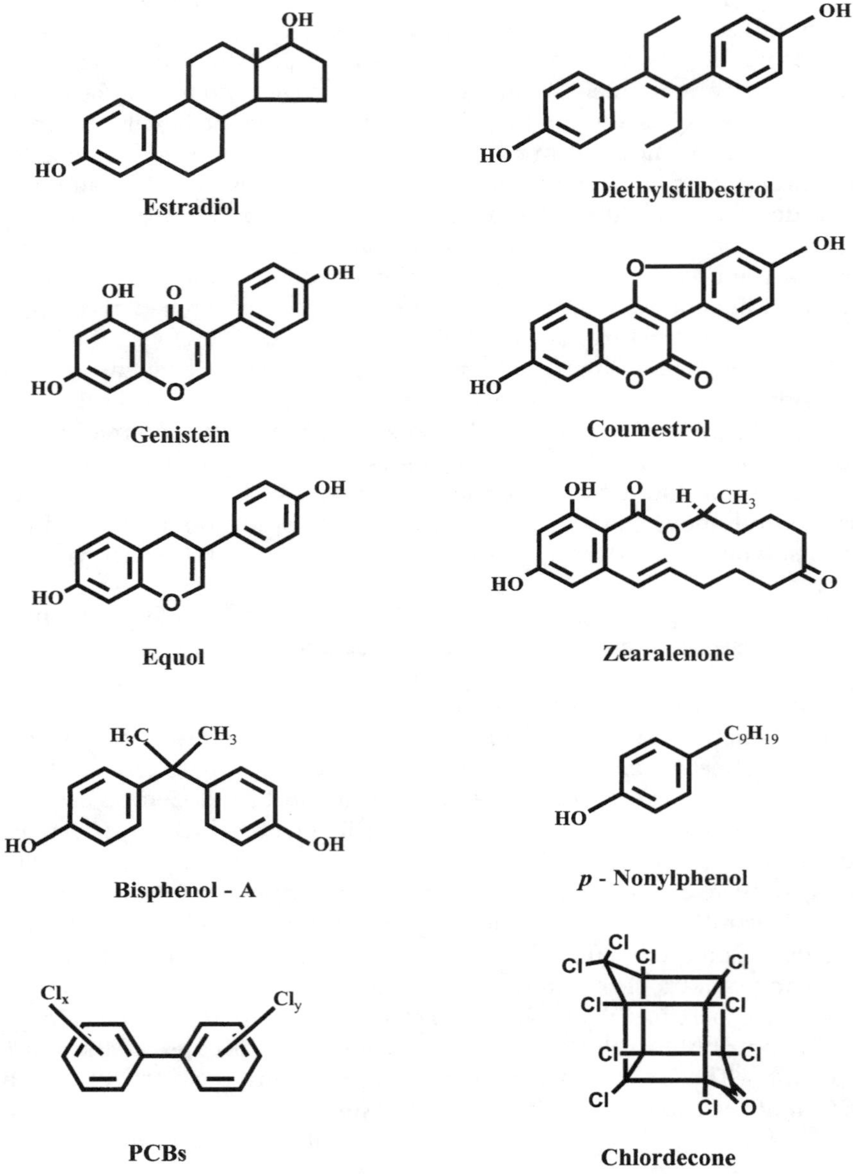

FIGURE 6.1
Structures of environmental estrogens. The structures of selected phytoestrogens (genistein, coumestrol, and equol), a mycoestrogen (zearalenone), and several xenoestrogens (bisphenol-A, p-nonylphenol, PCBs, and chlordecone) are illustrated, along with those of estradiol and diethylstilbestrol.

to a recent article by Soto and her colleagues,[13] who have focused on this area and to the references therein.

6.3 Receptor Interactions and Regulation of Gene Expression

In order to conceptualize molecular and cellular mechanisms for the potential untoward effects of environmental estrogens on proliferation, it is necessary to consider their actions in light of the mechanisms of estrogen-regulated gene expression and cell proliferation. Until quite recently, most models of estrogen-induced cell growth were conceptually very straightforward. An estrogen agonist was thought to bind to the ER to alter the transcription of "early response" genes, such as growth factors, their cognate receptors, cellular oncogenes, etc., which would in turn initiate a cascade of cellular events, including the activation of "intermediate" and "late" genes that would culminate in DNA replication and cell division. In such a model, all estrogens produce the same basic response if one allows for differences in their receptor affinities and pharmacokinetic properties. However, recent data on the basic mechanisms of estrogen action have indicated that the activity of different estrogenic agonists and antagonists may be cell type and gene specific.[19,20] This raises even greater concern about the potential toxicity of environmental estrogens, because as we discuss below, their actions may lead to patterns of growth factor and proto-oncogene gene expression that are fundamentally different or "unbalanced" relative to those produced by estradiol and other natural estrogens. For this reason this chapter reviews traditional models of hormone actions and newly emerging concepts.

6.3.1 Traditional Models of Hormone Action and Environmental Estrogen Toxicity

Until quite recently, the actions of estrogens were analyzed primarily as a simple 2-component or "bipartite" type of response system with the two components being the estrogenic ligand and its receptor, i.e., the ER.[19] The receptor was viewed as basically an "on/off" switch that was activated by the binding of an agonist. Until very recently, it was thought that the same ER encoded by a single gene was responsible for regulating the expression of estrogen-responsive genes in all target tissues, and since all estrogens (endogenous and environmental) are quite lipophilic, they freely enter all target tissues and occupy receptor sites therein. The activated receptor in turn was thought to regulate the transcription of target genes, such as growth factors or proto-oncogenes, by interacting with regulatory sequences termed

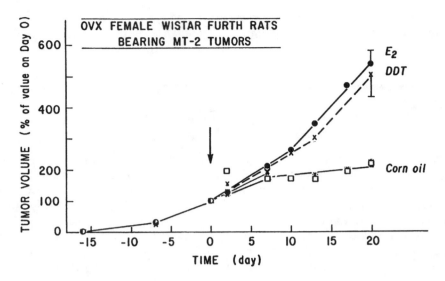

FIGURE 6.2

DDT drives the growth of an estrogen-responsive rat mammary tumor. At day 15, intact female rats were given a flank injection of 2.5 million MT-2 tumor cells grown in tissue culture, and tumors were allowed to grow for approximately 2 weeks. At day 0, animals were ovariecto-mized and then treated with daily injections of o,p'-DDT (100 mg/kg) or the corn oil vehicle alone. As a positive control, another group was given a pellet implant of estradiol (27 mg of hormone). Tumor volume was then measured as a function of time. (From Robison, A. K., Sirbasku, D. A., and Stancel, G. M., *Toxicol. Lett.*, 27, 109, 1985. With permission.)

estrogen response elements (EREs) in the promoter region of the target genes. The first ERE identified was that found in the vitellogenin gene.[21,22] This element is a perfect palindrome, with the sequence GGTCAnnnTGACC, and it was generally assumed that all estrogen-responsive genes would have very similar if not identical EREs.

In such a model, the overall control of biological function is exerted primarily by ligand binding, which "switches" the ER from the "off" to the "on" state so that its interaction with a common ERE triggers expression of all target genes in a similar manner. In this situation, an environmental estrogen would produce a "toxic" response simply by occupying the ER and triggering proliferation of target cells by increasing the synthesis of growth promoting genes. In other words, the toxicity of an environmental estrogen would result from a simple extension of its estrogenicity and would be similar in nature to the toxicity produced by endogenous or therapeutically administered estrogens. For example, an environmental estrogen might stimulate the growth of a hormone-responsive tumor.

An example of such an effect is shown in Figure 6.2, which represents data from an early study demonstrating that the pesticide o,p'-DDT stimulates the growth of an estrogen-dependent rat mammary tumor in a manner similar to that of estradiol.[23] DDT was thought to produce this effect via the ER, since many workers have shown it binds directly to the receptor (see

TABLE 6.1

Relative Binding Affinity of Selected Environmental Estrogens
to Estrogen Receptor-α

Compound	ER Source	RBA (Estradiol = 100%)
Genistein	M, S, H	0.25–5%
Equol	S	0.2–0.9%
Daidzen	M, S, H	0.01–0.1%
Coumestrol	R, S, H	5–94%
Zearalenone	R, H	1.8–3.3%
Zearalanol	R	10–100%
o,p′-DDT	R, H	0.1% or less
Chlordecone	R, C, T	0.1% or less
Various PCBs	R, M	0.1% or less
3,4,3′,4′-tetra-chlorobiphenyl	H	5%
Octylphenol	T	0.07%
Nonylphenol	T, H	0.02–0.03%
Bisphenol A	R, H	0.05–0.1%

Note: Species abbreviations: H — human, S — sheep, R — rat, M —
mouse, C — chicken, T — trout. References to original articles
may be found in a recent review. See Reference 6.

Reference 6 and references therein for a complete review), and we showed in
another early study that the growth-promoting actions of o,p′-DDT in the
uterus correlated well with its occupancy of nuclear ERs in the tissue.[24] In
this relatively straightforward situation, any differences in the actions of
endogenous and environmental estrogens are due primarily to differences in
their affinities for the ER or their pharmacokinetic properties as they alter the
fractional degree of receptor saturation and duration of receptor occupancy.

6.3.2 ER Binding of Environmental Estrogens and Activation of Gene Expression

Most studies of the effects of environmental estrogens on gene expression
have been performed in the context of relatively straightforward occupancy
models of ER-mediated gene expression at a time when all EREs were
thought to be quite similar to the vitellogenin element. Not surprisingly, the
emphasis of such studies has been on measuring the affinity of the ER for
environmental estrogens and on studying the regulation of single genes by
these compounds.

A number of studies have measured the affinity of the ER from various
sources for environmental estrogens, and we have summarized a number of
these studies in Table 6.1. While there is obviously a great range of relative
binding activities of environmental estrogens to the ER, a few generalities
are apparent. The mycoestrogen zearalanol (also referred to as zeranol) has
been found consistently to have a very high receptor affinity. In fact, two
reports that used radiolabeled compound to obtain a Kd value directly found
affinities essentially the same as that of estradiol,[25,26] and several other studies

using competitive binding found affinities 10-33% that of the endogenous hormone. The relative affinity of coumestrol for the ER from various sources is approximately 10% that of estradiol; that of zearalenone is roughly 2% that of the hormone, and several flavonoids display relative binding affinities of 0.1–1% that of estradiol. Special note should be made, however, of a recent report using *in vitro* translated human ER-α that found the relative binding affinities of coumestrol and genistein to be 94% and 5% of estradiol, respectively.[27] This is much higher than has been found in previous studies, which most often used tissue or cell homogenates rather than highly purified receptor. As a group, the xenoestrogens have by far the lowest relative binding, although several compounds in this class (e.g., phenolic metabolites of methoxychlor, bisphenol A, and the PCB 3,4,3',4'-tetrachlorobiphenyl) are reported to have affinities in the range of some phytoestrogens.

Despite these relatively low binding affinities, however, it is important to note that the relationships between *in vivo* dose–response curves and receptor affinities are not always straightforward or predictable. For example, a recent study reported that developmental defects caused by DES exposure display an inverted U-shaped dose–response curve.[28] It is not known whether other effects of environmental estrogens also display such relationships, but if they do, the extrapolation from receptor-binding effects to the production of *in vivo* actions may be very complex and quite important to understand in order to assess the true toxicity of these compounds.

There have been numerous reports of the effects of environmental estrogens on gene expression, which are summarized in Table 6.2. In general, most of these studies have found that the environmental estrogens tested produce changes in gene expression quantitatively similar to those produced by estradiol or DES, and the potency of environmental estrogens is generally in line with their measured affinities for the ER. However, even a casual examination of Table 6.2 reveals that the great majority have focused on induction of a very small number of endogenous genes (the progesterone receptor, pS2, creatine kinase, or vitellogenin genes) or transfection experiments using reporter constructs, such as CAT or luciferase, containing the consensus ERE most often linked to a strong heterologous promoter. However, there are absolutely no studies on the regulation of growth factor expression by environmental estrogens; there are only two reports[29,30] demonstrating acute induction of nuclear proto-oncogenes by phytoestrogens; and there are no studies that have examined the expression patterns of multiple genes in target cells by environmental estrogens. Since the effects of estrogens on cell proliferation and cancer are thought to be due to regulation of multiple proto-oncogenes and growth factors, this absence of data on regulation of such genes by environmental estrogens represents a very serious deficiency in our knowledge of the actions of these compounds.

Despite this deficiency, a simple occupancy-effect model is one plausible basis for the potential toxicity of environmental estrogens, and the above studies do indicate that a number of environmental estrogens can bind to the ER and stimulate expression of some estrogen-responsive genes. However,

TABLE 6.2

Genes Regulated by Environmental Estrogens

Compound	Responsive Genes
Genistein	ERE, fos, pS2
Coumestrol	ERE, fos, pS2
Equol	ERE
Enterodiol, Enterolactone	ERE, PR, pS2
Zearalenone, Zearalanol	ERE, CK, pS2
o,p'-DDT	ERE, pS2, PR, ER, CK
Methoxychlor	ERE, CK
Kepone	PR, ER, VIT, OVAL, CON
PCBs	ERE, pS2, ER, VIT
Octylphenol, Nonylphenol	ERE, VIT, PR, ER, pS2, MUC-1
Bisphenol A	ERE, PR

Note: Gene Abbreviations: ERE — reporter constructs with the consensus ERE, GGTCAnnnTGACC; *fos* — the proto-oncogene c-*fos*, PR — progesterone receptor, CK — creatine kinase, ER — estrogen receptor, VIT — vitellogenin, OVAL — ovalbumin, CON — conalbumin. References to individual studies may be found in a recent review. See Reference 6.

we suspect that a number of other factors could also contribute to the toxicity of environmental estrogens in more subtle ways. To understand these potential factors and how they could contribute to toxicity, one must appreciate advances in the understanding of the basic mechanism of estrogen action which have occurred very recently.

6.3.3   Hormonal Regulation of Endogenous Gene Expression Involves Diverse *cis*- and *trans*-Acting Elements

As part of our studies of estrogen-induced proliferation, our group was interested in the regulation of "immediate early" genes, such as the AP-1 components c-*fos* and c-*jun*, which we[18] and others[31] showed were rapidly induced in growth responsive tissues. While investigating the mechanisms involved, we defined the EREs for the rodent *fos*[32] and *jun*[33] genes. To our surprise, both of these genes contained regulatory elements that differed in sequence and location from the vitellogenin sequence, which is considered to be the consensus ERE (sequence = GGTCAnnnTGACC). The mouse c-*fos* gene contains an ERE with the sequence GGTCAnnn**CAG**CC in the 3'-flanking region of the gene well beyond the poly A addition signal, and the rat c-*jun* gene contains an ERE with the sequence **GCAG**AnnnTGACC in its single exon. Despite the considerable sequence variability from the consensus ERE, both

TABLE 6.3

Examples of Selected Estrogen Response Elements (EREs)

Consensus (i.e., vitellogenin) ERE	GGTCAnnnTGACC
Rodent Genes	
c-*fos* (mouse)	GGTCAnnn**CAG**CC
c-*jun* (rat)	G**CAG**AnnnTGACC
calbindin (rat)	GGTCAnnnTGAT**C**
creatine kinase (rat)	GGTCA(n)$_{21}$**GG**C**GG**
c-*myc* (rat)	G**G**GCA(n)$_{22}$**GG**C**GG**
prolactin (rat)	GGTCAnnnTG**T**CC
Human Genes	
pS2	GGTCAnnnTG**G**CC
c-*myc*	G**G**GCA(n)$_{17}$**GG**C**GG**
cathepsin D	G**G**GCA(n)$_{23}$**GG**C**GG**
RARα-1	GGTCA(n)$_{10}$**GG**C**GG**
progesterone receptor	GGTC**G**nnnTGAC**T**

Note: Base sequences different from the consensus element are printed in bold. Note also that the spacing between the half-sites of the creatine kinase, myc, cathepsin D, and RARα-1 genes is also different than the 3 nucleotide spacer in the consensus element. See accompanying text for literature references to ERE sequences.

these elements conferred estrogen inducibility to reporter constructs containing either homologous or heterologous promoters, and both bound the ER in cell free studies using band-shift assays. Interestingly, however, the three regulatory sequences appear to have different affinities for the ER,[34] and as discussed in a subsequent section, this difference may have the potential to contribute to the toxicity of both endogenous and environmental estrogens.[35,36]

In addition to our studies on the rodent c-*fos* and c-*jun* genes, other workers have now identified the EREs in a number of estrogen-responsive genes; representative examples are shown in Table 6.3. It is interesting to note that to date the so-called consensus ERE has only been identified in nature in a single gene, the vitellogenin gene. It is now clear that a diversity of sequences are involved in controlling the expression of estrogen target genes, and the implications of these differences are only now starting to be considered. References to most of the EREs listed in Table 6.3 may be found in a recent review,[35] and additional references for these elements are as follows: c-*myc*,[37] cathepsin D,[38] and RARα-1.[39,40]

A second recent realization has been that the regulation of transcription by the ER and other steroid receptors involves interactions with a very large number of protein factors. These include both general transcription factors (e.g., the TATA binding protein and other TFIID components)[41] as well as more specific factors, including steroid receptor coactivators and corepressors.[42] These accessory proteins interact with the ER domains responsible for transcriptional activation (the so-called TAFs or AFs) to control gene expression, and the accessory proteins required for transcriptional activation are likely to be gene specific. Furthermore, the steroid receptors are known to contain multiple TAFs, and it is now clear that some ligands (e.g., estradiol) may activate all TAFs, while others (e.g., tamoxifen) may activate some but not others (see References 19 and 20 and references therein). This raises the possibility that environmental estrogens may affect the receptor's TAF domains differentially than endogenous estrogens and hence may produce a different set of interactions between the ER, coactivators/corepressors, and other proteins involved in transcription control. As discussed below, this provides another potential mechanism by which environmental and ovarian estrogens potentially could produce different patterns of gene expression, which might result in abnormal tissue responses.

Finally, it is now clear that multiple estrogen receptors exist in humans and animals. Since the pioneering discoveries of estrogen receptors in the laboratories of Elwood Jensen and Jack Gorski in the 1960s, it has been thought that only a single type of estrogen receptor was present in hormone target cells. However, in 1996 a second form of ER, termed ER-β to distinguish it from the traditional receptor (now referred to as ER-α) was identified in both rodent[43] and human cells.[44] While the affinity of ER-α and ER-β is essentially the same for estradiol, the receptors appear to exhibit different relative affinities for at least two environmental estrogens, genistein and coumestrol, and the two proteins display different tissue distributions.[27] If the overall response of an organism to a particular estrogen is due to the net effect of its actions at these receptor sites in multiple tissues, then differential affinities of the receptors for an environmental estrogen represent another potential basis for toxicity, since it could lead to uncoordinated responses of different organs in the intact organism.

6.4   Selective Gene Responses to Estrogen Agonists and Antagonists

6.4.1   Selective Induction of Target Genes by a Single Estrogen

As mentioned in a previous section, we determined that the proto-oncogene c-*fos*[32] and c-*jun*[33] contained ERE sequences with multiple base differences from those in the consensus element. Using a competitive binding assay that examined the ability of oligonucleotides containing these two elements in their native context to compete with the vitellogenin ERE for receptor binding, we were then able to show that the affinity of the ER for the *fos* element was approximately four- to five-fold greater than that of the *jun* element.[34] This caused us to wonder if there were any biological ramifications of this difference. One obvious possibility was that the *fos* gene would be more sensitive to induction than the *jun* gene in target tissues.

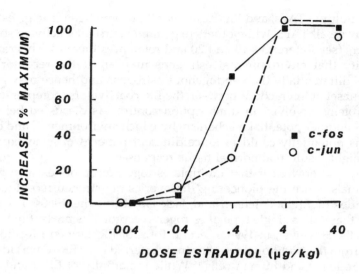

FIGURE 6.3

Dose–response curves for induction of uterine c-*fos* and c-*jun* mRNA by estradiol. Immature female rats were injected with estradiol 3 hours before sacrifice; total uterine RNA was prepared; and oncogene transcript levels were determined in aliquots of the same RNA preparations by blot analysis and densitometry. (From Chiapetta, C., Kirkland, J. L., Loose-Mitchell, D. S., Murthy, L., and Stancel, G. M., *J. Steroid Biochem. Mol. Biol.*, 41, 113, 1992. With permission.)

To examine this possibility, we performed the experiment shown in Figure 6.3 which illustrates data we obtained in a previous study.[45] In this study, immature rats were treated with increasing doses of estradiol and uterine RNA was prepared. Aliquots of the same RNA samples were then analyzed for the levels of both proto-oncogene transcripts by Northern analysis, and the results were quantitated by densitometry. The results illustrate that in the same animals, the dose–response curve for *fos* induction is shifted to the left of that for *jun* induction, that is, two genes in the same tissue are differentially sensitive to estrogenic induction. While it is impossible to state unequivocally that this difference is due to the different affinities of the ERE sequences for the ER in the cell-free experiments noted above, it is interesting to note that the relative differences are the same magnitude (i.e., four- to five-fold) for both parameters. In addition, a similar result has been obtained more recently by others who found that the induction of vitellogenin and pS2 reporter constructs in cultured cells occurs at different doses of estradiol, and there was a corresponding difference in the affinity of the EREs of the two genes for the ER *in vitro*.[46]

6.4.2 Differential Antagonism of Hormone-Induced Gene Expression

Environmental compounds that bind to the ER could act either as estrogen agonists or antagonists. We[47] and others[48] had shown previously that estrogen

TABLE 6.4

Selective Antagonism of Estrogen-Responsive Genes
by the Antagonist ICI 182,780

Dose of ICI 182,780 (mg/kg)	%Inhibition of mRNA Induction	
	c-*fos*	VEGF
1 mg/kg	82 ± 1.8%	21 ± 10%
3 mg/kg	98 ± 2.0%	60 ± 6%

Note: Immature rats were treated with estradiol alone or
the hormone plus the indicated doses of ICI 182,780.
Uterine mRNA was then isolated and analyzed by
blot analysis and densitometry and the % inhibition
of induction of the two transcripts by the antiestrogen
was calculated. Values in this table have been obtained from scans of data presented in Reference 49.

antagonists such as nafoxidine could selectively antagonize gross tissue
responses (e.g., uterine weight increases) in intact animals. This implied that
ER-antagonist complexes could selectively occupy ERE sites in target cell
nuclei, but to our knowledge no one had ever demonstrated such selective
blockade of individual hormone-responsive genes *in vivo*. Since the studies
described in the preceding section showed that a given estrogen could induce
one estrogen-regulated gene vs. another differentially, we also wondered if
an estrogen antagonist could selectively block hormonal induction of one
gene vs. another. To test this idea we examined the ability of the pure estrogen
receptor antagonist ICI 182,780 to block the induction of two estrogen-regulated genes, c-*fos* and vascular endothelial growth factor or VEGF, *in vivo*.[49]

In this study, animals were treated with a dose of estradiol (40 μg/kg),
which yields maximum induction of both genes. Other groups of animals
were then injected with the hormone, and either a low (1 mg/kg) or high
(3 mg/kg) dose of the ICI compound. Three hours after the hormone treatments, animals were sacrificed, and uterine RNA was obtained. Aliquots of
the RNA samples were then analyzed for expression of both genes by Northern analyses and densitometry. As seen in Table 6.4, the low dose of the
antagonist inhibited the induction of c-*fos* by 82% but inhibited the level of
VEGF transcript induction by only 21%. The higher dose of 3 mg/kg ICI
182,780 completely blocked the induction of c-*fos* and blocked VEGF mRNA
induction by 60%. To our knowledge this was the first demonstration that
an estrogen receptor antagonist could selectively block the induction of one
hormone-responsive gene vs. another in an estrogen-responsive tissue.[49]

This result implied that the ER-agonist complex might interact preferentially with the VEGF regulatory elements relative to the *fos* regulatory elements. In other words, since more antagonist is needed to blunt the VEGF
response, this response is presumably stimulated with fewer functional ER
complexes. If this is so, one might also predict that some estrogen agonists
would be able to activate VEGF transcription preferentially relative to *fos*

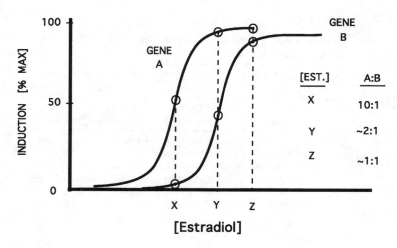

FIGURE 6.4

Hypothetical illustration of the levels of expression of two estrogen-induced genes A and B, with different dose–response curves. Note that the ratio of gene products varies with the total dose of estrogens from all sources.

transcription. Interestingly, we have observed that clomiphene and nafoxidine, which both have agonist activity in the uterus, preferentially induce VEGF mRNA levels vs. *fos* transcript levels in that tissue,[50] although we have not yet established this theoretical mechanism for the effect we have observed on induction of these two genes.

6.4.3 Implications of Selective Induction and Antagonism of Hormone Responsive Genes for Toxicity of Estrogens

The ability of estrogen agonists and antagonists to affect gene expression selectively raises the possibility of a type of toxicity that is more subtle than simple hormonal agonism or antagonism, an "imbalanced" production of growth regulatory substances in target cells. To appreciate this possibility, consider the hypothetical induction of two estrogen-responsive genes A and B, which display different dose–response curves, and the manner in which any given estrogen, either endogenous or environmental, might affect the ratio of their gene products. This is illustrated schematically in Figure 6.4, where the point noted as "Y" on the x-axis is meant to represent induction of the two genes by some concentration of estradiol alone; as drawn, the ratio of the gene products of A:B would be 2:1 at this estrogen concentration. The point marked "Z" is meant to illustrate the effect of adding more estradiol, or another estrogen from either environmental or other sources, to the system. Because the two dose–response curves are offset, the ratio of the two gene products would now be 1:1. Conversely, point "X" is meant to illustrate the situation in the presence of an estrogen receptor antagonist; again because the two curves are offset, the ratio of the gene products changes to

10:1. If an antagonist selectively antagonized induction of one of the genes, (such as the relative effect of ICI 182,780 on c-*fos* and VEGF expression), then the change in the ratio of the resultant gene products could be even greater than illustrated. We have discussed previously the toxicological implications of such different dose–response curves in somewhat more detail in several recent references.[35,36]

In target tissues, such as the endometrium and mammary gland, estrogens are known to induce a substantial number of growth factors and proto-oncogenes.[16-18,31] It seems quite reasonable to suggest that if these growth regulatory factors were produced in the wrong ratios, one might cause abnormal effects on cell proliferation and differentiated functions. In the hypothetical situation we have depicted in Figure 6.4, this could occur by an abnormal production of exogenous ovarian estrogens, administration of synthetic estrogens used therapeutically, exposure to environmental estrogens, or exposure to antiestrogens used therapeutically or present in the environment.

When considering these possibilities, it is important to ask whether results such as we have obtained for induction and antagonism of c-*fos* and c-*jun* are unique for estradiol or are common to other estrogens. In this regard it is important to note the work of Korach and Brooks and their colleagues. Korach and colleagues found, for example, that a series of DES analogs produced differential uterine responses, including DNA synthesis, glucose-6-phosphate dehydrogenase induction, and increased progesterone receptor levels, when administered to mice *in vivo*.[51-53] They suggested that "the ability of a particular response to be increased may depend on the chemical nature of the ligand receptor complex and its interaction at genomic sites."[51] In other studies, Brooks and his colleagues found that a series of estrogen analogs showed differential patterns of induction of endogenous genes (progesterone receptor, pS2, and cathepsin D) and reporter constructs containing the consensus ERE.[54-56] We noted above that others have also found differential induction of reporter constructs containing EREs from the vitellogenin and pS2 promoters.[46] Finally, in preliminary studies currently ongoing in our lab, we have some evidence that o,p'-DDT differentially induces a series of estrogen-responsive genes *in vivo*, including c-*fos*, c-*jun*, VEGF, and creatine kinase B. Collectively, these findings suggest that the differential induction of hormone-responsive genes may be more common than previously recognized and may occur with many if not all estrogens. Given the extremely diverse structures of environmental estrogens (see Figure 6.1), they may induce conformational changes in the ER that could elicit very different patterns of gene activation than those produced by endogenous hormones.

6.4.4 Differential Patterns of Gene Expression Produced by Different Estrogens

The experiments and discussion in the preceding section were based upon the differential induction of multiple genes by a single estrogen. In addition, we wished to expand the concept of differential induction of gene expression to investigate the possibility that different estrogenic ligands might produce different patterns of gene expression. Since the [ER-ligand] complex interacts with a nuclear site, including an ERE and a number of nuclear proteins, one may view such nuclear sites as the pharmacological "receptors" for the [ER-ligand] complex, which may be viewed as the "agonist" (or "antagonist") for that site. We consider such nuclear sites containing the ERE, all associated nuclear proteins, and other DNA sites they may contact as a functional hormone response unit or HRU. Since it is now clear that the HRUs in different hormone-responsive genes contain different ERE sequences and associated proteins,[19–21,41,42] we considered the possibility that complexes between the ER and different ligands might produce different patterns of gene expression. We believe this is a very likely possibility, since recent crystallographic studies have illustrated that there are major differences in ER conformation when it is occupied by different estrogenic ligands.[57]

A functional test of this hypothesis would be to compare the pattern of gene expression produced by two different ligands in a single biological system. As an initial test of this possibility, we decided to compare the induction of a set of proto-oncogenes in the uterus to estradiol and tamoxifen.[58] Tamoxifen generally is considered to be an antiestrogen in the breast, but we chose it for this study because it is known to have agonist activity in the uterus. Furthermore, there have been reports that women receiving tamoxifen therapy for breast cancer have an increased risk of endometrial cancer,[59,60] suggesting that the drug might be producing an aberrant uterine response, and the drug has been shown to cause the formation of DNA-adducts in the livers of experimental animals.[61]

In an initial series of experiments, we investigated the induction of c-*fos* in the immature rat uterus by estradiol and tamoxifen. These studies revealed that the two compounds had different time courses of action, estradiol showing peak induction of the gene in 3 h but tamoxifen requiring 6 h for maximum effect, as well as different potencies. These differences were consistent with the known pharmacokinetics and ER affinities of the two compounds, but when we studied both compounds at maximally effective doses and times of peak induction, they produced exactly the same magnitude of c-*fos* mRNA induction (see Table 6.5). We next investigated the induction of three other nuclear proto-oncogenes by the two compounds under similar conditions. The three cellular oncogenes tested were c-*jun*, *jun*B, and c-*myc*, which are known to be estrogen regulated.[18,31,45] The results are illustrated in Figure 6.5 and were very striking — under conditions where estradiol and tamoxifen induced one oncogene (i.e., *fos*) to exactly the same degree, tamoxifen induced two other oncogenes (c-*jun* and c-*myc*) to roughly half the extent as estradiol and showed essentially no induction of a third oncogene (*jun*B), which was dramatically induced by the hormone.[58] Other workers also have found major differences in the transcriptional responses seen in the rodent uterus following tamoxifen vs. estradiol treatment.[62,63]

TABLE 6.5

Induction of c-*fos* Transcription by Estradiol and Tamoxifen

Treatment	c-*fos* mRNA level	Determinations
Vehicle control	4.59 ± 1.1	26
Estradiol (3 h)	100 ± 6.4	20
Tamoxifen (6 h)	101 ± 5.8	25

Note: Immature female rats were treated with estradiol or tamoxifen for 3 or 6 h, which are the respective times for maximum *fos* induction. Total uterine RNA was then analyzed by blot analysis and densitometry to determine the level of c-*fos* mRNA, which is given in arbitrary densitometric units. Taken from Reference 58 with permission.

From Kirkland, J. L., Murthy, L., and Stancel, G. M., *Mol. Pharmacol.*, 43, 709, 1993. With permission.

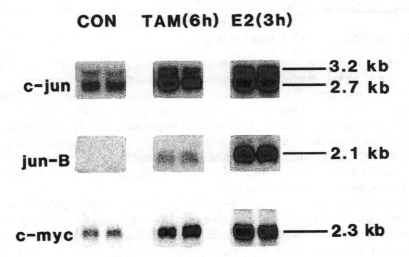

FIGURE 6.5

Uterine patterns of proto-oncogene mRNAs produced by treatment of immature female rats with either estradiol or tamoxifen. Immature female rats were treated with tamoxifen for 6 h (TAM), estradiol for 3 h (E2), or the vehicle alone (CON), and total uterine RNA was isolated. Replicate aliquots of the same samples were analyzed by Northern blots for the indicated proto-oncogene transcripts. The illustrated bands represent the levels of the 3.2 and 2.7 kb c-*jun* transcripts (top), the 2.1 kb *jun*-B transcript (middle), and the 2.3 kb c-*myc* transcript (bottom) in the same RNA samples. (From Kirkland, J. L., Murthy, L., and Stancel, G. M., *Mol. Pharmacol.*, 43, 709, 1993. With permission.)

At present we do not know whether these differences in responses of the four genes to tamoxifen and estradiol are due to different orders of potency of the two ligands (i.e., the order of the dose-response curves of the four genes is different for the two compounds) or whether they represent differences in the efficacy of the compounds (i.e., tamoxifen is a full agonist for c-*fos* induction but a partial agonist for induction of c-*myc* and c-*jun* and inactive for the induction of *jun*B). In either case, however, it is clear that the two compounds produce very different ratios of the transcripts for the four genes tested. Since the dimers formed by various combinations of these nuclear proteins are thought to produce different transcriptional effects,[18,31] their production in different ratios suggests that this may be a potential basis for the uterine toxicity reported in some patients receiving tamoxifen therapy. We have now initiated a series of similar studies to compare the patterns of gene expression caused by environmental estrogens such as o,p'-DDT to those produced by endogenous estrogens such as estradiol to see if they also show substantial differences.

6.5   Summary and Conclusions

Estrogenic hormones are thought to stimulate cell proliferation, in large part by regulating the expression of growth factors and proto-oncogenes at the transcriptional level. It is clear that environmental estrogens can bind to the ER and stimulate transcription of some estrogen-responsive genes and reporter constructs. This straightforward hormonal activity represents one molecular basis for the potential toxicity of environmental estrogens, although almost nothing is known about the effects of these compounds on the specific growth factors and cellular oncogenes thought to be involved in estrogen-mediated cell proliferation.

In addition, a single estrogen may display different dose–response curves for induction of different genes, a single antiestrogen may selectively antagonize hormonal effects on transcription, and different estrogen ligands may produce different patterns of gene expression in target cells. The net result of such differences could be an imbalanced production of growth factors, growth factor receptors, proto-oncogenes, and other cell regulatory molecules by environmental estrogens relative to estradiol. Such an altered profile of regulatory molecules could lead to abnormal proliferative and differentiative properties of hormone target cells, especially at critical times in development. While these suggestions admittedly are speculative, they stem from concepts that have emerged recently about the basic molecular actions of steroid receptors. We thus offer them here to stimulate discussion and experimentation on possible mechanisms of toxicity of environmental estrogens. We also emphasize that our experiments and others discussed here are laboratory based. Thus, while the results raise genuine concerns about the potential toxicity of environmental estrogens the effects we have observed cannot be extrapolated directly to humans and wildlife without additional information about the levels and duration of real world exposures.

Acknowledgments

Research in our laboratories described in this article was supported by NIH grants HD-08615 and ES-06995, grants from the Texas Affiliate of the American Heart Association, and the John P. McGovern Foundation.

References

1. McLachlan, J. A., *Estrogens in the Environment*, Elsevier/North-Holland, New York, 1980.
2. McLachlan, J. A., *Estrogens in the Environment. II. Influences on Development*, Elsevier, New York, 1985.
3. McLachlan, J. A. and Korach, K. S., Estrogens in the environment. III. Global health implications, *Environ. Health Perspect.*, 103 (Suppl. 7), 1995.
4. Kurzer, M. S. and Xu, X., Dietary phytoestrogens, *Annu. Rev. Nutr.*, 17, 353, 1997.
5. Adlercreutz, H. and Mazur, W., Phyto-estrogens and western diseases, *Ann. Med.*, 29, 95, 1997.
6. Makela, S., Hyder, S. M., and Stancel, G. M., Environmental estrogens, in *Handbook of Experimental Pharmacology — Estrogens and Antiestrogens*, Oettel, M. and Schillinger, G., Eds., Springer-Verlag, Heidelberg, 1998, (in press).
7. Colborn, T. and Clement, C., Chemically-induced alterations in sexual and functional development: the wildlife/human connection, in *Advances in Modern Experimental Toxicology*, Vol. 21, Princeton Scientific Publ., Princeton, 1992.
8. Daston, G. P., Gooch, J. W., Breslin, W. J., Shuey, D. L., Nikiforov, A. I., Fico, T. A., and Gorsuch, J. W., Environmental estrogens and reproductive health — a discussion of the human and environmental data, *Reprod. Toxicol.*, 11, 465, 1997.
9. Safe, S. H., Environmental and dietary estrogens and human health: is there a problem? *Environ. Health Perspect.*, 103, 346, 1995.
10. Akiyama, T., Ishida, J., Nakagawa, S., Ogawara, H., Watanabe, S., Itoh, N. M., Shibuya, M., and Fukami, Y., Genistein, a specific inhibitor of tyrosine-specific protein kinases, *J. Biol. Chem.*, 262, 5592, 1987.
11. Jobling, S., Reynolds, T., White, R., Parker, M. G., and Sumpter, J. P., A variety of environmentally persistent chemicals, including some phthalate plasticizers, are weakly estrogenic, *Environ. Health Perspect.*, 103 (Suppl. 7), 582, 1995.
12. Sharpe, R. M., Fisher, J. S., Millar, M. M., Jobling, S., and Sumpter, J. P., Gestational and lactational exposure of rats to xenoestrogens results in reduced testicular size and sperm production, *Environ. Health Perspect.*, 103, 1136, 1995.

13. Soto, A. M., Sonnenschein, C., Chung, K. L., Fernandez, M. F., Olea, N., and Serrano, F. O., The E-SCREEN assay as a tool to identify estrogens: an update on estrogenic environmental pollutants, *Environ. Health Perspect.*, 103, 113, 1995.

14. Herbst, A. L. and Bern, H. A., *The Developmental Effects of Diethylstilbestrol (DES) in Pregnancy*, Thieme-Stratton, New York, 1981.

15. Shapiro, S., Kelly, J. P., Rosenberg, L., Kaurman, D. W., Helmrich, S. P., Rosenshein, N. B., Lewis, J. L., Jr., Knapp, R. C., Stolley, P. D., and Schottenfeld, D., Risk of localized and widespread endometrial cancer in relation to recent and discontinued use of conjugated estrogens, *N. Engl. J. Med.*, 313, 969, 1985.

16. Khan, S. A. and Stancel, G. M., *Protooncogenes and growth factors in steroid hormone induced growth and differentiation*, CRC Press, Boca Raton, FL, 1994.

17. Stancel, G. M., Baker, V. V., Hyder, S. M., Kirkland, J. L., and Loose-Mitchell, D. S., Oncogenes and uterine function, *Oxford Rev. Reprod. Biol.*, 15, 1, 1993.

18. Hyder, S. M., Stancel, G. M., and Loose-Mitchell, D. S., Steroid hormone-induced expression of oncogene encoded nuclear proteins, *Crit. Rev. Eukaryotic Gene Expression*, 4, 55, 1994.

19. Katzenellenbogen, J. A., O'Malley, B. W., and Katzenellenbogen, B. S., Tripartite steroid hormone receptor pharmacology: interaction with multiple effector sites as a basis for the cell- and promoter-specific action of these hormones, *Mol. Endocrinol.*, 10, 119, 1996.

20. Katzenellenbogen, B. S., Estrogen receptors: bioactivities and interactions with cell signaling pathways, *Biol. Reprod.*, 54, 287, 1996.

21. Klein-Hitpass, L., Ryffel, G. U., Heitlinger, E., and Cato, A. C. B., A 13 bp palindrome is a functional estrogen responsive element and interacts specifically with estrogen receptor, *Nucl. Acids Res.*, 16, 647, 1988.

22. Burch, J. B. E., Evans, M. I., Friedman, T. M., and O'Malley, B. W., Two functional estrogen response elements are located upstream of the major chicken vitellogenin gene, *Mol. Cell. Biol.*, 8, 1123, 1988.

23. Robison, A. K., Sirbasku, D. A., and Stancel, G. M., DDT supports the growth of an estrogen responsive tumor, *Toxicol. Lett.*, 27, 109, 1985.

24. Robison, A. K. and Stancel, G. M., The estrogenic activity of DDT: correlation of estrogenic effect with nuclear levels of estrogen receptor, *Life Sci.*, 31, 2479, 1982.

25. Mastri, C., Mistry, P., and Lucier, G. W., *In vivo* oestrogenicity and binding characteristics of alpha-zearalanol (P-1496) to different classes of oestrogen binding proteins in rat liver, *J. Steroid Biochem.*, 23, 279, 1985.

26. Katzenellenbogen, B. S., Katzenellenbogen, J. A., and Mordecai, D., Zearalenones: characterization of the estrogenic potencies and receptor interactions of a series of fungal beta-resorcylic acid lactones, *Endocrinology*, 105, 33, 1979.

27. Kuiper, G. G. J. M., Carlsson, B., Grandien, K., Enmark, E., Haggblad, J., Nilsson, S., and Gustafsson, J. A., Comparison of the ligand binding specificity and transcript tissue distribution of estrogen receptors alpha and beta, *Endocrinology*, 138, 863, 1997.

28. vom Saal, F. S., Timms, B. G., Montano, M. M., Palanza, P., Thayer, K. A., Nagel, S. C., Dhar, M. D., Ganjam, V. K., Parmigiani, S., and Welshons, W. W., Prostate enlargement in mice due to fetal exposure to low doses of estradiol or diethylstilbestrol and opposite effects at high doses, *Proc. Natl. Acad. Sci. U.S.A.*, 94, 2056, 1997.

29. Makela, S., Santti, R., Salo, L., and McLachlan, J. A., Phytoestrogens are partial estrogen agonists in the adult male mouse, *Environ. Health Perspect.*, 103, 123, 1995.

30. Santell, R. C., Chang, Y. C., Nair, M. G., and Helferich, W. G., Dietary genistein exerts estrogenic effects upon the uterus, mammary gland and the hypothalamic/pituitary axis in rats, *J. Nutr.*, 127, 263, 1997.

31. Weisz, A. and Bresciani, F., Estrogen regulation of proto-oncogenes coding for nuclear proteins, *Crit. Rev. Oncogenes*, 4, 361, 1993.

32. Hyder, S. M., Stancel, G. M., Nawaz, Z., McDonnell, D. P., and Loose-Mitchell, D. S., Identification of an estrogen response element in the 3'-flanking region of the murine c-*fos* protooncogene, *J. Biol. Chem.*, 267, 18047, 1992.

33. Hyder, S. M., Nawaz, Z., Chiappetta, C., Yokoyama, K., and Stancel, G. M., The protooncogene c-*jun* contains an unusual estrogen-inducible enhancer within the coding sequence, *J. Biol. Chem.*, 270, 8506, 1995.

34. Hyder, S. M. and Stancel, G. M., *In vitro* interaction of uterine estrogen receptor with the estrogen response element present in the 3'-flanking region of the murine c-*fos* protooncogene, *J. Steroid Biochem. Mol. Biol.*, 48, 69, 1994.

35. Stancel, G. M., Boettger-Tong, H. L., Chiappetta, C., Hyder, S. M., Kirkland, J. L., Murthy, L., and Loose-Mitchell, D. S., Toxicity of endogenous and environmental estrogens: what is the role of elemental interactions? *Environ. Health Perspect.*, 103, 29, 1995.

36. Stancel, G. M., Boettger-Tong, H. L., Chiappetta, C., Hyder, S. M., Kirkland, J. L., Murthy, L., and Loose-Mitchell, D. S., Estrogen regulation of uterine proliferation: how many ERRs are required?, in *Molecular and Cellular Aspects of Periimplantation Processes*, Dey, S. K., Ed., Springer-Verlag, New York, 1995, 236.

37. Dubik, D. and Shiu, R. P., Mechanism of estrogen activation of c-*myc* oncogene expression, *Oncogene*, 7, 1587, 1992.

38. Krishnan, V., Wang, X., and Safe, S., Estrogen receptor-Sp1 complexes mediate estrogen induced cathepsin D gene expression in MCF-7 human breast cancer cells, *J. Biol. Chem.*, 269, 15912, 1994.

39. Elgort, M. G., Zou, A., Marschke, K. B., and Allegretto, E. A., Estrogen and estrogen receptor antagonists stimulate transcription from the human retinoic acid receptor alpha-1 promoter via a novel sequence, *Mol. Endocrinol.*, 10, 477, 1996.

40. Rishi, A. K., Shao, Z. M., Baumann, R. G., Li, S. X., Sheiky, S., Kimura, S., Bashirelahi, N., and Fontana, J. A., Estradiol regulation of the human retinoic acid receptor alpha gene in human breast carcinoma cells is mediated via an imperfect half-palindromic estrogen response element and Sp1 motifs, *Canc. Res.*, 55, 4999, 1995.

41. Beato, M. and Sanchez-Pacheco, S., Interaction of steroid hormone receptors with the transcription initiation complex, *Endocr. Rev.*, 17, 587, 1996.

42. Horwitz, K. B., Jackson, T. B., Bain, D. L., Richer, J. K., Takimoto, G. S., and Tung, L., Nuclear receptor coactivators and corepressors, *Mol. Endocrinol.*, 10, 1167, 1996.

43. Kuiper, G. G. J. M., Enmark, E., Pelto-Huikko, M., Nilsson, S., and Gustafsson, J. A., Cloning a novel estrogen receptor expressed in rat prostate and ovary, *Proc. Natl. Acad. Sci. U.S.A.*, 93, 5925, 1996.

44. Mosselman, S., Polman, J., and Dijkema, R., ER Beta: identification and characterization of a novel human estrogen receptor, *FEBS Lett.*, 392, 49, 1996.

45. Chiappetta, C., Kirkland, J. L., Loose-Mitchell, D. S., Murthy, L., and Stancel, G. M., Estrogen regulates expression of the *jun* family of protooncogenes in the uterus, *J. Steroid Biochem. Mol. Biol.*, 41, 113, 1992.

46. Nardulli, A. M., Romine, L. E., Carpo, C., Greene, G. L., and Rainish, B., Estrogen receptor affinity and location of consensus and imperfect estrogen response elements influence transcription activation of simplified promoters, *Mol. Endocrinol.*, 10, 694, 1996.

47. Gardner, R. M., Kirkland, J. L., and Stancel, G. M., Selective blockade of uterine responses to estrogen by the antiestrogen nafoxidine, *Endocrinology*, 103, 1583, 1978.

48. Galand, P., Mairesse, N., Rooryck, J., and Flandroy, L., Differential blockade of estrogen-induced uterine responses by the anti-estrogen nafoxidine, *J. Steroid Biochem.*, 19, 1259, 1983.

49. Hyder, S. M., Chiappetta, C., Murthy, L., and Stancel, G. M., Selective inhibition of estrogen-regulated gene expression *in vivo* by the pure antiestrogen ICI 182,780, *Canc. Res.*, 57, 2547, 1997.

50. Hyder, S. M., Chiappetta, C., and Stancel, G. M., Triphenylethylene antiestrogens induce uterine vascular endothelial growth factor expression via their partial estrogen agonist activity, *Canc. Lett.*, 120, 165, 1997.

51. Korach, K. S., Fox-Davies, C., Quarmby, V. E., and Swaisgood, M. H., Diethylstilbestrol metabolites and analogs. Biochemical probes for differential stimulation of uterine estrogen responses, *J. Biol. Chem.*, 260, 15420, 1985.

52. Korach, K. S., Chae, K., Gibson, M., and Curtis, S., Estrogen receptor stereochemistry: ligand binding and hormonal responsiveness, *Steroids*, 56, 263, 1991.

53. Metzger, D. A., Curtis, S., and Korach, K. S., Diethylstilbestrol metabolites and analogs: differential ligand effects on estrogen receptor interactions with nuclear matrix sites, *Endocrinology*, 128, 1875, 1991.

54. Pilat, M. J., Hafner, M. S., Kral, L. G., and Brooks, S. C., Differential induction of pS2 and cathepsin D mRNAs by structurally altered estrogens, *Biochemistry*, 32, 7009, 1993.

55. VanderKuur, J. A., Wiese, T., and Brooks, S. C., Influence of estrogen structure on nuclear binding and progesterone receptor induction by the receptor complex, *Biochemistry*, 32, 7002, 1993.

56. VanderKuur, J. A., Hafner, M. S., Christman, J. K., and Brooks, S. C., Effects of estradiol-17 beta analogs on activation of estrogen response element regulated chloramphenicol acetyltransferease expression, *Biochemistry*, 32, 7016, 1993.

57. Brzozowski, A. M., Pike, A. C. W., Dauter, Z., E., Hubbard, R. E., Bonn, T., Engstrom, O., Ohman, L., Greene, G. L., Gustafsson, J.-A., and Carlquist, M., Molecular basis of agonism and antagonism in the oestrogen receptor, *Nature*, 389, 753, 1997.

58. Kirkland, J. L., Murthy, L., and Stancel, G. M., Tamoxifen stimulates expression of the c-*fos* proto-oncogene in rodent uterus, *Mol. Pharmacol.*, 43, 709, 1993.

59. Anderson, M., Storm, H., and Mouridsen, H. T., Incidence of new primary tumors after adjuvant tamoxifen therapy and radiotherapy for early breast cancer, *J. Natl. Canc. Inst.*, 83, 1013, 1991.

60. Malfetano, J. H., Tamoxifen-associated endometrial carcinoma in postmenopausal breast cancer patients, *Gynecol. Oncol.*, 39, 82, 1990.

61. Han, X. L. and Liehr, J. G., Induction of covalent DNA adducts in rodents by tamoxifen, *Canc. Res.*, 52, 1360, 1992.

62. Nephew, K. P., Polek, T. C., and Khan, S. A., Tamoxifen-induced proto-oncogene expression persists in uterine endometrial epithelium, *Endocrinology*, 137, 219, 1996.

63. Nephew, K. P., Polek, T. C., Akcali, K. C., and Khan, S. A., The antiestrogen tamoxifen induces c-*fos* and *jun*-B, but not c-*jun* and *jun*-D, protooncogenes in the rat uterus, *Endocrinology*, 133, 419, 1993.

7

2,3,7,8-Tetrachlorodibenzo-p-dioxin (TCDD) and Related Environmental Antiestrogens: Characterization and Mechanism of Action

Stephen H. Safe

CONTENTS

0-8493-3164-1/99/$0.00+$.50
© 1999 by CRC Press LLC

7.1   Aryl Hydrocarbon Receptor Agonists: Biochemical and Toxic Responses

7.1.1   Introduction

Organochlorine industrial chemicals have been extensively used in the production of plastics, flame retardants, dielectric fluids, pesticides, drugs, and a host of other commercial products. Some of these chemicals, such as the organochlorine insecticides, which include DDT, are both highly stable and lipophilic, and trace residues have been detected as pollutants in air, water, sediments, fish, wildlife, human adipose tissue, blood, and milk.[1] Other halogenated aromatic compounds, such as the polychlorinated biphenyls (PCBs), dibenzo-*p*-dioxins (PCDDs) and dibenzofurans (PCDFs) exhibit comparable widespread environmental distribution profiles.[2,3] After initial identification of DDT, its metabolite DDE, and PCBs as environmental pollutants, regulatory agencies have either banned or restricted use of most persistent organochlorine compounds, and residue levels for most of these chemicals have declined dramatically over the past 20 to 30 years.[1]

Organochlorine contaminants exhibit multiple species-dependent effects, and these pollutants have been linked to reproductive and developmental failures of some wildlife populations in contaminated regions such as the Great Lakes.[4] Some of these adverse effects may be related to the endocrine-like activity of some organochlorine compounds. There has been considerable scientific and public controversy regarding the potential wildlife and human health effects associated with exposure to endocrine disruptors, particularly those compounds that exhibit estrogenic activity (i.e., xenoestrogens).[4-6] Wolff and co-workers initially reported that adipose tissue PCB levels were higher in a cohort of women with breast cancer (in Connecticut), and in a nested case-control study in New York serum DDE levels were higher in breast patients than controls.[7,8] Their analysis showed that women with the highest levels of DDE had a four-fold increased risk for breast cancer, and it was concluded that "environmental contamination with organochlorine residues may be an important etiologic factor in breast cancer."[7] It was later hypothesized that xenoestrogens were a preventable cause of breast cancer,[9-11] and there has been considerable research on testing the validity of the reported correlational studies. Recent studies on women from the San Francisco Bay area, five European countries, the Nurses Health Study (comprising 121,700 women from 11 states), and three Mexico City hospitals have compared serum or tissue DDE, and in some cases, PCB levels in breast cancer in patients and controls.[12-15] The results (Table 7.1) showed that levels of DDE/PCBs were not significantly different in breast cancer patients vs. controls, indicating that correlational studies do not support a role for these compounds as etiologic factors for breast cancer in women.

The xenoestrogen-breast cancer hypothesis was challenged on several counts, including the authors' failure to account for diverse organochlorine compounds that exhibit antiestrogenic activity.[16,17] For example, women in Seveso, Italy, accidentally exposed in 1976 to high levels of 2,3,7,8-tetrachlorodibenzo-*p*-dioxin (TCDD) exhibited a lower incidence of breast and endometrial cancer in the early 1990s.[18] TCDD is the most toxic member of a class of compounds that includes other PCDDs, PCDFs, and PCBs, and this review will describe their inhibition of 17β-estradiol (estrogen, E2)-induced responses, the molecular mechanism of action of these chemicals, and the development of a new class of mechanism-based indirect antiestrogens for treatment of breast cancer.[19]

7.1.2 TCDD and Related Compounds: Biochemical and Toxic Responses

TCDD has been used extensively as a prototype for investigating the biochemical and toxic responses elicited by halogenated aromatic hydrocarbons (HAHs).[19-24] TCDD induces a diverse spectrum of phase I and phase II drug-metabolizing enzymes, including CYP1A1, CYP1A2, CYP1B1, and their dependent activities,[25] glutathione S-transferase,[26,27] glucuronosyl transferase,[28] and NAD(P)H quinone:oxidoreductase.[29] TCDD also increases expression of other genes/gene products, including aldehyde-3-dehydrogenase,[30] transforming growth factor α (TGFα),[31,32] δ-aminolevulinic acid synthetase,[33] plasminogen activator inhibitor 2,[34] interleukin 1β,[34] c-*fos* and c-*jun* protooncogenes,[35] and prostaglandin endoperoxide H synthase-2.[36] It has also been reported that TCDD decreases expression of several genes/gene products, such as c/EBPα,[37] peroxisome proliferator receptor γ,[37] lipoprotein lipase,[37] estrogen receptor, urophorphyrinogen decarboxylase,[38,39] rat liver aldolase B,[40] phosphoenol pyruvate carboxykinase,[41] pyruvate carboxylase,[42] hydroxysteroid sulfotransferase a,[43] and adenosine deaminase.[44] The list of genes and/or gene products which are modulated after treatment with TCDD is continually expanding; however, these responses are highly tissue-specific. For example, although TCDD induces interleukin 1β and plasminogen activator inhibitor-2 in human keratinocytes,[34] no induction was observed in Sprague-Dawley rat liver.[45]

TCDD and related compounds also elicit a diverse spectrum of toxic responses, which include acute lethality, a wasting syndrome, tissue-/cell-specific hypo- and hyperplastic effects, immunotoxicity, thymic atrophy, developmental and reproductive toxicity, carcinogenesis, hepatotoxicity, porphyria, chloracne and related dermal lesions.[19-25] The acute lethal toxicity of TCDD and related compounds are observed in most species; however, the LD_{50} values vary from 2.0 µg/kg for the highly responsive guinea pig to 5051 and 7200 µg/kg for the resistant hamster and Hann/Wistar rat, respectively. In contrast, many other toxic responses are highly species-, sex-, and age-specific. For example, long-term dietary exposure to male and female Sprague-Dawley rats to TCDD (0.001, 0.01 and 0.1 µg/kg/d) resulted in development of hepatocellular carcinomas in females but not male rats. This type of response variability is typical for halogenated aromatics, and the mechanisms associated with tissue-/species-specific responsiveness or nonresponsiveness are poorly understood.

7.1.3   Identification of the Aryl Hydrocarbon Receptor (AhR)

Poland, Nebert, and coworkers extensively investigated induction of hepatic CYP1A1-dependent aryl hydrocarbon hydroxylase (AHH) activity in genetically inbred strains of mice by TCDD and 3-methylcholanthrene (MC).[46-48] Both TCDD and MC induced hepatic microsomal AHH activity in Ah-responsive mice typified by the C57BL/6 strain, and TCDD was approximately 10^4 times more potent than MC. The differences in potency were attributed to the higher rate of metabolism of MC. In contrast, TCDD but not MC induced the same response in DBA/2 mice, a prototypical Ah-nonresponsive strain; however, the effective dose of TCDD was at least ten times higher. It was suggested that these strain differences may be related to differential expression or structure of an intracellular receptor or acceptor protein. Support for the role of a receptor protein was derived from other studies, which showed that for a number of halogenated aromatics, there was a correlation between structure-induction (AHH activity) vs. other structure-activity relationships.[49] Poland and co-workers were the first to identify a hepatic cytosolic protein in C57BL/6 mice which bound [^{3}H]TCDD with high affinity.[50] Subsequent studies identified the AhR in multiple species/tissues and photoaffinity labeling using 2-azido-3[^{125}I]iodo-7,8-dibromodibenzo-*p*-dioxin, and hepatic cytosol from various species gave the following apparent molecular masses for the AhR: 95-kD (mouse), 101-kD (chicken), 103-kD (guinea pig), 104-kD (rabbit), 106-kD (rat and human), 113-kD (monkey), and 124-kD (hamster).[51]

Treatment of Ah-responsive cells/animals with TCDD results in the rapid formation of a liganded 190- to 210-kD nuclear AhR complex, which contains the AhR and a second protein, which has been identified as the AhR nuclear translocator (Arnt) protein.[52,53] Genes for both the AhR and Arnt have been

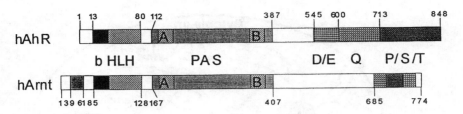

FIGURE 7.1
Structural domains of the AhR and Arnt proteins.

cloned, and sequence analysis has demonstrated that both proteins are members of the basic helix-loop-helix (bHLH) family of nuclear transcription factors.[54-59] The AhR and Arnt genes encode for proteins that exhibit several common structural domains (Figure 7.1), which include the DNA-binding bHLH region, two A/B repeats, a PAS domain common to the Per, Arnt and Sim proteins, a ligand-binding domain (within the AhR), and Q-rich transactivation domains in the C-terminal region of both proteins. There is high sequence homology in the bHLH (N-terminal) and PAS domain of AhR proteins from different species and considerable variability in the C-terminal Q-rich regions. For example, Ema and co-workers compared the sequence of the AhR from Ah-responsive C57BL/6 and less responsive DBA/2 mice and humans.[55] The major differences between the two strains of mice were associated with the length of the C-terminal regions and a critical alanine[375]-valine change in the ligand-binding domain, which is associated with the decreased binding affinity for TCDD for the AhR from DBA/2 mice. Interestingly, the ligand-binding region from the human AhR resembles that described for the less Ah-responsive DBA/2 mouse strain.[55] Recent studies by Wilson and co-workers have identified a 39-kD Arnt splice variant expressed in several estrogen receptor (ER)-negative human breast cancer cell lines and in some human mammary tumors.[60] This splice variant contains a large deletion in the transactivation domain and has been designated as TAD⁻Arnt.

7.1.4 Molecular Mechanisms of AhR-Mediated Transactivation

The heterodimeric nuclear AhR complex is a ligand-induced transcription factor, and *cis*-genomic sequences were initially identified by several groups in the 5′-promoter regions of the rodent and human CYP1A1 genes.[61-67] The CYP1A1 gene promoter contains one or more copies of dioxin or xenobiotic responsive elements (DREs or XREs) which contain the following core binding sequence:

$$5' - T - GCGTG - 3'$$

$$3' - A - CGCAC - 5''$$

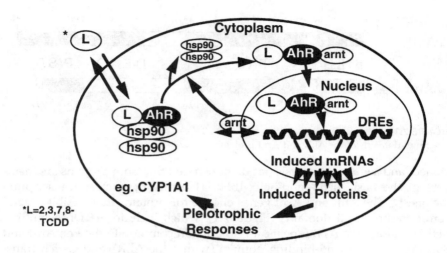

FIGURE 7.2
Proposed mechanism of ligand-induced AhR-mediated genes based on the CYP1A1 model.

The core binding sequence is required for binding the nuclear AhR complex and transactivation; however, additional nucleotides are required for transactivation, and the following sequence has been proposed for a functional DRE/XRE.[68,69]

$$5' - \text{T/G N } \textit{GCGTG} \text{ A/C N G/C NNN} - 3'$$

$$3' - \text{A/C N } \textit{CGCAC} \text{ T/G N C/G NNN} - 5'$$

These enhancer elements have been identified in promoter regions of several Ah-responsive genes including CYP1A2,[70] CYP1B1,[71] NAD(P) quinone:oxidoreductase,[29] aldehyde-3-dehydrogenase,[30] glutathione S-transferase,[26,27] and glucuronyl transferase.[28] The generally accepted mechanism of AhR-mediated transactivation (Figure 7.2) is comparable to that described for other ligand-induced transcription factor complexes, namely, initial binding of ligand to the AhR, heterodimer formation, binding of the nuclear AhR complex with promoter elements (XRE/DRE), and interaction of the DNA-bound transcription factor complex with general transcription factors, coactivators, and other nuclear proteins required for transactivation (Figure 7.2).

  Studies with Arnt- or AhR-defective mouse Hepa-1 cells have demonstrated that both proteins are required for induction of CYP1A1 gene expression by TCDD;[72-75] however, many other factors may play an important role in Ah-responsiveness. For example, proteins that bind a negative regulatory element (NRE) may modulate AhR-mediated transactivation in some cell lines.[76,77] Superinduction of CYP1A1 after treatment with cycloheximide

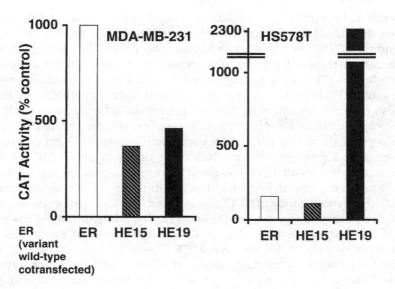

FIGURE 7.3

Cell-type specific restoration of Ah-responsiveness in MDA-MB-231 and Hs578T human breast cancer cells treated with TCDD and transiently transfected with pRNH11c and wild-type (ER) or variant (HE15 or HE19) ER expression plasmids.

suggests that labile inhibitory proteins may regulate induction of CYP1A1 in some cells.[78]

7.1.5 Modulation of Ah-Responsiveness by the ER in Human Breast Cancer Cell Lines

Initial studies with both ER-negative and ER-positive breast cancer cell lines showed that while both cell lines express the AhR and Arnt and form a nuclear AhR complex after treatment with TCDD, induction of CYP1A1 was observed only in cells expressing the ER.[79,80] The requirement for ER expression on Ah-responsiveness was further investigated in transient transfection studies in both ER-negative MDA-MB-231[81] and Hs578T[82] cells transiently transfected with pRNH11c, a construct containing the –1142 to +2434 region of the CYP1A1 gene promoter linked to a bacterial chloramphenicol acetyl transferase (CAT) gene. The results (Figure 7.3) illustrate the cell-type specific restoration of Ah-responsiveness in cells cotransfected with pRNH11c and expression plasmids for the wild-type ER (hER), an N-terminal deletion variant containing the ligand-binding domain and activator function-2 (AF-2, HE19), and a C-terminal deletion variant containing AF-1 (HE15). TCDD induces CAT activity in MDA-MB-231 cells cotransfected with hER, HE15 or HE19; however, only HE19 restored inducibility in Hs578T cells.

Crosstalk between the ER and AhR-mediated responses was further investigated in MDA-MBA-231 cells stably transfected with the ER. TCDD did not induce CYP1A or GST-P gene expression or their dependent activities; moreover, in transient transfection assays using pRNH11c or a construct containing a GST-P gene promoter insert, TCDD did not induce reporter gene activity.[83] These data suggest that cellular factors in addition to the ER are also required for restoring Ah-responsiveness in breast cancer cells.

The complexity of ER-AhR crosstalk was further complicated by results showing that there was not a strict correlation between ER expression and AhR-mediated gene expression. Treatment of ER-negative MDA-MB-468 breast cancer cells with TCDD resulted in formation of a nuclear AhR complex, which also bound [^{32}P]DRE in a gel mobility shift assay to form an AhR-DRE retarded band.[84] TCDD also induced CYP1A1 gene expression and dependent activity, and the results showed that MDA-MB-468 cells represented the first ER-negative Ah responsive human breast cancer cell line. Long-term culture of ER-positive MCF-7 cells in 1 μM benzo[a]pyrene resulted in isolation of resistant clones, which exhibited altered genotypes.[85] BaP-resistant cells were E2-responsive and expressed the AhR and Arnt; however, TCDD did not induce CYP1A1 gene expression in this variant cell line. The nuclear AhR complex for BaP-resistant MCF-7 cells did not exhibit DNA binding in gel mobility shift assays; the reasons for this defective binding are currently being investigated.

Wang and co-workers[86] extensively characterized the AhR from seven human cancer cell lines, including both ER-positive MCF-7 and ER-negative MDA-MB-231 breast cancer cells. Photoaffinity labeling studies identified a 110-kD protein in all cell lines; however, the sedimentation coefficient for the nuclear AhR complex from MDA-MB-231 cells was significantly lower (6.62 S) than observed for MCF-7 cells (7.23 S). Subsequent RT-PCR analysis for Arnt mRNA in MDA-MB-231 cells identified a major 1.3 kb transcript, whereas the expected 2.6 kb transcript was detected in MCF-7 cells.[60] The truncated Arnt protein was also observed by Western blot analysis using Arnt antibodies, and sequence analysis of the gene indicated that a splice variant transcript was expressed in which a major region of the C-terminal transactivation domain (TAD) had been deleted. The 36-kDa TAD-Arnt variant binds the AhR and forms a nuclear heterodimer, which interacts with [^{32}P]DRE in gel mobility shift assay. However, the results indicate that deletion of the TAD region of Arnt results in loss of Ah-responsiveness. In contrast, the TAD-Arnt protein binds H1F1α, and growth of MDA-MB 231 cells under conditions of hypoxia results in upregulation of hypoxia-responsive genes.[87] Thus, the TAD-Arnt protein interacts with H1F1α to form a functional heterodimer; therefore, the TAD is not required for hypoxia-responsiveness. Ongoing studies are probing the tissue- and cell-specific expression of TAD-Arnt to delineate the biological role of the Arnt variant.

7.2 Inhibition of ER-Mediated Responses by AhR Agonists: A New Class of Antiestrogens

7.2.1 Introduction

Several studies have reported that TCDD and related compounds inhibit diverse hormone/growth factor-mediated responses in animal and cellular models.[19] For example, TCDD inhibits epidermal growth factor (EGF) receptor binding and/or autophosphorylation in multiple species/tissues; however, the role of this response in AhR-mediated toxicity has not been determined.[88-93] Treatment of human keratinocytes[34] or MDA-MB-468[84] human breast cancer cells with TCDD increases TGFα mRNA and protein levels, and this is also accompanied by inhibition of MDA-MB-468 cell growth.[84] Subsequent studies showed that the growth inhibitory response by TCDD was directly related to induction of TGFα, which exhibits antimitogenic activity in this cell line. In contrast, TCDD inhibits the mitogenic activity of TGFα, EGF, and insulin-like growth factor-1 (IGF-1) in MCF-7 or T47D cells.[94-96] TCDD modulates several steps in metabolism of cholesterol to various steroid hormones,[97,98] and induction of CYP1A1, CYP1A2, and CYP1B1 is associated with increased 2- and 4-steroid hydroxylase activities.[99-102] The antiestrogenic activity of AhR agonists has been investigated intensively in several laboratories. This chapter will focus primarily on this response, which involves complex interactions between the AhR and ER signaling pathways.

7.2.2 Antiestrogenic and Antimitogenic Activity of AhR Agonists

7.2.2.1 Inhibition of Mammary Tumor Growth by TCDD

Kociba and co-workers[103] first reported that female Sprague-Dawley rats that were administered TCDD (0.1, 0.01 or 0.001 μg/kg/d) developed hepatocellular carcinomas, whereas this response was not observed in male rats. A high incidence of spontaneous mammary and endometrial tumors was observed in control female rats; however, in animals treated with TCDD, there was a dose-dependent decrease in both tumors. Since formation of rodent mammary and endometrial cancer is E2-dependent, these results suggest that TCDD exhibits antiestrogenic activity, and this has been confirmed in rodent models. TCDD inhibited 7,12-dimethylbenzanthracene (DMBA)-induced mammary tumor formation and growth in female Sprague-Dawley rats,[104] and similar results were reported in animals initiated with diethylnitrosamine.[105] Gierthy and co-workers also reported that TCDD inhibited mammary tumor growth in athymic B6D2F1 mice implanted with E2 pellets and bearing MCF-7 cell xenografts.[106] The antiestrogenic activity of TCDD observed in rodent tumor models has also been reported in individuals exposed to TCDD after an industrial accident in Seveso, Italy, in

1976. Serum levels of TCDD in some Seveso residents were among the highest ever reported (>70,000 ppt). Severe chloracne was observed in many of the more highly exposed groups, and there was a high mortality in the exposed rodent population. Health surveys in Seveso have not shown significant long-term adverse health effects, although a recent study reported a higher female-to-male ratio in offspring of highly exposed individuals.[107,108] In addition, the incidence of both endometrial and breast cancer was lower than expected in women exposed to TCDD in the Seveso accident.[18] These results were consistent with rodent studies.

7.2.2.2   Antiestrogenic Activity of TCDD and Related Compounds in Laboratory Animals

The rodent uterus is particularly sensitive to both estrogens and antiestrogens and is extensively utilized as an *in vivo* bioassay. Gallo and co-workers first reported the antiestrogenic activity of TCDD and related compounds in the CD-1 mouse uterus, showing that TCDD blocked E2-induced uterine wet weight increase and decreased cytosolic and nuclear ER levels.[109-112] Johnson and co-workers also showed that while TCDD alone did not affect implantation in the hypophysectomized female rat, there was a 35% inhibition of estrone-induced implantation in animals cotreated with the hormone plus TCDD.[113] Brown and Lamartiniere also showed that after treatment of pubertal female Sprague-Dawley rats with TCDD, proliferation and development of the mammary gland were inhibited.[114]

Research in this laboratory has focused on the antiestrogenic activity of halogenated aromatic hydrocarbons in the immature 25-day-old female Sprague-Dawley rat.[91,115-119] TCDD alone decreased gene expression/activities of several E2-regulated responses, including uterine wet weight, peroxidase activity, cytosolic PR binding, c-*fos* mRNA and EGF receptor mRNA levels. TCDD-induced effects were dose-dependent, with the following order of sensitivity: EGF receptor mRNA > c-*fos* mRNA > peroxidase activity > uterine wet weight > cytosolic PR binding. The dose-dependent antiestrogenic activity of TCDD for these same responses was not determined over a range of doses; however, the antiestrogenic potency of TCDD followed a comparable response-dependent order of sensitivity. The results were similar to those recently reported by Hyder and co-workers using the direct-acting antiestrogen ICI 182,780.[120] Their studies showed that E2 induced both vascular endothelial growth factor (VEGF) and c-*fos* gene expression in the rodent uterus, and ICI 182,780 inhibited both responses but at different doses.

7.2.2.3   Antiestrogenic Activity of TCDD and Related Compounds in Human Breast Cancer Cells

7.2.2.3.1   MCF-7 and T47D Cells

MCF-7 human breast cancer cells have been used extensively as an *in vitro* model for investigating E2-regulated responses and gene expression, effects, and mechanism of action of antiestrogens.[121,122] MCF-7 cells express relatively high levels of ERα, and E2 induces cell proliferation and expression of several genes and related activities. Both the AhR and Arnt proteins are also expressed in MCF-7 cells and, after treatment with TCDD and related HAHs, a nuclear AhR complex is rapidly formed, resulting in induction of CYP1A1 mRNA levels and CYP1A1-dependent activities.[86,123] Based on the Ah- and E2-responsiveness of this cell line, studies on the crosstalk between the AhR- and ER-mediated signaling pathways have been investigated. Gierthy and co-workers first showed that TCDD inhibited E2-induced secretion of tissue plasminogen activator activity and postconfluent focus production in MCF-7 cells.[124,125] Subsequent studies have shown that TCDD and related compounds inhibit E2-induced cell proliferation in ER-positive MCF-7 and T47D cells, and a diverse spectrum of other responses were also inhibited by AhR agonists. TCDD inhibits E2-induced secretion of tissue plasminogen activator activity, pS2, 160-, 52- and 34-kD proteins; progesterone receptor (PR) binding; lactate formation; pS2, cathepsin D, prolactin receptor, and PR mRNA levels; postconfluent focus production; cell proliferation; reporter gene activity in cells transiently transfected with plasmids containing inserts derived from the pS2, cathepsin D and vitellogenin A2 genes.[123-136] Ongoing studies in this laboratory have shown that several other E2-induced genes and/or their derived E2-responsive plasmids are inhibited after cotreatment with TCDD, which include TGFα, bcl-2, insulin-like growth factor binding protein 4 (IGFBP-4), c-*fos*, retinoic acid receptor α1, cyclin D1, E2F1, heat shock protein 27 (Hsp 27), and creatine kinase B (unpublished results). These data clearly demonstrate that crosstalk between the AhR and ER results in inhibition of diverse E2-regulated genes and responses, which is comparable to that observed for direct-acting "pure antiestrogens" such as ICI 164,384 and 182,780.[137]

7.2.2.3.2 Inhibition of Growth Factor-Induced Responses

Research in this laboratory also has shown that TCDD inhibits TGFα, EGF, IGF-1, and insulin-induced proliferation of MCF-7 and/or T47D human breast cancer cells and E2-induced IGFBP-4 expression in MCF-7 cells.[94-96,138] Figure 7.4 illustrates results of recent studies that demonstrate both the antiestrogenic and antimitogenic activities of TCDD using MCF-7 cells. Although mechanisms of growth factor-AhR crosstalk are unknown, TCDD modulates components of growth factor signaling. For example, TCDD alone did not affect IGF-1 receptor mRNA levels or K_D values; however, TCDD significantly decreased IGF-1-induced IGF receptor binding sites.[96] TCDD alone did not affect K_D and B_{max} values for binding of [^{125}I]insulin to the insulin receptor (IR) but decreased the K_D value for IR-ligand binding and increased B_{max} in cells cotreated with TCDD and insulin.[138] TCDD also inhibited insulin-induced phosphorylation of the IR. Current studies focus on determining the mechanism of growth factor-AhR crosstalk and the role of the ER in mediating these interactions.

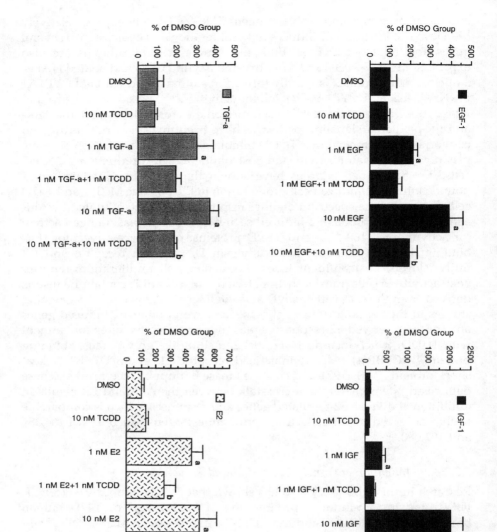

FIGURE 7.4
Effects of EGF, IGF-1, TGF-α, and E2 on proliferation of MCF-7 cells and the growth inhibitory activity of TCDD.

7.2.2.3.3   Inhibition of MDA-MB-468 Breast Cancer Cell Growth by TCDD[84]

The antiestrogenic activities of AhR agonists have been investigated primarily in E2-responsive human breast cancer cell lines, and most studies have demonstrated a correlation between Ah- and E2-responsiveness. These results suggest that the potential clinical utility of AhR agonists for treatment of breast cancer would be limited to ER-positive tumors. However, after screening a number of ER-negative breast cancer cell lines, it was shown that ER-negative MDA-MB-468 cells expressed the AhR, and TCDD induced CYP1A1 gene expression, ethoxyresorufin O-deethylase (EROD) activity, and CAT activity in cells transiently transfected with pRNH11c. These data established MDA-MB-468 cells as the first ER-negative Ah-responsive breast cancer cell line. Previous studies showed that cytotoxic drugs and EGF inhibited growth of MDA-MB-468 cells, and the unusual antimitogenic activity of EGF was accompanied by increased expression of EGF receptor, c-*myc* and c-*fos* protooncogene levels, and increased apoptosis. TCDD also significantly decreased growth of MDA-MB-468 cells and increased EGF receptor mRNA levels; however, TCDD did not induce c-*fos* or *myc* gene expression and was significantly less active than EGF as an inducer of apoptosis. EGF protein and mRNA levels are expressed at low levels in this cell line, and TCDD did not significantly modulate this response. Subsequent studies showed that TCDD increased TGFα mRNA and immunoreactive protein levels in MDA-MB-468 cells, and antibodies directed against the EGF receptor blocked the antimitogenic activity of TCDD. Since TGFα protein alone also inhibited proliferation of MDA-MB-468 cells, the results of this study showed that the antimitogenic activity of TCDD in this ER-negative cell line was associated with induction of TGFα protein. These data illustrate the unusual breast cancer cell-specific antimitogenic activity of TCDD, which inhibits TGFα and growth factor-induced proliferation of ER-positive breast cancer cells (Figure 7.4) but induces TGFα protein, which is antimitogenic in ER-negative MDA-MB-468 cells.

7.2.2.3.4   *Inhibition of E2-Induced Cell Cycle Enzymes by TCDD*

Recent studies in this laboratory also have focused on ER-AhR crosstalk associated with cell cycle enzymes. Several studies have reported that E2 decreases cells in G0/G1 and increases cells in S phase,[139-142] and the pure antiestrogen ICI 182,780 inhibits many of these estrogenic responses. The specific cell cycle enzymes in MCF-7 cells that are modulated by E2 show some variability between studies; however, cyclin dependent kinase 2 (cdk2) and cdk4-associated activities are increased, and retinoblastoma (RB) protein phosphorylation, E2F1 protein, cyclin D1 mRNA, and protein levels are elevated. Results of recent studies in this laboratory showed that in addition to these responses, E2 also affected the cdk-activating kinase (CAK) that contains cyclin H/cdk7 proteins and plays an important role in phosphorylation (and activation) of both cdk2 and cdk4 at threonine-160 and threonine-170, respectively.[143] Although E2 did not affect levels of cyclin H protein, cdk7 levels were increased 2.1-fold 24 h after treatment. Activation of cdk2/cdk4 is also dependent on cdc25 phosphatase-mediated hydrolysis of tyrosine 15, and in MCF-7 cells treated with E2 there was a significant increase (>two-fold) in cdc 25 protein. Thus, treatment of cells with E2 activates multiple cell cycle proteins and related activity and thereby offers multiple targets for the indirect antiestrogenic activity of TCDD. Like ICI 182,780, TCDD inhibits cells from E2-induced progression into S phase, and, in MCF-7 cells cotreated with E2 plus TCDD, there was selective inhibition of hormone-induced effects on cell cycle enzymes. For example, TCDD significantly inhibited the following E2-induced responses in MCF-7 cells: E2F1 protein, cyclin D protein and mRNA levels, phosphorylation of RB, and inhibition of cdk2-, cdk4-, and cdk7-associated kinase activities. Interestingly, TCDD alone had minimal effects on most cell cycle enzymes; however, in cells cotreated with E2 plus TCDD, there was a significant increase in p21 levels; this response may contribute to decreased cdk2- and cdk4-associated activities. Ongoing studies in this laboratory are focused on delineating the molecular mechanisms of AhR crosstalk with hormone-regulated cell cycle enzymes in both *in vitro* and *in vivo* models.

7.2.2.4   *Mechanisms of AhR-Mediated Antiestrogenicity*

7.2.2.4.1   *Role of the AhR*

Several different approaches have been utilized to demonstrate that the antiestrogenic activities of TCDD and related compounds are mediated via binding to the AhR and formation of a functional nuclear AhR complex. Structure-antiestrogenicity relationships have been observed for several *in vivo* and *in vitro* responses, including inhibition of E2-induced uterine wet weight increase, uterine PR binding and peroxidase activity (*in vivo*), downregulation of the ER, and secretion of procathepsin D in MCF-7 breast cancer cells.[91,116,132,133,136,144] In all of these studies, there was an excellent rank order correlation between structure-antiestrogenicity and structure receptor binding affinities (or AhR-mediated activities) for several HAHs. Cell lines with known defects in AhR signaling have also been utilized in these studies. For example, TCDD inhibited E2-induced reporter gene activity in wild-type Ah-responsive mouse Hepa-1 cells transiently cotransfected with an hER expression plasmid and E2-responsive constructs derived from the vitellogenin A2, cathepsin D, or pS2 genes.[129,133,136] In contrast, antiestrogenic activities were not observed in Ah-defective Hepa-1 variant cell lines. Gillesby and co-workers also showed that TCDD did not affect reporter gene activity induced by E2 in Hepa-1 C4 (Arnt-defective) or C12 (AhR-defective) cells transiently transfected with an E2-responsive pS2-luc plasmid.[133] However, the antiestrogenic activity of TCDD in C4 and C12 cells was restored in these cells after cotransfection with Arnt or AhR expression plasmids, respectively.

BaP^r MCF-7 cells express both the AhR and Arnt; however, this cell line is Ah-nonresponsive due to failure of the nuclear AhR to bind DNA as determined in gel mobility shift assays using [^{32}P]DRE.[85] Utilizing both wild-type and variant BaP^r MCF-7 cells, it was shown that E2 induced cell proliferation, secretion of cathepsin D, and CAT activity (in cells transiently transfected with a plasmid containing an E2-responsive vitellogenin A2 gene promoter insert); however, in cells treated with TCDD plus E2, antiestrogenic responses were observed only in wild-type but not BaP[r] cells. Results from both structure-activity relationships and Ah-defective cell lines strongly support a role for the nuclear AhR in mediating the antiestrogenic activity of TCDD and related HAHs.

7.2.2.4.2 Induction of E2 Hydroxylase Activities

TCDD induces CYP1A1 and CYP1B1 gene expression in MCF-7 cells, which is accompanied by an increased rate of E2 metabolism and E2 2-, 4-, 15α-, and 16-hydroxylase activities.[99-102,145] Spink and co-workers[99-102,145] suggested that induced hormone metabolism and subsequent depletion of cellular E2 levels may be responsible for the antiestrogenic activity of TCDD. While this response may contribute to AhR-mediated antiestrogenic activity in cell culture studies, there is ample evidence showing antiestrogenic responses that are independent of induced E2 metabolism. For example, (1) several weak AhR agonists, such as 6-methyl-1,3,8-triCDF (6-MCDF) and indole-3-carbinol (I3C), exhibit antiestrogenic activity at concentrations that do not induce CYP1A1;[119] (2) TCDD induces cathepsin D gene expression and glucose → lactate conversion at time points (≤2 h) that precede induction of CYP1A1 protein-dependent activities;[130] (3) induction of ERE-regulated reporter gene activities in a transient transfection experiment are not inhibited by TCDD, indicating that increased oxidative metabolism of E2 is not accompanied by an antiestrogenic response;[136] (4) transient transfection studies using a construct derived from the pS2 gene promoter and various ligand (E2)-dependent or -independent chimeric ERs showed that TCDD inhibited reporter gene activity using ligand independent chimeras (HE15 and ER$_c$VP16);[133] (5) circulating E2 levels were not affected after *in vivo* treatment of rodents with TCDD. These results and additional data from mechanistic studies suggest that induced oxidative metabolism of E2 is not a primary mechanism of AhR-mediated antiestrogenicity.[146]

7.2.2.4.3 Inhibitory DREs (iDREs) as Genomic Targets for the AhR

Results of preliminary screening studies in this laboratory showed that some E2-inducible genes or constructs containing promoter inserts were inhibited by TCDD within 2 to 4 h after treatment, suggesting that the inhibitory response was probably not related to induction of a new gene product. For example, in nuclear run-on assays with nuclei from cells treated with E2 for 24 h and TCDD for 60 min, there was a >70% decrease in cathepsin D mRNA levels induced by E2.[129] These results suggested that the inhibitory response may be mediated directly by the nuclear AhR complex, which is formed rapidly after treatment of MCF-7 cells with TCDD. Subsequent studies in this laboratory identified three E2-responsive enhancer sequences in the proximal region of the cathepsin D gene promoter, including an Sp1(N)$_{23}$ERE-half site at –199 to –165, an imperfect palindromic ERE at –119 to –107 and a GC-rich Sp1 binding site –145 to –135 (Figure 7.5A).[129,147,148] Two unusual

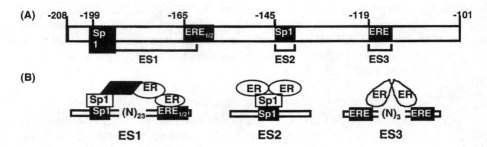

FIGURE 7.5
Identification of three E2 responsive enhancer elements in the cathepsin D gene promoter (A), and characteristics of the core iDRE (-175 to -181) in the same promoter (B).

motifs, which involve formation of a transcriptionally active ER/Sp1 protein complex, mediate E2-induced transactivation. The $Sp1(N)_{23}ERE(1/2)$ sequence binds nuclear extracts from MCF-7 cells to form a protein-DNA complex that requires intact Sp1 and ERE(1/2) sequences; the GC-rich site binds only the Sp1 protein; however, the ER mediates transactivation via ER-Sp1 (protein–protein) interactions, which may involve other proteins that stabilize ER/Sp1 complex formation. Studies in this laboratory have identified other E2-responsive GC-rich sites on the c-*fos* proto-oncogene and retinoic acid receptor α1 gene promoters. The Sp1 binding site within the −145 to −135 region of the cathepsin D gene promoter forms an ER/Sp1-DNA complex (binding to the GC-rich site) but also requires cooperative interactions with an adjacent core DRE site, which binds unliganded nuclear AhR complex. Results of transient transfection and gel mobility shift assays using wild-type and mutant oligonucleotides show that E2-responsiveness of this region of the promoter involves an ER/Sp1-AhR/Arnt complex interacting with an $Sp1(N)_4DRE$ motif.[148]

At least two functional iDREs have been identified within the −200 to −100 region of the cathepsin D gene promoter; and iDRE1 has been characterized extensively using the wild-type $Sp1(N)_{23}ERE(1/2)$ oligonucleotide in gel mobility shift and transient transfection assays (see Figure 7.5B). Interaction of the liganded AhR complex with iDRE1 results in disruption of the ER/Sp1-DNA complex and loss of transactivation in transient transfection assays. Moreover, using a bromodeoxyuridine-substituted $Sp1(N)_{23}ERE(1/2)$ oligonucleotide, the AhR complex could be crosslinked to the DNA sequence.[129] In contrast, an $Sp1(N)_{23}ERE(1/2)$ oligonucleotide containing a mutant iDRE motif bound nuclear extracts to form an ER/Sp1-DNA complex and was E2-responsive in transient transfection assays; however, the inhibitory effects of the AhR complex were not observed in these studies. A comparable approach also has been utilized for characterizing other functional iDREs in the pS2, Hsp 27, and c-*fos* gene promoters. Current research is focused on identifying functional iDREs in other genes and investigating alternative mechanisms associated with AhR-mediated antiestrogenic activity.

7.2.3 Development of AhR-Based Antiestrogens for Treatment of Breast Cancer

7.2.3.1 Introduction

Results reported in this review clearly demonstrate that AhR agonists exhibit antiestrogenic activities in the rodent uterus/mammary and in human breast cancer cell lines. There is also evidence from human studies that the AhR agonists exhibit antiestrogenic activities. For example, women in Seveso, Italy, exposed to TCDD following an industrial accident in 1976 exhibit a lower incidence of mammary and endometrial tumors.[18] Epidemiology studies have shown that the incidence of endometrial cancer is reduced significantly among cigarette smokers,[149,150] which corresponds to their exposure to AhR agonists such as polycyclic aromatic hydrocarbons (PAHs).[151] The effects of cigarette smoking in breast cancer incidence are variable and this may be due to protective (antiestrogenic) effects of PAHs in smoke and the genotoxicity of the same compounds. The major problems for development of clinically useful AhR-based antiestrogens are comparable to the design of other drugs, namely the compounds should exhibit maximal efficacy in target organs (breast and endometrium) but minimal toxic side-effects in nontarget tissues. Two classes of AhR-based antiestrogens have been developed in this laboratory, namely, alternate-substituted alkyl PCDFs and substituted diindolylmethanes (DIMs), their low toxicity and high antitumorigenic activity indicate that these compounds are promising new drugs for treatment of breast cancer in women.

7.2.3.2 Alternate Substituted PCDFs

A series of 6-alkyl-1,3,8-trichlorodibenzofurans (triCDFs) was originally synthesized for investigating their activities as partial AhR antagonists, and 6-methyl-1,3,8-trichlorodibenzofuran (6-MCDF) was used as a prototype for this series of compounds. 6-MCDF competitively bound with moderate affinity to the rodent cytosolic AhR but was a relatively weak agonist for several AhR-mediated biochemical and toxic responses, including induction of CYP1A1 and CYP1A2 in rats and cells in culture; porphyria, immunotoxicity, and cleft palate (teratogenicity) in mice.[117,152-155] Since 6-MCDF was a weak AhR agonist, it was hypothesized that 6-MCDF may be a partial AhR antagonist. This was confirmed in several studies that showed that 6-MCDF inhibited induction of CYP1A1 and CYP1A2 by TCDD in rats and fetal cleft palate, porphyria, and immunotoxicity in C57BL/6 mice.

Results of preliminary studies showed that 6-MCDF did not antagonize TCDD-induced antiestrogenicity in the female rat uterus but appeared to be a relatively potent antiestrogen. Astroff and Safe[117] reported that both TCDD and 6-MCDF caused a dose-dependent decrease in nuclear and cytosolic ER and PR binding in 21- to 25-d-old female Sprague-Dawley rats and that 6-MCDF was only 300 to 570 times less active than TCDD as an antiestrogen. In contrast, TCDD was >157,000 times more potent than 6-MCDF as an inducer of hepatic CYP1A1 in the same animals (a surrogate for toxic potency). Subsequent studies showed that 6-MCDF and related compounds inhibited E2-induced hypertrophy, peroxidase activity, cytosolic ER and PR binding, and EGF receptor and c-*fos* mRNA levels in the rat uterus.[91,117,118,156] 6-MCDF is also active in MCF-7 human breast cancer cells and, at concentrations of 10^{-7} to 10^{-6} M, inhibits a diverse spectrum of E2-induced responses.[157] An extensive structure-antiestrogenicity study of 15 alternate substituted (2,4,6,8- and 1,3,6,8-) alkyl-PCDFs was carried out in MCF-7 cells using three E2-induced responses, namely cell proliferation, induction of CAT activity in cells transiently transfected with an E2-responsive Vit-CAT plasmid, and induction of EROD activity.[158] The results showed that the antiestrogenic activities of these congeners were response-specific, and ten of the compounds were active in only one of the assays for antiestrogenicity (i.e., inhibition of E2-induced cell growth or CAT activity). Five compounds were active in both assays, including 6-MCDF, 6-ethyl-1,3,8-triCDF, 6-isopropyl-1,3,8-triCDF, 3-isopropyl-6-methyl-1,8-diCDF, and 6-methyl-2,4,8-triCDF.

The *in vivo* antiestrogenic activity of a series of alkyl-substituted PCDFs has been investigated in the immature female Sprague-Dawley rat uterus.[159] The compounds utilized in this study contain two, three, or four lateral substituents and include 6-MCDF, 6-ethyl-1,3,8-triCDF, 6-*n*-propyl-1,3,8-triCDF, 6-*i*-propyl-1,3,8-triCDF, 6-*t*-butyl-1,3,8-triCDF, 8-MCDF (two lateral substituents); 6-methyl-2,3,8-triCDF, 6-methyl-2,3,4,8-tetraCDF, 8-methyl-1,3,7-triCDF, and 8-methyl-1,2,4,7-tetraCDF (three lateral substituents); 8-methyl-2,3,7-triCDF, 8-methyl-2,3,4,7-tetraCDF (four lateral substituents). Two additional compounds, 8-methyl-2,3,7-trichlorodibenzo-*p*-dioxin and 8-methyl-2,3,7-tribromodibenzo-*p*-dioxin (four lateral substituents), were also investigated. All alkyl-substituted compounds inhibited estrogen-induced uterine wet weight increase and cytosolic and nuclear PR and ER binding. Quantitative structure-antiestrogenicity relationships were determined using 6-*i*-propyl-1,3,8-triCDF, 6-methyl-2,3,4,8-tetraCDF, and 8-methyl-2,3,4,7-tetraCDF as representative congeners containing two, three, and four lateral substituents, respectively. The ED_{50} values for antiestrogenicity were similar for the three compounds; however, the ED_{50} values for induction of hepatic CYP1A1-dependent activity were 73,600 (estimated), 8.52, and 5.31 µmol/kg for 6-*i*-propyl-1,3,8-triCDF, 6-methyl-2,3,4,8-tetraCDF, and 8-methyl-2,3,4,7-tetraCDF, respectively. Based on results of previous studies, CYP1A1 can be used as a surrogate for toxic potency in the rat; therefore, high ED_{50} (induction)/ED_{50} (antiestrogenicity) ratios would be indicative of low toxicity and high antiestrogenic potency. The ratio was 13,990 to 17,100 for 6-*i*-propyl-1,3,8-triCDF, whereas corresponding ratios for the compounds with three and four lateral substituents varied from 0.64 to 3.34. These data suggest that alternate 1,3,6,8-substituted alkyl PCDFs are useful structural models for developing new AhR-mediated antiestrogens for treatment of breast cancer.

The *in vivo* antitumorigenic activity of 6-MCDF, 8-MCDF, and 6-cyclohexyl-1,3,8-triCDF (6-CHDF) were investigated in the DMBA rat mammary

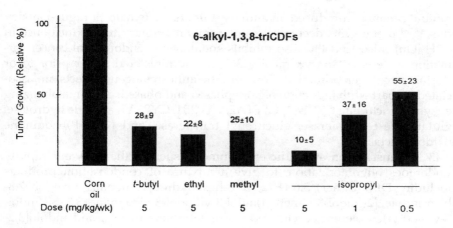

FIGURE 7.6

Comparative activities of 6-alkyl-1,3,8-triCDFs as inhibitors of DMBA-induced mammary tumor growth administered at a dose of 5 mg/kg/week.

tumor model.[160] At doses of 5, 10, or 25 mg/kg/week, 6- and 8-MCDF significantly inhibited mammary tumor growth, and at the 5 mg/kg/week dose, >50% growth inhibition was observed for both isomers. In contrast, 6-CHDF was inactive at the 5 mg/kg/week dose, and the structure-antitumorigenicity relationships (6-/8-MCDF » 6-CHDF) correlated with structure-antiestrogenicity (rat uterus) studies and the relative binding affinities of these compounds for the AhR. The antitumorigenic activity of 6- or 8-MCDF in the mammary was not accompanied by any significant changes in liver/body weight ratios, liver morphology, or induction of hepatic CYP1A1-dependent activity, which is one of the most sensitive indicators of exposure to AhR agonists. RT-PCR and Western blot analysis of mammary tumor mRNA and protein extracts, respectively, confirmed the presence of the AhR, suggesting that AhR-mediated signaling pathways are functional in rat mammary tumors. The effects of other alternate-substituted PCDFs have also been investigated. The results (Figure 7.6) clearly demonstrate that CH_3-substituted 1,3,6,8- and 2,4,6,8-PCDFs and other 6-alkyl PCDFs were potent antitumorigenic compounds. Dose-response studies with 6-isopropyl-1,3,8-triCDF showed that inhibition of mammary tumor growth was observed at doses as low as 0.5 mg/kg/week. Ongoing studies are investigating other alternate-substituted PCDFs to delineate specific congeners, which can be further developed for clinical applications.

7.2.3.3 Substituted DIMs

Indole-3-carbinol (I3C) is found as a conjugate in cruciferous vegetables such as broccoli, Brussels sprouts, and cauliflower;[161] results of several studies indicate that I3C is both anticarcinogenic and antiestrogenic in several bioassays.[162-171] For example, I3C, related compounds, and Brussels sprouts inhibit carcinogen-induced mammary tumors in female Sprague-Dawley rats;[168,169] dietary I3C decreases spontaneous mammary tumor incidence in C3H/OuJ mice, and I3C also inhibits spontaneous endometrial cancer formation in female Donryu rats.[171] I3C was administered either prior to or during carcinogen administration, and the anticarcinogenic effects are associated, in part, with induction of both phase I and phase II drug-metabolizing enzymes, including CYP1A1, CYP1A2, CYP2B1, CYP3A1, epoxide hydrolase, glutathione S-transferase, glucuronyl transferase, and NAD(P)H:quinone oxidoreductase.[169,172-186]

I3C is unstable in an acidic environment (such as the gut) and rapidly undergoes oligomerization, to give a mixture of condensation products including DIM (dimer), 5,6,11,12,17,18-hexahydrocyclononal[1,2-b:4,5-b':7,8-b"]triindole, [2-(indol-3-ylmethyl)indol-3-yl]indol-3-ylmethane, 3,3'-bis(indol-3-ylmethyl)indolenine, cyclic and linear tetramers of I3C, and indolo[3,2-b]carbazole (ICZ).[173,177,182,186,187] I3C binds weakly to the AhR, and the higher molecular weight condensation products exhibit increased binding affinity for this receptor.[181,186]

Previous studies have demonstrated that incubation of I3C with breast cancer cells results in formation of DIM, and both compounds induce CYP1A1 gene expression;[182-184] however, the concentrations required for an induction response were >30 (DIM) or >100 μM (I3C).[188] Ongoing studies in this laboratory have focused on the AhR agonist activities of DIM in MCF-7 cells.[189] The results show that after treatment of cells with DIM, there is depletion of cytosolic AhR, which rapidly translocates into the nucleus and forms an AhR-[^{32}P]DRE complex in a gel mobility shift assay; nuclear extracts form a 200-kD crosslinked band after photoinduced crosslinking with bromodeoxyuridine-substituted DRE. These results are consistent with a ligand-induced AhR-mediated response (e.g., Figure 7.2). However, it is clear from the results that antiestrogenic responses are observed at concentrations lower (0.1 to 60 μM) than required for induction of CYP1A1 gene expression (30 to 100 μM). Moreover, at a concentration of 10 μM, nuclear extracts from cells treated with DIM form a retarded band with [^{32}P]DRE and, like MCDF, DIM forms a nuclear AhR complex at concentrations that exhibit antiestrogenic activity but do not induce CYP1A1.

The antitumorigenic activity of DIM in the DMBA-induced rat mammary tumor model[189] was similar to that previously observed for alternate-substituted alkyl PCDFs.[160] At an oral dose of 5 mg/kg every second day, DIM significantly inhibited mammary tumor growth (Figure 7.7), but this was not accompanied by any changes in body or organ weights and histopathology (kidney, spleen, heart, uterus, or liver). Moreover, DIM did not induce hepatic microsomal EROD activity. Results of preliminary studies with other substituted-DIM and some I3C analogs show that these compounds inhibit rat mammary tumor growth at doses between 1 to 5 mg/kg (every other day), and current studies are focused on development of substituted-I3C/DIM compounds, which can be used for clinical treatment of breast cancer in women.

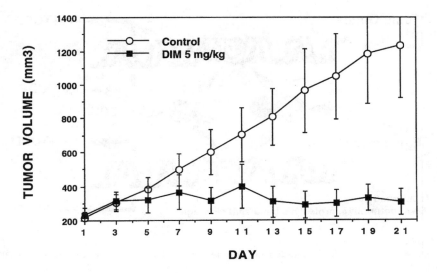

FIGURE 7.7
Inhibition of mammary tumor growth in vehicle (○) or DIM (■, 5 mg/kg every second day) treated female Sprague-Dawley rats initiated with DMBA.

The antiestrogenic/antitumorigenic activity of alternate-substituted PCDFs and DIM analogs is observed *in vivo* at doses that do not induce hepatic CYP1A1, which is one of the most sensitive indicators of exposure to toxic AhR agonists such as HAHs. Ligand-dependent differences in activity have been observed for other compounds that bind steroid hormone, such as the ER. A possible mechanism for AhR ligand-dependent differences is illustrated in Figure 7.8 using MCDF and TCDD as models. Both ligands induce rapid formation of a nuclear AhR complex, and TCDD induces a complete spectrum of AhR-mediated responses, including antiestrogenicity, induction of CYP1A1, and toxicity. In contrast, MCDF (or DIM) exhibits antiestrogenic activity at doses/concentrations that do not induce CYP1A1 and are not toxic. This suggests that MCDF (or DIM) induces conformational changes in the nuclear AhR complex, which allow binding to iDREs associated with inhibition of E2-induced genes; in contrast, the MCDF-AhR complex exhibits ineffective binding to DREs in promoters of CYP1A1 and other genes that play a role in toxic response pathways. Santostefano and Safe[190] studied ligand-dependent (e.g., TCDD vs. MCDF) differences in properties of the transformed cytosolic or nuclear AhR complex using a proteolytic clipping band shift assay. The results showed that there were significant differences in the pattern of degraded protein-DNA products using nuclear AhR complexes derived from mouse Hepa 1c1c7 cells treated with TCDD or MCDF, confirming ligand-dependent differences in the conformation of the nuclear AhR complex. Moreover, results of *in vivo* DNA footprinting studies show that in Hepa 1c1c7 cells treated with TCDD, a footprint was observed in the CYP1A1 gene promoter DRE, whereas 6-MCDF and I3C did

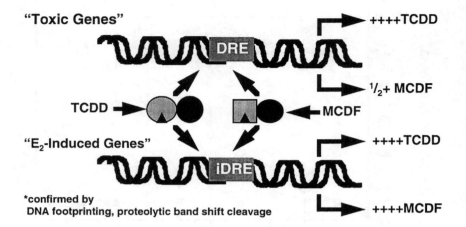

FIGURE 7.8
Proposed mechanism for ligand-dependent differences in the mechanisms of action of TCDD and MCDF.

not induce this footprint.[191] Current studies are focused on further development of relatively nontoxic AhR-based antiestrogens for clinical applications and studies, which delineate mechanisms of crosstalk between AhR- and ER-mediated signaling pathways.

Acknowledgments

The financial assistance of the National Institutes of Health (CA-64801 and ESO4176), Avax Technologies (Kansas City), the State of Texas Advanced Technology Program, and the Texas Agricultural Experiment Station is gratefully acknowledged. S. Safe is a Sid Kyle Professor of Toxicology.

References

1. Kutz, F. W., Wood, P. H., and Bottimore, D. P., Organochlorine pesticides and polychlorinated biphenyls in human adipose tissue, *Rev. Environ. Contamin. Toxicol.*, 120, 1, 1991.
2. Rappe, C., Dietary exposure and human levels of PCDDs and PCDFs, *Chemosphere*, 25, 231, 1992.
3. Rappe, C., Sources of exposure, environmental concentrations and exposure assessment of PCDDs and PCDFs, *Chemosphere*, 27, 211, 1993.

4. Colborn, T., Vom Saal, F. S., and Soto, A. M., Developmental effects of endocrine-disrupting chemicals in wildlife and humans, *Environ. Health Perspect.,* 101, 378, 1993.
5. Sharpe, R. M. and Skakkebaek, N. F., Are oestrogens involved in falling sperm counts and disorders of the male reproductive tract? *Lancet,* 341, 1392, 1993.
6. Sharpe, R. M., Reproductive biology. Another DDT connection, *Nature,* 375, 538, 1995.
7. Wolff, M. S., Toniolo, P. G., Leel, E. W., Rivera, M., and Dubin, N., Blood levels of organochlorine residues and risk of breast cancer, *J. Natl. Canc. Inst.,* 85, 648, 1993.
8. Falck, F., Ricci, A., Wolff, M. S., Godbold, J., and Deckers, P., Pesticides and polychlorinated biphenyl residues in human breast lipids and their relation to breast cancer, *Arch. Environ. Health,* 47, 143, 1992.
9. Davis, D. L., Bradlow, H. L., Wolff, M., Woodruff, T., Hoel, D. G., and Anton-Culver, H., Medical hypothesis: xenoestrogens as preventable causes of breast cancer, *Environ. Health Perspect.,* 101, 372, 1993.
10. Davis, D. L. and Bradlow, H. L., Can environmental estrogens cause breast cancer? *Sci. Am.,* 273, 166, 1995.
11. Wolff, M. S., Pesticides — how research has succeeded and failed in informing policy: DDT and the link with breast cancer, *Environ. Health Perspect.,* 103 (Suppl. 6), 87, 1995.
12. Krieger, N., Wolff, M. S., Hiatt, R. A., Rivera, M., Vogelman, J., and Orentreich, N., Breast cancer and serum organochlorines: a prospective study among white, black, and Asian women, *J. Natl. Canc. Inst.,* 86, 589, 1994.
13. López-Carrillo, L., Blair, A., López-Cervantes, M., Cebrián, M., Rueda, C., Reyes, R., Mohar, A., and Bravo, J., Dichlorodiphenyltrichloroethane serum levels and breast cancer risk: a case-control study from Mexico, *Canc. Res.* 57, 3728, 1997.
14. Van't Veer, P., Lobbezoo, I. R., Martin-Moreno, J. M., Guallar, F., Gomez-Aracena, J., Kardinaal, A. F. M., Kohlmeier, L., Martin, B. C., Strain, J. J., Thumm, M., Van Zoonen, P., Baumann, B. A., Huttunen, J. K., and Kok, F. J., DDT (dicophane) and postmenopausal breast cancer in Europe: case control study, *Br. J. Med.,* 315, 81, 1997.
15. Hunter, D. J., Hankinson, S. E., Laden, F., Colditz, G., Munson, J. E., Willett, W. C., Speizer, F. E., and Wolff, M. S., Plasma organochlorine levels and the risk of breast cancer, *N. Engl. J. Med.,* 337, 1253, 1997.
16. Safe, S., Environmental and dietary estrogens and human health — is there a problem? *Environ. Health Perspect.,* 103, 346, 1995.
17. Safe, S., Is there an association between exposure to environmental estrogen and breast cancer? *Environ. Health Perspect.,* 105(Suppl. 3), 675, 1997.
18. Bertazzi, P. A., Pesatori, A. C., Consonni, D., Tironi, A., Landi, M. T., and Zocchetti, C., Cancer incidence in a population accidentally exposed to 2,3,7,8-tetrachlorodibenzo-*p*-dioxin, *Epidemiology,* 4, 398, 1993.
19. Safe, S., Modulation of gene expression and endocrine response pathways by 2,3,7,8-tetrachlorodibenzo-*p*-dioxin and related compounds, *Pharmacol. Therap.,* 67, 247, 1995.
20. Goldstein, J. A. and Safe, S., Mechanism of action and structure-activity relationships for the chlorinated dibenzo-*p*-dioxins and related compounds, in *Halogenated Biphenyls, Naphthalenes, Dibenzodioxins and Related Compounds,* Kimbrough, R. D. and Jensen, A. A., Eds., Elsevier-North Holland, Amsterdam, 1989, 239.

21. Poland, A., Greenlee, W. F., and Kende, A. S., Studies on the mechanism of action of the chlorinated dibenzo-*p*-dioxins and related compounds, *Annu. N.Y. Acad. Sci.*, 320, 214, 1979.
22. Poland, A. and Knutson, J. C., 2,3,7,8-Tetrachlorodibenzo-*p*-dioxin and related halogenated aromatic hydrocarbons. Examinations of the mechanism of toxicity, *Annu. Rev. Pharmacol. Toxicol.*, 22, 517, 1982.
23. Safe, S., Comparative toxicology and mechanism of action of polychlorinated dibenzo-*p*-dioxins and dibenzofurans, *Annu. Rev. Pharmacol. Toxicol.*, 26, 371, 1986.
24. Whitlock, J. P., Jr., Mechanistic aspects of dioxin action, *Chem. Res. Toxicol.*, 6, 754, 1993.
25. Whitlock, J. P., Okino, S. T., Dong, L., Ko, H. P., Clarke-Katzenberg, R., Ma, Q., and Li, H., Induction of cytochrome P4501A1: a model for analyzing mammalian gene transcription, *FASEB J.*, 10, 809, 1996.
26. Rushmore, T. H. and Pickett, C. B., Glutathione *S*-transferases, structure, regulation, and therapeutic implications, *J. Biol. Chem.*, 268, 11475, 1993.
27. Pimental, R. A., Liang, B., Yee, G. K., Wilhelmsson, A., Poellinger, L., and Paulson, K. E., Dioxin receptor and C/EBP regulate the function of the glutathione S-transferase Ya gene xenobiotic response element, *Mol. Cell. Biol.*, 13, 4365, 1993.
28. Emi, Y., Ikushiro, S., and Iyanagi, T., Xenobiotic responsive element-mediated transcriptional activation in the UDP glucuronosyl transferase family 1 gene complex, *J. Biol. Chem.*, 271, 3952, 1996.
29. Jaiswal, A. K., Human NAD(P)H:quinone oxidoreductase: gene structure, activity and tissue-specific expression, *J. Biol. Chem.*, 269, 14502, 1994.
30. Asman, D. C., Takimoto, K., Pitot, H. C., Dunn, T. J., and Lindahl, R., Organization and characterization of the rat class 3 aldehyde dehydrogenase gene, *J. Biol. Chem.*, 268, 12530, 1993.
31. Choi, E. J., Toscano, D. G., Ryan, J. A., Riedel, N., and Toscano, W. A., Dioxin induced transforming growth factor-a in human keratinocytes, *J. Biol. Chem.*, 266, 9591, 1991.
32. Gaido, K. W., Maness, S. C., Leonard, L. S., and Greenlee, W. F., 2,3,7,8-Tetrachlorodibenzo-*p*-dioxin-dependent regulation of transforming growth factors-a and b_2 expression in a human keratinocyte cell line involves both transcriptional and post-transcriptional control, *J. Biol. Chem.*, 267, 24591, 1992.
33. Poland, A. and Glover, E., 2,3,7,8-Tetrachlorodibenzoo-*p*-dioxin: a potent inducer of d-aminolevulinic acid synthetase, *Science*, 179, 476, 1973.
34. Sutter, T. R., Guzman, K., Dold, K. M., and Greenlee, W. F., Targets for dioxin: genes for plasminogen activator inhibitor-2 and interleukin-1b, *Science*, 254, 415, 1991.
35. Puga, A., Nebert, D. W., and Carrier, F., Dioxin induces expression of c-*fos* and c-*jun* proto-oncogenes and a large increase in transcription factor AP-1, *DNA Cell Biol.*, 11, 269, 1992.
36. Kraemer, S. A., Arthur, K. A., Denison, M. S., Smith, W. L., and DeWitt, D. L., Regulation of prostaglandin endoperoxide H synthase-2 expression by 2,3,7,8,-tetrachlorodibenzo-p-dioxin, *Arch. Biochem. Biophys.*, 330, 319, 1996.
37. Liu, P. C., Phillips, M. A., and Matsumura, F., Alteration by 2,3,7,8-Tetrachlorodibenzo-p-dioxin of CCAAT/enhancer binding protein correlates with suppression of adipocyte differentiation in 3T3-L1 cells, *Mol. Pharmacol.*, 49, 989, 1996.

38. Wang, X., Porter, W., Krishnan, V., Narasimhan, T. R., and Safe, S., Mechanism of 2,3,7,8-tetrachlorodibenzo-*p*-dioxin (TCDD)-mediated decrease of the nuclear estrogen receptor in MCF-7 human breast cancer cells, *Mol. Cell. Endocrinol.*, 96, 159, 1993.

39. Lu, Y.-F., Wang, X., and Safe, S., Interaction of 2,3,7,8-tetrachlorodibenzo-*p*-dioxin and retinoic acid in MCF-7 human breast cancer cells, *Toxicol. Appl. Pharmacol.*, 127, 1, 1994.

40. Ishii, Y., Kato, H., Hatsumura, M., Ishida, T., Ariyoshi, N., and Oguri, K., Significant suppression of rat liver aldolase B by a toxic coplanar polychlorinated biphenyl, 3,3′,4,4′,5-pentachlorobiphenyl, *Toxicology*, 116, 193, 1997.

41. Stahl, B. U., 2,3,7,8-Tetrachlorodibenzo-p-dioxin blocks the physiological regulation of hepatic phosphoenolpyruvate carboxykinase activity in primary rat hepatocytes, *Toxicology*, 103, 45, 1995.

42. Ryu, B. W., Roy, S., Sparrow, B. R., Selivonchick, D. P., and Schaup, H. W., Ah receptor involvement in mediation of pyruvate carboxylase levels and activity in mice given 2,3,7,8-tetrachlorodibenzo-*p*-dioxin, *J. Biochem. Toxicol.*, 10, 103, 1995.

43. Runge-Morris, M. and Wilusz, J., Suppression of hydroxysteroid sulfotransferase-a gene expression by 3-methylcholanthrene, *Toxicol. Appl. Pharmacol.*, 125, 133, 1994.

44. Muralidhara, M., Matsumura, F., and Blankenship, A., 2,3,7,8-Tetrachlorodibenzo-*p*-dioxin (TCDD)-induced reduction of adenosine deaminase activity *in vivo* and *in vitro*, *J. Biochem.*, 9, 249, 1994.

45. Fox, T. R., Best, L. L., Goldsworthy, S. M., Mills, J. J., and Goldsworthy, T. L., Gene expression and cell proliferation in rat liver after 2,3,7,8-tetrachlorodibenzo-*p*-dioxin exposure, *Canc. Res.*, 53, 2265, 1993.

46. Poland, A., Glover, E., Robinson, J. R., and Nebert, D. W., Genetic expression of aryl hydrocarbon hydroxylase activity. Induction of monooxygenase activities and cytochrome, P-450 formation by 2,3,7,8-tetrachlorodibenzo-*p*-dioxin in mice generally 'nonresponsive' to other aromatic hydrocarbons, *J. Biol. Chem.*, 249, 5599, 1975.

47. Poland, A. and Glover, E., Genetic expression of aryl hydrocarbon hydroxylase by 2,3,7,8-tetrachlorodibenzo-*p*-dioxin: evidence for a receptor mutation in genetically nonresponsive mice, *Mol. Pharmacol.*, 11, 389, 1975.

48. Nebert, D. W., Robinson, J. R., Niwa, A., Kumaki, K., and Poland, A. P., Genetic expression of aryl hydrocarbon hydroxylase activity in the mouse, *J. Cell. Physiol.*, 85, 393, 1976.

49. Poland, A. and Glover, E., Chlorinated dibenzo-*p*-dioxins: potent inducer of d-aminolevulinic acid synthetase and aryl hydrocarbon hydroxylase. II. A study of the structure-activity relationship, *Mol. Pharmacol.*, 9, 736, 1973.

50. Poland, A., Glover, E., and Kende, A. S., Stereospecific, high affinity binding of 2,3,7,8-tetrachlorodibenzo-*p*-dioxin by hepatic cytosol: evidence that the binding species is receptor for induction of aryl hydrocarbon hydroxylase, *J. Biol. Chem.*, 251, 4936, 1976.

51. Poland, A. and Glover, E., Variation in the molecular mass of the Ah receptor among vertebrate species and strains of rats, *Biochem. Biophys. Res. Commun.*, 146, 1439, 1987.

52. Elferink, C. J., Gasiewicz, T. A., and Whitlock, J. P., Jr., Protein–DNA interactions at a dioxin-responsive enhancer. Evidence that the transformed Ah receptor is heteromeric, *J. Biol. Chem.*, 265, 20708, 1990.

53. Gasiewicz, T. A., Elferink, C. J., and Henry, E. C., Characterization of multiple forms of the Ah receptor: recognition of a dioxin-responsive enhancer involves heteromer formation, *Biochemistry,* 30, 2909, 1991.
54. Ema, M., Sogawa, K., Watanabe, N., Chujoh, Y., Matsushita, N., Gotoh, O., Funae, Y., and Fujii-Kuriyama, Y., cDNA cloning and structure of the putative Ah receptor, *Biochem. Biophys. Res. Commun.,* 184, 246, 1992.
55. Ema, M., Ohe, N., Suzuki, M., Mimura, J., Sogawa, K., Ikawa, S., and Fujii-Kuriyama, Y., Dioxin binding activities of polymorphic forms of mouse and human aryl hydrocarbon receptors, *J. Biol. Chem.,* 269, 27337, 1994.
56. Dolwick, K. M., Schmidt, J. V., Carver, L. A., Swanson, H. I., and Bradfield, C. A., Cloning and expression of a human Ah receptor cDNA, *Mol. Pharmacol.,* 44, 911, 1993.
57. Schmidt, J. V., Carver, L. A., and Bradfield, C. A., Molecular characterization of the murine *Ahr* gene: organization, promoter analysis, and chromosomal assignment, *J. Biol. Chem.,* 268, 22203, 1993.
58. Burbach, K. M., Poland, A. B., and Bradfield, C. A., Cloning of the Ah-receptor cDNA reveals a distinctive ligand-activated transcription factor, *Proc. Natl. Acad. Sci. U.S.A.,* 89, 8185, 1992.
59. Hoffman, E. C., Reyes, H., Chu, F., Sander, F., Conley, L. H., Brooks, B. A., and Hankinson, O., Cloning of a factor required for activity of the Ah (dioxin) receptor, *Science,* 252, 954, 1991.
60. Wilson, C. L., Thomsen, J., Hoivik, D. J., Wormke, M. T., Stanker, L., Holtzapple, C., and Safe, S. H., Aryl hydrocarbon (Ah)-nonresponsiveness in estrogen receptor-negative MDA-MB-231 cells is associated with expression of a variant Arnt protein, *Arch. Biochem. Biophys.,* 346, 65, 1997.
61. Gonzalez, F. J. and Nebert, D. W., Autoregulation plus upstream positive and negative control regions associated with transcriptional activation of the mouse cytochrome P_1-450 gene, *Nucl. Acids Res.,* 13, 7269, 1985.
62. Jones, P. B., Galeazzi, D. R., Fisher, J. M., and Whitlock, J. P., Jr., Control of cytochrome P_1-450 gene expression by dioxin, *Science,* 227, 1499, 1985.
63. Jones, P. B., Durrin, L. K., Galeazzi, D. R., and Whitlock, J. P., Jr., Control of cytochrome P_1-450 gene expression: analysis of a dioxin-responsive enhancer system, *Proc. Natl. Acad. Sci. U.S.A.,* 83, 2802, 1986.
64. Jones, P. B., Durrin, L. K., Fisher, J. M., and Whitlock, J. P., Jr., Control of gene expression by 2,3,7,8-tetrachlorodibenzo-*p*-dioxin: multiple dioxin-responsive domains 5'-ward of the cytochrome P_1-450 gene, *J. Biol. Chem.,* 261, 6647, 1986.
65. Neuhold, L. A., Shirayoshi, Y., Ozato, K., Jones, J. E., and Nebert, D. W., Regulation of mouse CYP1A1 gene expression by dioxin: requirement of two *cis*-acting elements during induction, *Mol. Cell. Biol.,* 9, 2378, 1989.
66. Sogawa, K., Fujisawa-Sehara, A., Yamane, M., and Fuji-Kuriyama, Y., Location of regulatory elements responsible for drug induction in the rat cytochrome P-450c gene, *Proc. Natl. Acad. Sci. U.S.A.,* 83, 8044, 1986.
67. Fujisawa-Sehara, A., Sogawa, K., Nishi, C., and Fujii-Kuriyama, Y., Regulatory DNA elements localized remotely upstream from the drug-metabolizing cytochrome P-450c gene, *Nucl. Acids Res.,* 14, 1465, 1986.
68. Yao, E. F. and Denison, M. S., DNA sequence determinants for binding of transformed Ah-receptor to a dioxin-responsive enhancer, *Biochemistry,* 31, 5060, 1992.

69. Shen, E. S. and Whitlock, J. P., Protein-DNA interactions at a dioxin-responsive enhancer — mutational analysis of the DNA-binding site for the liganded Ah receptor, *J. Biol. Chem.*, 267, 6815, 1992.

70. Quattrochi, L. C., Vu, T., and Tukey, R. H., The human *CYP1A2* gene and induction by 3-methylcholanthrene: a region of DNA that supports Ah-receptor binding and promoter-specific induction, *J. Biol. Chem.*, 269, 6949, 1994.

71. Wo, Y. P., Stewart, J., and Greenlee, W. F., Functional analysis of the promoter for the CYP1B1 gene, *J. Biol. Chem.*, 272, 26702, 1997.

72. Hankinson, O., Single-step selection of clones of a mouse hepatoma line deficient in aryl hydrocarbon hydroxylase, *Proc. Natl. Acad. Sci. U.S.A.*, 76, 373, 1979.

73. Hankinson, O., Unstable aryl hydrocarbon hydroxylase-deficient variants of a rat hepatoma line, *Somatic Cell Genet.*, 6, 751, 1980.

74. Hankinson, O., Dominant and recessive aryl hydrocarbon hydroxylase-deficient mutants of mouse hepatoma line, Hepa-1, and assignment of recessive mutants to three complementation groups, *Somatic Cell Genet.*, 9, 497, 1983.

75. Israel, D. I. and Whitlock, J. P., Jr., Induction of mRNA specific for cytochrome P_1-450 in wild type and variant mouse hepatoma cells, *J. Biol. Chem.*, 258, 10390, 1983.

76. Boucher, P. D., Ruch, R. J., and Hines, R. N., Specific nuclear protein binding to a negative regulatory element on the human *CYP1A1* gene, *J. Biol. Chem.*, 268, 17384, 1993.

77. Sterling, K., Weaver, J., Ho, K. L., Xu, L. C., and Bresnick, E., Rat *CYP1A1* negative regulatory element: biological activity and interaction with a protein from liver and hepatoma cells, *Mol. Pharmacol.*, 44, 560, 1993.

78. Israel, D. I., Estolano, M. G., Galeazzi, D. R., and Whitlock, J. P., Jr., Superinduction of cytochrome P_1-450 gene transcription by inhibition of protein synthesis in wild type and variant mouse hepatoma cells, *J. Biol. Chem.*, 260, 5648, 1985.

79. Vickers, P. J., Dufresne, M. J., and Cowan, K. H., Relation between cytochrome P4501A1 expression and estrogen receptor content of human breast cancer cells, *Mol. Endocrinol.*, 3, 157, 1989.

80. Thomsen, J. S., Nissen, L., Stacey, S. N., Hines, R. N., and Autrup, H., Differences in 2,3,7,8-tetrachlorodibenzo-*p*-dioxin-inducible CYP1A1 expression in human breast carcinoma cell lines involve altered transacting factors, *Eur. J. Biochem.*, 197, 577, 1991.

81. Thomsen, J. S., Wang, X., Hines, R. N., and Safe, S., Restoration of Ah responsiveness in MDA-MB-231 human breast cancer cells by transient expression of the estrogen receptor, *Carcinogenesis*, 15, 933, 1994.

82. Wang, W. L., Thomsen, J. S., Porter, W., Moore, M., and Safe, S., Effect of transient expression of the estrogen receptor on constitutive and inducible CYP1A1 in Hs578T human breast cancer cells, *Br. J. Canc.*, 73, 316, 1996.

83. Hoivik, D., Wilson, C., Wang, W., Willett, K., Barhoumi, R., Burghardt, R., and Safe, S., Studies on the relationship between estrogen receptor content, glutathione S-transferase p expression and induction by 2,3,7,8-tetrachlorodibenzo-*p*-dioxin and drug resistance in human breast cancer cells, *Arch. Biochem. Biophys.*, 348, 174, 1997.

84. Wang, W., Porter, W., Burghardt, R., and Safe, S., Mechanism of inhibition of MDA-MB-468 breast cancer cell growth by 2,3,7,8-tetrachlorodibenzo-*p*-dioxin, *Carcinogenesis*, 18, 925, 1997.

85. Moore, M., Wang, X., Lu, Y.-F., Wormke, M., Craig, A., Gerlach, J., Burghardt, R., and Safe, S., Benzo[a]pyrene resistant (BaP^R) human breast cancer cells: a unique aryl hydrocarbon (Ah)-nonresponsive clone, *J. Biol. Chem.*, 269, 11751, 1994.

86. Wang, X., Thomsen, J. S., Santostefano, M., Rosengren, R., Safe, S., and Perdew, G. H., Comparative properties of the nuclear Ah receptor complex from several human cell lines, *Eur. J. Pharmacol.*, 293, 191, 1995.

87. Wilson, C. L., Identification and Characterization of an Aryl Hydrocarbon Receptor Nuclear Translocator Protein Variant, Ph.D. diss., Texas A&M University, College Station, TX, 1997.

88. Kärenlampi, S. O., Eisen, H. J., Hankinson, O., and Nebert, D. W., Effects of cytochrome P_1-450 inducers on the cell-surface receptors for epidermal growth factor, phorbol 12,13-dibutyrate, or insulin of cultured mouse hepatoma cells, *J. Biol. Chem.*, 258, 10378, 1983.

89. Madhukar, B. V., Brewster, D. W., and Matsumura, F., Effects of *in vivo*-administered 2,3,7,8-tetrachlorodibenzo-*p*-dioxin on receptor binding of epidermal growth factor in the hepatic plasma membrane of rat, guinea pig, mouse, and hamster, *Proc. Natl. Acad. Sci. U.S.A.*, 81, 7407, 1984.

90. Madhukar, B. V., Ebner, K., Matsumura, F., Bombick, D. W., Brewster, D. W., and Kawamoto, T., 2,3,7,8-Tetrachlorodibenzo-*p*-dioxin causes an increase in protein kinases associated with epidermal growth factor receptor in the hepatic plasma membrane, *J. Biochem. Toxicol.*, 3, 261, 1988.

91. Astroff, B. and Safe, S., 2,3,7,8-Tetrachlorodibenzo-*p*-dioxin as an antiestrogen: effect on rat uterine peroxidase activity, *Biochem. Pharmacol.*, 39, 485, 1990.

92. Lin, F. H., Stohs, S. J., Birnbaum, L. S., Clark, G., Lucier, G. W., and Goldstein, J. A., The effects of 2,3,7,8-tetrachlorodibenzo-*p*-dioxin (TCDD) on the hepatic estrogen and glucocorticoid receptors in congenic strains of Ah-responsive and Ah-nonresponsive C57BL/6 mice, *Toxicol. Appl. Pharmacol.*, 108, 129, 1991.

93. Sunahara, G. I., Lucier, G. W., McCoy, Z., Bresnick, E. H., Sanchez, E. R., and Nelson, K. G., Characterization of 2,3,7,8-tetrachlorodibenzo-*p*-dioxin-mediated decreases in dexamethasone binding to rat hepatic cytosolic glucocorticoid receptor, *Mol. Pharmacol.*, 36, 239, 1989.

94. Fernandez, P. and Safe, S., Growth inhibitory and antimitogenic activity of 2,3,7,8-tetrachlorodibenzo-*p*-dioxin (TCDD) in T47D human breast cancer cells, *Toxicol. Lett.*, 61, 185, 1992.

95. Fernandez, P., Burghardt, R., Smith, R., Nodland, K., and Safe, S., High passage T47D human breast cancer cells: altered endocrine and 2,3,7,8-tetrachlorodibenzo-*p*-dioxin responsiveness, *Eur. J. Pharmacol.*, 270, 53, 1994.

96. Liu, H., Biegel, L., Narasimhan, T. R., Rowlands, C., and Safe, S., Inhibition of insulin-like growth factor-I responses in MCF-7 cells by 2,3,7,8-tetrachlorodibenzo-*p*-dioxin and related compounds, *Mol. Cell. Endocrinol.*, 87, 19, 1992.

97. Mebus, C. A. and Piper, W. N., Decreased rat adrenal 21-hydroxylase activity associated with decreased adrenal microsomal cytochrome P-450 after exposure to 2, 3,7,8-tetrachlorodibenzo-*p*-dioxin, *Biochem. Pharmacol.*, 35, 4359, 1986.

98. Kleeman, J. M., Moore, R. W., and Peterson, R. E., Inhibition of testicular steroidogenesis in 2,3,7,8-tetrachlorodibenzo-*p*-dioxin-treated rats: evidence that the key lesion occurs prior to or during pregnenolone formation, *Toxicol. Appl. Pharmacol.*, 106, 112, 1990.

99. Spink, D. C., Lincoln, D. W., Dickerman, H. W., and Gierthy, J. F., 2,3,7,8-Tetra-chlorodibenzo-*p*-dioxin causes an extensive alteration of 17b-estradiol metabolism in human breast cancer cells, *Proc. Natl. Acad. Sci. U.S.A.*, 87, 6917, 1990.

100. Spink, D. C., Eugster, H., Lincoln, D. W., II, Schuetz, J. D., Schuetz, E. G., Johnson, J. A., Kaminsky, L. S., and Gierthy, J. F., 17b-Estradiol hydroxylation catalyzed by human cytochrome P4501A1: a comparison of the activities induced by 2,3,7,8-tetrachlorodibenzo-*p*-dioxin in MCF-7 cells with those from heterologous expression of the cDNA, *Arch. Biochem. Biophys.*, 293, 342, 1992.

101. Spink, D. C., Johnson, J. A., Connor, S. P., Aldous, K. M., and Gierthy, J. F., Stimulation of 17b-estradiol metabolism in MCF-7 cells by bromochloro- and chloromethyl-substituted dibenzo-*p*-dioxins and dibenzofurans: correlations with antiestrogenic activity, *J. Toxicol. Environ. Health*, 41, 451, 1994.

102. Hayes, C. L., Spink, D. C., Spink, B. C., Cao, J. Q., Walker, N. J., and Sutter, T. R., 17b-Estradiol hydroxylation catalyzed by human cytochrome P450 1B1, *Proc. Natl. Acad. Sci. U.S.A.*, 93, 9776, 1996.

103. Kociba, R. J., Keyes, D. G., Beger, J. E., Carreon, R. M., Wade, C. E., Dittenber, D. A., Kalnins, R. P., Frauson, L. E., Park, C. L., Barnard, S. D., Hummel, R. A., and Humiston, C. G., Results of a 2-year chronic toxicity and oncogenicity study of 2,3,7,8-tetrachlorodibenzo-*p*-dioxin (TCDD) in rats, *Toxicol. Appl. Pharmacol.*, 46, 279, 1978.

104. Holcomb, M. and Safe, S., Inhibition of 7,12-dimethylbenzanthracene-induced rat mammary tumor growth by 2,3,7,8-tetrachlorodibenzo-*p*-dioxin, *Canc. Lett.*, 82, 43, 1994.

105. Tritscher, A. M., Clark, G. C., Sewall, C., Sills, R. C., Maronpot, R., and Lucier, G. W., Persistence of TCDD-induced hepatic cell proliferation and growth of enzyme altered foci after chronic exposure followed by cessation of treatment in DEN initiated female rats, *Carcinogenesis*, 16, 2807, 1995.

106. Gierthy, J. F., Bennett, J. A., Bradley, L. M., and Cutler, D. S., Correlation of *in vitro* and *in vivo* growth suppression of MCF-7 human breast cancer by 2,3,7,8-tetrachlorodibenzo-*p*-dioxin, *Canc. Res.*, 53, 3149, 1993.

107. Reggiani, G., Acute human exposure to TCDD in Seveso, Italy, *J. Toxicol. Environ. Health*, 6, 27, 1980.

108. Mocarelli, P., Brambilia, P., Gerthoux, P. M., Patterson, D. G., and Needham, L. I., Change in sex ratio with exposure to dioxin, *Lancet*, 348, 409, 1996.

109. Umbreit, T. H. and Gallo, M. A., Physiological implications of estrogen receptor modulation by 2,3,7,8-tetrachlorodibenzo-*p*-dioxin, *Toxicol. Lett.*, 42, 5, 1988.

110. Umbreit, T. H., Hesse, E. J., MacDonald, G. J., and Gallo, M. A., Effects of TCDD-estradiol interactions in three strains of mice, *Toxicol. Lett.*, 40, 1, 1988.

111. Umbreit, T. H., Scala, P. L., MacKenzie, S. A., and Gallo, M. A., Alteration of the acute toxicity of 2,3,7,8-tetrachlorodibenzo-*p*-dioxin (TCDD) by estradiol and tamoxifen, *Toxicology*, 59, 163, 1989.

112. Gallo, M. A., Hesse, E. J., MacDonald, G. J., and Umbreit, T. H., Interactive effects of estradiol and 2,3,7,8-tetrachlorodibenzo-*p*-dioxin on hepatic cytochrome P-450 and mouse uterus, *Toxicol. Lett.*, 32, 123, 1986.

113. Johnson, D. C., Sen, M., and Dey, S. K., Differential effects of dichlorodiphenyltrichloroethane analogs, chlordecone, and 2,3,7,8-tetrachlorodibenzo-*p*-dioxin on establishment of pregnancy in the hypophysectomized rat, *Proc. Soc. Exp. Biol. Med.*, 199, 42, 1992.

114. Brown, N. M. and Lamartiniere, C. A., Xenoestrogens alter mammary gland differentiation and cell proliferation in the rat, *Environ. Health Perspect.*, 103, 708, 1995.

115. Romkes, M. and Safe, S., Comparative activities of 2,3,7,8-tetrachlorodibenzo-*p*-dioxin and progesterone on antiestrogens in the female rat uterus, *Toxicol. Appl. Pharmacol.*, 92, 368, 1988.

116. Romkes, M., Piskorska-Pliszczynska, J., and Safe, S., Effects of 2,3,7,8-tetrachlorodibenzo-*p*-dioxin on hepatic and uterine estrogen receptor levels in rats, *Toxicol. Appl. Pharmacol.*, 87, 306, 1987.

117. Astroff, B. and Safe, S., Comparative antiestrogenic activities of 2,3,7,8-tetrachlorodibenzo-*p*-dioxin and 6-methyl-1,3,8-trichlorodibenzofuran in the female rat, *Toxicol. Appl. Pharmacol.*, 95, 435, 1988.

118. Astroff, B., Rowlands, C., Dickerson, R., and Safe, S., 2,3,7,8-Tetrachlorodibenzo-*p*-dioxin inhibition of 17b-estradiol-induced increases in rat uterine EGF receptor binding activity and gene expression, *Mol. Cell. Endocrinol.*, 72, 247, 1990.

119. Astroff, B., Eldridge, B., and Safe, S., Inhibition of 17b-estradiol-induced and constitutive expression of the cellular protooncogene c-*fos* by 2,3,7,8-tetrachlorodibenzo-*p*-dioxin (TCDD) in the female uterus, *Toxicol. Lett.*, 56, 305, 1991.

120. Hyder, S. M., Chiappetta, C., Murthy, L., and Stancel, G. M., Selective inhibition of estrogen-regulated gene expression *in vivo* by the pure antiestrogen ICI 182,780, *Canc. Res.*, 57, 2547, 1997.

121. Brooks, S. C., Locke, E. R., and Soule, H. D., Estrogen receptor in a human cell line (MCF-7) from breast carcinoma, *J. Biol. Chem.*, 248, 6251, 1973.

122. Levenson, A. S. and Jordan, V. C., MCF-7: the first hormone-responsive breast cancer cell line, *Canc. Res.*, 57, 3071, 1997.

123. Harris, M., Piskorska-Pliszczynska, J., Zacharewski, T., Romkes, M., and Safe, S., Structure-dependent induction of aryl hydrocarbon hydroxylase in human breast cancer cell lines and characterization of the Ah receptor, *Canc. Res.*, 49, 4531, 1989.

124. Gierthy, J. F., Lincoln, D. W., Gillespie, M. B., Seeger, J. I., Martinez, H. L., Dickerman, H. W., and Kumar, S. A., Suppression of estrogen-regulated extracellular plasminogen activator activity of MCF-7 cells by 2,3,7,8-tetrachlorodibenzo-*p*-dioxin, *Canc. Res.*, 47, 6198, 1987.

125. Gierthy, J. F. and Lincoln, D. W., Inhibition of postconfluent focus production in cultures of MCF-7 breast cancer cells by 2,3,7,8-tetrachlorodibenzo-*p*-dioxin, *Breast Canc. Res.*, 12, 227, 1988.

126. Biegel, L. and Safe, S., Effects of 2,3,7,8-tetrachlorodibenzo-*p*-dioxin (TCDD) on cell growth and the secretion of the estrogen-induced 34-, 52- and 160-kDa proteins in human breast cancer cells, *J. Steroid Biochem. Mol. Biol.*, 37, 725, 1990.

127. Krishnan, V. and Safe, S., Polychlorinated biphenyls (PCBs), dibenzo-*p*-dioxins (PCDDs) and dibenzofurans (PCDFs) as antiestrogens in MCF-7 human breast cancer cells: quantitative structure-activity relationships, *Toxicol. Appl. Pharmacol.*, 120, 55, 1993.

128. Krishnan, V., Narasimhan, T. R., and Safe, S., Development of gel staining techniques for detecting the secretion of procathepsin D (52-kDa protein) in MCF-7 human breast cancer cells, *Anal. Biochem.*, 204, 137, 1992.

129. Krishnan, V., Porter, W., Santostefano, M., Wang, X., and Safe, S., Molecular mechanism of inhibition of estrogen-induced cathepsin D gene expression by 2,3,7,8-tetrachlorodibenzo-*p*-dioxin (TCDD) in MCF-7 cells, *Mol. Cell. Biol.*, 15, 6710, 1995.

130. Moore, M., Narasimhan, T. R., Wang, X., Krishnan, V., Safe, S., Williams, H. J., and Scott, A. I., Interaction of 2,3,7,8-tetrachlorodibenzo-*p*-dioxin, 12-*O*-tetradecanoylphorbol-13-acetate (TPA) and 17b-estradiol in MCF-7 human breast cancer cells, *J. Steroid Biochem. Mol. Biol.*, 44, 251, 1993.

131. Narasimhan, T. R., Safe, S., Williams, H. J., and Scott, A. I., Effects of 2,3,7,8-tetrachlorodibenzo-*p*-dioxin on 17b-estradiol-induced glucose metabolism in MCF-7 human breast cancer cells: ^{13}C-nuclear magnetic resonance studies, *Mol. Pharmacol.*, 40, 1029, 1991.

132. Harper, N., Wang, X., Liu, H., and Safe, S., Inhibition of estrogen-induced progesterone receptor in MCF-7 human breast cancer cells by aryl hydrocarbon (Ah) receptor agonists, *Mol. Cell. Endocrinol.*, 104, 47, 1994.

133. Zacharewski, T., Bondy, K., McDonell, P., and Wu, Z. F., Antiestrogenic effects of 2,3,7,8-tetrachlorodibenzo-*p*-dioxin on 17b-estradiol-induced pS2 expression, *Canc. Res.*, 54, 2707, 1994.

134. Lu, Y.-F., Sun, G., Wang, X., and Safe, S., Inhibition of prolactin receptor gene expression by 2,3,7,8-tetrachlorodibenzo-*p*-dioxin in MCF-7 human breast cancer cells, *Arch. Biochem. Biophys.*, 332, 35, 1996.

135. Gillesby, B., Santostefano, M., Porter, W., Wu, Z. F., Safe, S., and Zacharewski, T., Identification of a motif within the 5′-regulatory region on pS2 which is responsible for Ap1 binding and TCDD-mediated suppression, *Biochemistry*, 36, 6080, 1997.

136. Nodland, K. I., Wormke, M., and Safe, S., Inhibition of estrogen-induced activity by 2,3,7,8-tetrachlorodibenzo-*p*-dioxin (TCDD) in the MCF-7 human breast cancer and other cell lines transfected with vitellogenin A2 gene promoter constructs, *Arch. Biochem. Biophys.*, 338, 67, 1997.

137. Parker, M. G., Action of "pure" antiestrogens in inhibiting estrogen receptor action, *Breast Canc. Res., Treat.*, 26, 131, 1993.

138. Liu, H. and Safe, S., Effects of 2,3,7,8-tetrachlorodibenzo-*p*-dioxin (TCDD) on insulin-induced responses in MCF-7 human breast cancer cells, *Toxicol. Appl. Pharmacol.*, 138, 242, 1996.

139. Foster, J. S. and Wimalasena, J., Estrogen regulates activity of cyclin-dependent kinases and retinoblastoma protein phosphorylation in breast cancer cells, *Mol. Endocrinol.*, 10, 488, 1996.

140. Prall, O. W. J., Sarcevic, B., Musgrove, E. A., Watts, C. K. W., and Sutherland, R. L., Estrogen-induced activation of Cdk4 and Cdk2 during G_1-S phase progression is accompanied by increased cyclin D1 expression and decreased cyclin-dependent kinase inhibitor association with cyclin E-Cdk2, *J. Biol. Chem.*, 272, 10882, 1997.

141. Planas-Silva, M. D. and Weinberg, R. A., Estrogen-dependent cyclin E-cdk2 activation through p21 redistribution, *Mol. Cell. Biol.*, 17, 4059, 1997.

142. Musgrove, E. A., Hamilton, J. A., Lee, C. S., Sweeney, K. J., Watts, C. K., and Sutherland, R. L., Growth factor, steroid, and steroid antagonist regulation of cyclin gene expression associated with changes in T-47D human breast cancer cell cycle progression, *Mol. Cell. Biol.*, 13, 3577, 1993.

143. Wang, W., Smith, R., and Safe, S., Aryl hydrocarbon receptor-mediated antiestrogenicity in MCF-7 cells: modulation of hormone-induced cell cycle enzymes, *Arch. Biochem. Biophys.*, 356, 239, 1998.

144. Harris, M., Zacharewski, T., and Safe, S., Effects of 2,3,7,8-tetrachlorodibenzo-*p*-dioxin and related compounds on the occupied nuclear estrogen receptor in MCF-7 human breast cancer cells, *Canc. Res.*, 50, 3579, 1990.

145. Gierthy, J. F., Lincoln, D. W., Kampcik, S. J., Dickerman, H. W., Bradlow, H. L., Niwa, T., and Swaneck, G. E., Enhancement of 2- and 16a-estradiol hydroxylation in MCF-7 human breast cancer cells by 2,3,7,8-tetrachlorodibenzo-*p*-dioxin, *Biochem. Biophys. Res. Commun.*, 157, 515, 1988.

146. Shiverick, K. T. and Muther, T. F., Effects of 2,3,7,8-tetrachlorodibenzo-*p*-dioxin on serum concentrations and the uterotrophic actions of exogenous estrone in rats, *Toxicol. Appl. Pharmacol.*, 65, 170, 1982.

147. Wang, F., Porter, W., Xing, W., Archer, T. K., and Safe, S., Identification of a functional imperfect estrogen responsive element in the 5'-promoter region of the human cathepsin D gene, *Biochemistry*, 36, 7793, 1997.

148. Wang, F. and Safe, S., Functional and physical interactions between the estrogen receptor-Sp1 and the nuclear aryl hydrocarbon receptor complexes, *Nucl. Acids Res.*, 26, 3044, 1998.

149. Baron, J. A., La Vecchia, C., and Levi, F., The antiestrogenic effect of cigarette smoking in women, *Am. J. Obstet. Gynecol.*, 162, 502, 1990.

150. Lesko, S. M., Rosenberg, L., Kaufman, D. W., Helmrich, S. P., Miller, D. R., Strom, B., Schottenfeld, D., Rosenschein, N. B., Knapp, R. C., Lewis, J., and Shapiro, S., Cigarette smoking and the risk of endometrial cancer, *N. Engl. J. Med.*, 313, 593, 1985.

151. Chaloupka, K., Krishnan, V., and Safe, S., Polynuclear aromatic hydrocarbon carcinogens as antiestrogens in MCF-7 human breast cancer cells. Role of the Ah receptor, *Carcinogenesis*, 13, 2223, 1992.

152. Harris, M., Zacharewski, T., Astroff, B., and Safe, S. Partial antagonism of 2,3,7,8-tetrachlorodibenzo-*p*-dioxin-mediated induction of aryl hydrocarbon hydroxylase by 6-methyl-1,3,8-trichlorodibenzofuran: mechanistic studies, *Mol. Pharmacol.*, 35, 729, 1989.

153. Bannister, R., Biegel, L., Davis, D., Astroff, B., and Safe, S., 6-Methyl-1,3,8-trichlorodibenzofuran (MCDF) as a 2,3,7,8-tetrachlorodibenzo-*p*-dioxin antagonist in C57BL/6 mice, *Toxicology*, 54, 139, 1989.

154. Yao, C. and Safe, S., 2,3,7,8-Tetrachlorodibenzo-*p*-dioxin-induced porphyria in genetically inbred mice: partial antagonism and mechanistic studies, *Toxicol. Appl. Pharmacol.*, 100, 208, 1989.

155. Astroff, B., Zacharewski, T., Safe, S., Arlotto, M. P., Parkinson, A., Thomas, P., and Levin, W., 6-Methyl-1,3,8-trichlorodibenzofuran as a 2,3,7,8-tetrachlorodibenzo-*p*-dioxin antagonist: inhibition of the induction of rat cytochrome P-450 isozymes and related monooxygenase activities, *Mol. Pharmacol.*, 33, 231, 1988.

156. Astroff, B. and Safe, S., 6-Alkyl-1,3,8-trichlorodibenzofurans as antiestrogens in female Sprague-Dawley rats, *Toxicology*, 69, 187, 1991.

157. Zacharewski, T., Harris, M., Biegel, L., Morrison, V., Merchant, M., and Safe, S., 6-Methyl-1,3,8-trichlorodibenzofuran (MCDF) as an antiestrogen in human and rodent cancer cell lines: evidence for the role of the Ah receptor, *Toxicol. Appl. Pharmacol.*, 13, 311, 1992.

158. Sun, G. and Safe, S., Antiestrogenic activities of alternate substituted polychlorinated dibenzofurans in MCF-7 human breast cancer cells, *Canc. Chemother. Pharmacol.*, 40, 239, 1997.

159. Dickerson, R., Howie-Keller, L., and Safe, S., Alkyl polychlorinated dibenzofurans and related compounds as antiestrogens in the female rat uterus: structure-activity studies, *Toxicol. Appl. Pharmacol.*, 135, 287, 1995.

160. McDougal, A., Wilson, C., and Safe, S., Inhibition of 7,12-dimethyl-benz[a]antracene-induced rat mammary tumor growth by aryl hydrocarbon receptor agonists, *Canc. Lett.*, 120, 53, 1997.
161. Preobrazhenskaya, M. N., Bukhman, V. M., Korolev, A. M., and Efimov, S. A., Ascorbigen and other indole-derived compounds from *Brassica* vegetables and their analogs as anticarcinogenic and immunomodulating agents, *Pharmacol. Ther.*, 60, 301, 1993.
162. Wattenberg, L. W. and Loub, W. D., Inhibition of aromatic hydrocarbon-induced neoplasia by naturally occurring indoles, *Canc. Res.*, 38, 1410, 1978.
163. Nixon, J. E., Hendricks, J. D., Pawlowski, N. E., Pereira, C. B., Sinnhuber, R. O., and Bailey, G. S., Inhibition of aflatoxin B$_1$ carcinogenesis in rainbow trout by flavone and indole compounds, *Carcinogenesis*, 5, 615, 1984.
164. Kim, D. J., Lee, K. K., Han, B. S., Ahn, B., Bae, J. H., and Jang, J. J., Biphasic modifying effect on indole-3-carbinol on diethylnitrosamine-induced preneoplastic glutathione S-transferase placental form-positive liver cell foci in Sprague-Dawley rats, *Jpn. J. Canc. Res.*, 85, 578, 1994.
165. Morse, M. A., LaGreca, S. D., Amin, S. G., and Chung, F. L., Effects of indole-3-carbinol on lung tumorigenesis and DNA methylation induced by 4-(methylnitrosamino)-1-(3-pyridl)-1-butanone (NNK) and on the metabolism and disposition of NNK in A/J mice, *Canc. Res.*, 50, 1613, 1990.
166. Tanaka, T., Kojima, T., Morishita, Y., and Mori, H., Inhibitory effects of the natural products indole-3-carbinol and sinigrin during initiation and promotion phases of 4-nitroquinoline 1-oxide-induced rat tongue carcinogenesis, *Jpn. J. Canc. Res.*, 83, 835, 1992.
167. Tanaka, T., Mori, Y., Morishita, Y., Hara, A., Ohno, T., Kojima, T., and Mori, H., Inhibitory effect of sinigrin and indole-3-carbinol in diethylnitrosamine-induced hepatocarcinogenesis in male ACI/N rats, *Carcinogenesis*, 11, 1403, 1990.
168. Stoewsand, G. S., Anderson, J. L., and Munson, L., Protective effect of dietary brussels sprouts against mammary carcinogenesis in Sprague-Dawley rats, *Canc. Lett.*, 39, 199, 1988.
169. Grubbs, C. J., Steele, V. E., Casebolt, T., Juliana, M. M., Eto, I., Whitaker, L. M., Dragnev, K. H., Kelloff, G. J., and Lubet, R. L., Chemoprevention of chemically-induced mammary carcinogenesis by indole-3-carbinol, *Anticanc. Res.*, 15, 709, 1995.
170. Bradlow, H. L., Michnovicz, J. J., Telang, N. T., and Osborne, M. P., Effects of dietary indole-3-carbinol on estradiol metabolism and spontaneous mammary tumors in mice, *Carcinogenesis*, 12, 1571, 1991.
171. Kojima, T., Tanaka, T., and Mori, H., Chemoprevention of spontaneous endometrial cancer in female Donryu rats by dietary indol-3-carbinol, *Canc. Res.*, 54, 1446, 1994.
172. Stresser, D. M., Williams, D. E., McLellan, L. I., Harris, T. M., and Bailey, G. S., Indole-3-carbinol induces a rat liver glutathione transferase subunit (Yc2) with high activity toward aflatoxin B$_1$ *exo*-epoxide: association with reduced levels of hepatic aflatoxin-DNA adducts *in vivo*, *Drug Metab. Dispos.*, 22, 392, 1994.
173. Wortelboer, H. M., De Kruif, C. A., Van Iersel, A. J., Falke, H. E., Noordhoek, J., and Blaauboer, B. J., Acid reaction products of indole-3-carbinol and their effects on cytochrome P450 and phase II enzymes in rat and monkey hepatocytes, *Biochem. Pharmacol.*, 43, 1439, 1992.

174. Bradfield, C. A. and Bjeldanes, L. F., Effect of dietary indole-3-carbinol on intestinal and hepatic monooxygenase, glutathione *S*-transferase and epoxide hydrolase activities in the rat, *Food Chem. Toxicol.*, 22, 977, 1984.

175. Wortelboer, H. M., Van der Linder, E. C., de Truif, C. A., Noordhock, J., Blaaubar, B. J., Van Bladeren, P. J., and Falke, F. C., Effects of indole-3-carbinol on biotransformation enzymes in the rat: *in vivo* changes in liver and small intestinal mucosa in comparison with primary hepatocyte cultures, *Food Chem. Toxicol.*, 30, 589, 1992.

176. Baldwin, W. S. and LeBlanc, G. A., The anti-carcinogenic plant compound indole-3-carbinol differentially modulates P450-mediated steroid hydroxylase activities in mice, *Chem. Biol. Interact.*, 83, 155, 1992.

177. De Kruif, C. A., Marsman, J. W., Venekamp, J. C., Falke, H. E., Noordhoek, J., Blaauboer, B. J., and Wortelboer, H. M., Structure elucidation of acid reaction products of indole-3-carbinol: detection *in vivo* and enzyme induction *in vitro*, *Chem. Biol. Interact.*, 80, 303, 1991.

178. Tiwari, R. K., Guo, L., Bradlow, H. L., Telang, N. T., and Osborne, M. P., Selective responsiveness of breast cancer cells to indole-3-carbinol, a chemopreventative agent, *J. Natl. Canc. Inst.*, 86, 126, 1994.

179. Vang, O., Jensen, H., and Autrup, H., Induction of cytochrome P-450IA1, IA2, IIB1, IIB2 and IIE1 by broccoli in rat liver and colon, *Chem. Biol. Interact.*, 78, 85, 1991.

180. Vang, O., Jensen, M. B., and Autrup, H., Induction of cytochrome P450IA1 in rat colon and liver by indole-3-carbinol and 5,6-benzoflavone, *Carcinogenesis*, 11, 1259, 1990.

181. Jellinck, P. H., Forkert, P. G., Riddick, D. S., Okey, A. B., Michnovicz, J. J., and Bradlow, H. L., Ah receptor binding properties of indole carbinols and induction of hepatic estradiol hydroxylation, *Biochem. Pharmacol.*, 43, 1129, 1993.

182. Niwa, T., Swaneck, G., and Bradlow, H. L., Alterations in estradiol metabolism in MCF-7 cells induced by treatment with indole-3-carbinol and related compounds, *Steroids*, 59, 523, 1994.

183. Michnovicz, J. J. and Bradlow, H. L., Induction of estradiol metabolism by dietary indole-3-carbinol in humans, *J. Natl. Canc. Inst.*, 82, 947, 1990.

184. Jellinck, P. H., Michnovicz, J. J., and Bradlow, H. L., Influence of indole-3-carbinol on the hepatic microsomal formation of catechol estrogens, *Steroids*, 56, 446, 1991.

185. Jellinck, P. H., Newcombe, A., Forkert, P. G., and Martucci, C. P., Distinct forms of hepatic androgen 6b-hydroxylase induced in the rat by indole-3-carbinol and pregnenolone carbonitrile, *J. Steroid Biochem. Mol. Biol.*, 51, 219, 1994.

186. Bjeldanes, L. F., Kim, J. Y., Grose, K. R., Bartholomew, J. C., and Bradfield, C. A., Aromatic hydrocarbon responsiveness-receptor agonists generated from indole-3-carbinol *in vitro* and *in vivo* — comparisons with 2,3,7,8-tetrachlorodibenzo-*p*-dioxin, *Proc. Natl. Acad. Sci. U.S.A.*, 88, 9543, 1991.

187. Grose, K. R. and Bjeldanes, L. F., Oligomerization of indole-3-carbinol in aqueous acid, *Chem. Res. Toxicol.*, 5, 188, 1992.

188. Chen, I., Safe, S., and Bjeldanes, L., Indole-3-carbinol and diindolylmethane as aryl hydrocarbon (Ah) receptor agonists and antagonists in T47D human breast cancer cells, *Biochem. Pharmacol.*, 51, 1069, 1996.

189. Chen, I., McDougal, A., Wang, F., and Safe, S., Aryl hydrocarbon receptor-mediated antiestrogenic and antitumorigenic activity of diindolylmethane, in press, 1998.

190. Santostefano, M. and Safe, S., Characterization of the molecular and structural properties of the transformed and nuclear aryl hydrocarbon (Ah) receptor complexes by proteolytic digestion, *Chem. Biol. Interact.*, 100, 221, 1996.
191. Arellano-Johnson, L., unpublished results, 1997.
192. Chen, I., unpublished results, 1997.
193. McDougal, A., unpublished results, 1997.

Section II

Effect on the Male Reproductive System

8

Endocrine Disruptors and Male Infertility

Suresh C. Sikka and Rajesh K. Naz

CONTENTS

8.1 Introduction

Endocrine disruptors are estrogen-like and antiandrogenic chemicals in the environment that are potentially hazardous, not only to a variety of aquatic flora, wildlife, and humans but to our overall ecological well-being. These chemicals have been called "endocrine disruptors" because they are thought to mimic natural hormones, inhibit the action of hormones, or alter the normal regulatory function of endocrine systems. Reduced fertility in males is one of the major endpoints, in addition to testicular and prostate cancers, abnormal sexual development, alteration in pituitary and thyroid gland functions, immune suppression, and neurobehavioral effects. Interference with the action of androgen during development can cause male reproductive system abnormalities that include reduced sperm production capability.

Indeed, the evidence of the past twenty years has shown disturbing trends in male reproductive health. During a recent U.S. Congressional hearing, a startling but controversial finding reported that "each man in this room is half the man his grandfather was." Another report from Scotland revealed that men born after 1970 had a sperm count 25% lower than those born before 1959, an average decline of 2.1% a year. The lower sperm count was also associated with poor semen quality.[1,2] In contrast, Olsen et al., using several statistical models, found an actual increase in average sperm numbers.[3] Thus, while some environmentalists believe that the human species is approaching a fertility crisis, others think that the available data are insufficient to deduce worldwide conclusions.[4,5] Though these assertions have been disputed, the fact remains that one in six couples have trouble conceiving, with males equally responsible for their infertility.

When the reason for the poor quality of sperm cannot be identified, patients are treated using empirical methods. However, the development of intracytoplasmic sperm injection (ICSI), a technique introduced at the beginning of the 1990s, is beyond doubt the most important recent breakthrough in the treatment of male infertility. This research also has been made possible by many well-controlled clinical studies and basic scientific discoveries in the physiology, biochemistry, and molecular and cellular biology of the male reproductive system. This has helped in the identification of greater numbers of men with male factor problems. Newer tools for the detection of Y-chromosome deletions have further strengthened the hypothesis that the decline in male reproductive health and fertility may be related to the presence of certain toxic chemical compounds in the environment. These chemicals mimic or otherwise disrupt the estrogens or the androgen balance in the body by binding to hormone receptors during fetal and neonatal development. This may give rise to reproductive abnormalities, including low sperm counts.

Because of these effects, such endocrine disruptors are also popularly known as "gender benders." However, the evidence that such environmental chemicals cause infertility is still largely circumstantial. There are many missing links in the causal chain that would connect receptor binding to changes in reproductive health with decreased fertility. With recent discoveries of deformed frogs in Minnesota lakes and fertility problems in alligators found in Lake Apopka in Florida[6] attributed to embryonic exposure to pollutants, a myriad of environmental agents have been classified as male reproductive toxicants. This has been the subject of a number of reviews,[7-11] suggesting that etiology, diagnosis, and treatment of male factor infertility remains a real challenge.

8.2 Background

Several investigators have expressed serious concerns for the estrogenic effects of environmental xenobiotic chemicals, such as polychlorinated biphenyls (PCBs), dichlorodiphenyl-trichloroethane (DDT), dioxin, and some pesticides.[12-15] The potential hazards of these chemicals relative to human health and ecological well-being include reproductive tract cancers, reduced male fertility, and abnormality in sexual development.[14,16,17]

In the mid-1970s, it was determined that dibromochloropropane (DBCP) exposure impaired fertility in the absence of any other clinical signs of toxicity, suggesting that the male reproductive system was the most sensitive target organ. Reduced fertility, embryo/fetal loss, birth defects, childhood cancer, and other postnatal structural or functional problems were the most common outcomes from such exposures. However, the database for establishing safe exposure levels or risk assessment for such outcomes remains very limited. Declining semen quality is not the only indicator that human reproduction is at risk. A marked increase in the incidence of testicular cancer in young men has been associated with other abnormalities (including undescended testis, Sertoli-cell-only pattern, and hypospadias), which cause poor gonadal function and low fecundity rates.

The human male produces relatively fewer sperm on a daily basis compared with many of the animal species used for toxicity testing. A less dramatic decrease in sperm numbers or semen quality in humans can have serious consequences for reproductive potential. In fact, in many men over age 30, the lower daily sperm production rate already places them close to the subfertile or infertile range.[18,19] Decreased semen quality (low sperm number, motility, and structure) over the past 50 years has been attributed to environmental toxicants, many of which act as "estrogens".[20] This "estrogen hypothesis" has inspired a number of debates and serious investigations. Does that make men less fertile? After all, it takes only one sperm to fertilize an egg! Problems in the production, maturation, and fertilizing ability of sperm are the single most common cause of male infertility. Although produced in adequate numbers, sperm can have poor motility, viability, and morphology, be immature and lack acrosome, and display characteristics that will prevent them from fertilizing an oocyte. Normal sperm can also be produced in abnormally low numbers, thus diminishing the chances of fertilization. A dramatic increase in knowledge of reproductive toxicity and subsequent changes in fertility has resulted from advances in the understanding of gonadal function and dysfunction. Although any discussion of gonadal function and toxicity is of special relevance to man, much of this understanding has been obtained from research using animal species and various experimental models.

8.3   Endocrine Disruptors and Target Sites

An environmental agent could disrupt endocrine function in the male at several potential target sites, the most important being the testes, the male gonads, which usually exist in pairs and are the sites of spermatogenesis and androgen production. Spermatozoa are the haploid germ cells responsible for fertilization and species propagation. There are paracrine and autocrine regulations in various compartments of the testis that are under endocrine influences from the pituitary and hypothalamus. About 80% of the testicular mass consists of highly coiled seminiferous tubules within which spermatogenesis takes place. The remaining 20% consists of Leydig cells and Sertoli cells, whose main job is to establish normal spermatogenesis.

8.3.1   Leydig Cells

These cells arise from interstitial mesenchymal tissue between the tubules during the eighth week of human embryonic development. They are located in the connective tissue between the seminiferous tubules. Leydig cells are the endocrine cells in the testis that produce testosterone from cholesterol via a series of enzymatic pathways and steroidal intermediates under the control of luteinizing hormone (LH) from the pituitary.

8.3.2   Sertoli Cells

Within the testes are cells that envelope the developing sperm during spermatogenesis. These cells form a continuous and complete lining within the tubular wall and establish the blood-testis barrier by virtue of tight junctions. The luminal environment is both created and controlled by these Sertoli cells, also called "nurse cells," which are under the influence of follicle stimulating hormone (FSH) and inhibin. These Sertoli cells have several functions, including

1. Provide nourishment for the developing sperm cells
2. Destroy defective sperm cells

3. Secrete fluid that helps in the transport of sperm into the epididymis
4. Release the hormone inhibin, which helps regulate sperm production

The differentiation of Sertoli cells and the formation of a competent blood-testis barrier are essential to the establishment of normal spermatogenesis during puberty. Thus, many irregularities of spermatogenesis due to interference by endocrine disruptors may reflect changes in the function of the Sertoli cell population, not necessarily pathology in the germ cells themselves.

8.3.3 Establishment of Spermatogenesis

Spermatogenesis is a chronological process spanning about 42 d in the rodent and 72 d in man. During this period, relatively undifferentiated spermatogonia, the immature germ cells, cyclically develop into highly specialized spermatozoa. Spermatogonia undergo several mitotic divisions to generate a large population of cells called primary spermatocytes, which produce haploid germ cells by two meiotic cell divisions. Spermiogenesis is the transformation of spermatids into elongated flagellar germ cells capable of motility. The release of mature germ cells is known as spermiation. The germ cells comprise the majority of testicular volume, which diminishes if testicular damage has occurred. A significant characteristic of mitotic arrest is that the gonocyte becomes acutely sensitive to toxic agents, such as irradiation.[21] Low-dose irradiation may completely eradicate germ cells while causing little damage to developing Sertoli cells, thus creating Sertoli-cell-only testes.

8.4 Endocrine Disruptors That Affect Male Reproduction

Many endocrine disruptors, also termed estrogenic pollutants, from agricultural products (phytoestrogens), industrial chemicals, and heavy metals have significant environmental consequences due to their multiple routes of exposure, their widespread presence in the environment, and their ability to bioaccumulate and resist biodegradation. In addition, many pharmacological and biological agents, including radiation therapy, affect male reproduction via disrupting hormone influences. Table 8.1 lists the possible adverse effects caused by these agents described below.

8.4.1 Environmental Agents

8.4.1.1 Agricultural and Industrial Chemicals

Agricultural chemicals implicated in male reproductive toxicity include DDT (o,p-dichlorodiphenyl-trichloroethane), epichlorhydrin, ethylene dibromide, kepone, and the dioxins.[22] DBCP, a nematocide widely used in agriculture,

TABLE 8.1

Effects of Hormonal Disruptors on Male Reproduction

Class	Agent	Adverse Effects
(A) Environmental		
Organochemicals and pesticides	DBCP DDT PCBs Dioxins Methyl chloride	[↓ fertility, ↓ libido; embryo fetal loss, birth defects, cancer; estrogenic effects, poor semen quality]
Heavy metals	Lead Mercury Cadmium Cobalt Chromium	[↓ HPG-axis, ↓ spermatogenesis, CNS effects, testicular damage]
Ionizing radiations	α- and β-rays	[direct/indirect effect on gonads]
(B) Pharmacological		
Radiation therapy Drugs/Phytoestrogens	X-rays, γ-rays	[germ cell and Leydig cell damage]
	GnRH-analogs KTZ, leuprolide Cyclosporine Lithium, narcotics Anabolic steroids Ethanol, nicotine Flutamide Gossypol, marijuana	[↓ HPG-axis, ↓ sperm, ↓ libido, ↓ steroidogenesis]
(C) Biological		
	Hyperthermia	[↑ ROS, ↓ T biosynthesis, ↓ spermatogenesis, testicular damage, poor sperm morphology]
	Superoxide, and nitric oxide radicals	[↑ ROS, ↓ antioxidants, ↓ sperm function]
	Oxidative stress	[↑ ROS, ↑ LPO, ↑ cytokines, ↓ T, ↓ sperm function]

Note: Abbreviations: DBCP (dibromochloropropane); DDT (dichlorodiphenyl-trichloroethane); KTZ (ketoconazole); ROS (reactive oxygen species); LPO (lipid peroxidation).

is a testicular toxicant that induces hypergonadotropic hypogonadism.[23,24] DDT, a commonly used pesticide, and its metabolites (p,p′-DDT, and p,p′-DDE) have estrogenic effects in males by blocking the androgen receptors.[16] The levels of serum free/bound toxicant will influence the androgen-blocking capacity. The plasma/tissue concentration of an estrogenic toxicant depends upon the detoxification and elimination mechanisms in the organism. The fate and detoxification of these organochemicals have not been described, but these agents can disrupt the hypothalamic-pituitary-testicular axis, affecting the endocrine and reproductive functions. Methyl chloride, used in the production of organosilicates and gasoline antiknock additives, is a thoroughly studied industrial chemical.[25] Such organic solvents have been reported to induce changes in semen quality, testicular size, and serum gonadotropins.[26]

Polycyclic aromatic hydrocarbons (PAHs) are ubiquitous, undefined, complex mixtures encountered in the environment because of combustion as well as because of the use of tobacco products.[27] Since environmental exposures tend to be mixtures of various PAHs, the effect of their combined toxicity becomes more important but has not been examined in any detailed, well-designed study. A detrimental effect of endocrine disruptors on sperm concentration, motility, and morphology may be caused by impaired spermatogenesis secondary to various hormonal alterations.[28,29] A recent study has proposed that morphological sperm abnormalities due to secretory dysfunction of the Leydig and Sertoli cells may impair the sperm-fertilizing capacity.

8.4.1.2 Heavy Metals

Metals (e.g., lead, mercury, cadmium, aluminum, cobalt, chromium, arsenic, lithium, and antimony) have been noted to exert adverse reproductive effects in human and experimental animals. More reports are available on lead-induced toxicity than any other heavy metal. Historically, the fall of the Roman Empire has been attributed to lead poisoning.[30] Adverse effects on the reproductive capacity of men working in battery plants and exposed to toxic levels of lead have been reported.[31,32] In animals, lead exposure results in a dose-dependent suppression of serum testosterone and spermatogenesis.[33,34] Although testicular biopsies reveal peritubular fibrosis, vacuolation, and oligospermia, suggesting that lead is a direct testicular toxicant,[35] some mechanistic studies have revealed that lead exposure can disrupt the hormonal feedback mechanism at the hypothalamic-pituitary level.[8] Animal studies suggest that these effects can be reversed when lead is removed from the system. Such detailed evaluations in humans are under investigation.

Mercury exposure (during the manufacture of thermometers, thermostats, mercury vapor lamps, paint, electrical appliances, and in mining) can alter spermatogenesis and has been found to decrease fertility in experimental animals. Boron (extensively used in the manufacture of glass, cements, soaps, carpets, crockery, and leather products) has a major adverse reproductive effect on the testes and the hypothalamic-pituitary axis in a manner similar to lead. Oligospermia and decreased libido were reported in men working in boric acid-producing factories.[36] Cadmium, another heavy metal used widely in industries (electroplating, battery electrode production, galvanizing, plastics, alloys, paint pigments) and present in soil, coal, water, and cigarette smoke, is a testicular toxicant.[37] In animal studies, cadmium has been shown to cause strain-dependent severe testicular necrosis in mice.[38]

Cadmium-DNA binding and inhibition of sulfhydryl-containing proteins mediate cadmium toxicity directly or through transcription mechanisms. It can also induce the expression of heat shock proteins, oxidative stress response genes, and heme oxygenase induction mechanisms.[39] Further study is needed to delineate the specific gonadotoxic mechanisms involved. Clinical studies have associated cadmium exposure with testicular toxicity, altered libido, and infertility.

8.4.2   Pharmacological Agents

Many pharmacological drugs, chemotherapeutic agents, and radiation therapy are known to adversely affect male reproduction.

8.4.2.1   *Anabolic Steroids*

Anabolic steroids, which are mostly synthetic pharmacological agents, affect normal endocrine functions. The use/abuse of these anabolic steroids, mainly among athletes, has grown to epidemic proportions. This has resulted in severe oligozoospermia and decreased libido. Hypogonadotropic hypogonadism due to feedback inhibition of the hypothalamus-pituitary axis is the most common cause of severe impairment of normal sperm production in this population.[40] These defects can be reversed within 4 months of nonuse; however, sporadic azoospermia has been reported in some young men even 1 year after cessation of chronic anabolic steroid use.[41]

8.4.2.2   *Chemotherapeutic Agents*

Many antimicrobials (e.g., tetracycline derivatives, sulfa drugs, nitrofurantoin, and macrolide agents, like erythromycin) impair spermatogenesis and spermatozoal function.[42,43] As early as 1954, antibacterial agents were reported to be toxic to spermatozoa. Cancer chemotherapy usually damages the germinal epithelium.[44] Mechlorethamine, extensively used as nitrogen mustard during World War II, causes spermatogenic arrest.[45] Many common cytotoxic agents cause a dose-dependent progressive decrease in sperm count, leading to azoospermia.[46] Postmeiotic germ cells are sensitive specifically to cyclophosphamide treatment, with abnormalities observed in progeny.[47] Chronic low-dose cyclophosphamide treatment in men may affect the decondensation potential of spermatozoa, due to the alkylation of nuclear proteins or DNA. This is likely to affect pre- and postimplantation loss or contribute to congenital abnormalities in offspring.[48] Combination therapy with alkylating agents has been shown to improve survival in the treatment of Hodgkin's disease, lymphoma, and leukemia. However, such combination therapy has induced sterility in most adults, as revealed by complete germinal aplasia in testicular biopsy specimens.[49]

In general, the severity of testicular damage is related to the category of chemotherapeutic agent used, the dose and duration of therapy, and the developmental stage of the testis. The recovery of spermatogenesis is variable and depends upon the total therapeutic dose and duration of treatment.[50] The effects of cytotoxic drugs on the testicular function of children are inconclusive, due to the relative insensitivity in detecting such damage with available technology; however, the prepubertal and adolescent testes are reportedly affected less by chemo- and radiation therapy than is the postpubertal testis.[51] The use of testicular biopsy, semen analysis, and assessment of the HPG axis[44] commonly can achieve the evaluation of testicular toxicity.

8.4.2.3   Radiation Therapy

Radiotherapy is used alternatively for the treatment of seminomatous germ cell tumors and lymphomas. Testicular damage due to radiation exposure (X-rays, neutrons, and radioactive materials) is generally more severe and difficult to recover from than that induced by chemotherapy. Radiation effects on the testes depend on the schedule (total dose, number of fractions, duration) of the delivered irradiation, as well as the developmental stage of the germ cell in the testes at the time of exposure.[51] In general, germ cells are the most radiosensitive. A direct dose of irradiation to the testes greater than 0.35 Gy causes aspermia. The time taken for recovery increases with larger doses, and doses in excess of 2 Gy will likely lead to permanent azoospermia. At higher radiation doses (>15 Gy), Leydig cells will also be affected.[52] Vulnerability of the testis to irradiation depends upon the age and the pubertal status of the male. In addition to direct damage to the testes, whole body irradiation can also damage the hypothalamic-pituitary axis and affect reproductive capability.[53]

8.5   Mechanism(s) of Action of Endocrine Disruptors

Due to the complexity of the interactions involved in normal gonadal function and hormonal communication, any of these loci could be involved mechanistically in a toxicant's endocrine-related effect. Such impaired hormonal control could occur as a consequence of altered hormone synthesis, storage/release, transport/clearance, receptor recognition/binding, or post-receptor responses.

8.5.1   Altered Hormone Synthesis

A number of agents possess the ability to inhibit the synthesis of various hormones. Some of these agents inhibit specific enzymatic steps in the biosynthetic pathway of steroidogenesis (e.g., aminoglutethimide, cyanoketone, ketoconazole). Some fungicides block estrogen biosynthesis by inhibiting aromatase activity. Environmental estrogens and antiandrogens alter protein hormone synthesis induced by gonadal steroids. Both estrogen and testosterone have been shown to affect pituitary hormone synthesis directly or through changes in the glycosylation of LH and FSH.[54] A decrease in glycosylation of these glycoproteins reduces the biological activity of the hormones. Any environmental compound that mimics or antagonizes the action of these steroid hormones could presumably alter glycosylation.

8.5.2   Altered Hormone Storage and/or Release

Steroid hormones do not appear to be stored intracellularly within membranous secretory granules. For example, testosterone is synthesized by the Leydig cells of the testis and released on activation of the LH receptor. Thus, compounds that block the LH receptor or the activation of the 3',5'-cyclic AMP-dependent cascade involved in testosterone biosynthesis can alter rapidly the secretion of this hormone. The release of many protein hormones is dependent on the activation of second messenger pathways, such as cAMP, phosphatidylinositol 4,5-bisphosphate (PIP_2), inositol 1,4,5-trisphosphate (IP_3), tyrosine kinase, and Ca^{++}. Interference with these processes consequently will alter the serum levels (availability) of many hormones. Several metal cations have been shown to disrupt pituitary hormone release presumably by interfering with Ca^{++} flux.[55]

8.5.3   Altered Hormone Transport and Clearance

Hormones are transported from blood in the free or bound state. Steroid hormones are transported in the blood by specialized transport (carrier) proteins, known as sex-steroid hormone-binding globulin (SHBG) or testosterone-estrogen-binding globulin (TEBG). Regulation of the concentration of these binding globulins in the blood is of practical significance because there may be either increases or decreases that could affect steroid hormone availability. For example, DDT analogs are potent inducers of hepatic microsomal monooxygenase activities *in vivo*.[56] Induction of this monooxygenase activity by treatment with DDT analogs possibly could cause a decrease in testicular androgen as a result of enhanced degradation. Similarly, treatment with lindane (gamma-hexachlorocyclohexane) has been reported to increase the clearance of estrogen.[57]

8.5.4   Altered Hormone Receptor Recognition/Binding

Hormones elicit responses on their respective target tissues through direct interactions with either intracellular receptors or membrane-bound receptors. Specific binding of the natural ligand to its receptor is a critical step in hormone function. Intracellular (nuclear) receptors, such as those for sex steroids, adrenal steroids, thyroid hormones, vitamin D, and retinoic acid, regulate gene transcription in a ligand-dependent manner through their interaction with specific DNA sequences (response elements). A number of environmental agents may alter this process by mimicking the natural ligand and acting as an agonist or by inhibiting binding and acting as an antagonist. The best known examples are methoxychlor, chlordecone (kepone), DDT, some PCBs, and alkylphenols (e.g., nonylphenols and octylphenols), which can disrupt estrogen receptor function.[58,59] The antiandrogenic action of the dicarboximide fungicide vinclozolin is the result of an affinity of this compound's metabolites for the androgen receptor.[16] Interestingly, the DDT metabolite p,p'-DDE has been found to bind also to the androgen receptor and block testosterone-induced cellular responses *in vitro*.[60]

Many of the chemicals classified as environmental estrogens can actually inhibit binding to more than one type of intracellular receptor. For example, o,p-DDT and chlordecone can inhibit endogenous ligand binding to the estrogen and progesterone receptors, with each compound having IC50s that are nearly identical for the two receptors. Receptors for protein hormones are located on and in the cell membrane. When these hormones bind to their receptors, transduction of a signal across the membrane is mediated by the activation of second messenger systems. These may include (1) alterations in G-protein/cAMP-dependent protein kinase A (e.g., after LH stimulation of the Leydig cell); (2) phosphatidylinositol regulation of protein kinase C and inositol triphosphate (e.g., after GnRH stimulation of gonadotrophs, thyrotropin releasing hormone stimulation of thyrotrophs); (3) tyrosine kinase (e.g., after insulin binding to the membrane receptor); and (4) calcium ion flux. Xenobiotics thus can disrupt signal transduction of peptide hormones if they interfere with one or more of these processes.

8.5.5 Altered Hormone Postreceptor Activation

Once the endogenous ligand or an agonist binds to its receptor, a cascade of events is initiated indicative of the appropriate cellular response. This includes the response necessary for signal transduction across the membrane or, in the case of nuclear receptors, the initiation of transcription and protein synthesis. A variety of environmental compounds can interfere with the membrane's second messenger systems. For example, cellular responses that are dependent on the flux of calcium ions through the membrane (and the initiation of the calcium/Calmodulin-dependent cellular response) are altered by a variety of environmental toxicants. Interestingly, the well-known antiestrogen tamoxifen also inhibits protein kinase C activity.[61] Alternatively, the phorbol esters are known to mimic diacylglycerol and enhance protein kinase C activity.

Steroid hormone receptor activation can be modified by indirect mechanisms, such as a downregulation of the receptor (temporary decreased sensitivity to ligand) as seen after tetrachlorodibenzo-*p*-dioxin (TCDD) exposure (including the estrogen, progesterone, and glucocorticoid receptors).[62,63] Consequently, because of the diverse known pathways of endocrine disruption, any assessment must consider the net result of all influences on hormone receptor function and feedback regulation.

8.5.6 Induction of Oxidative Stress

"Oxidative stress" is a condition associated with an increased rate of cellular damage induced by oxygen and oxygen-derived free radicals, commonly known as reactive oxygen species (ROS), which belong to the class of free radicals. Chronic disease states, aging, toxin exposure, physical injury, and exposure to many types of environmental contaminants can enhance this oxidative process and cause gonadal damage.[64] Similarly, the generation of nitric oxide (NO·) and reactive nitrogen species (RNS) recently has been found to have an astounding range of biological roles, including vascular tone, inflammation, and mediation of many cytotoxic and pathological effects.[65] NO generation in response to toxic exposure associated with hormonal imbalance can contribute to poor sperm motility and function, leading to infertility.[66] Nitric oxide and superoxide radicals combine to form highly reactive peroxynitrite radicals, which induce endothelial cell injury.[67] This may result in altered blood flow to the testis and impaired testicular function.

The assumption that free radicals can influence male fertility has received substantial scientific support.[68] The proposed mechanism for loss of testicular and sperm function due to oxidative stress has been shown to involve excessive generation of ROS.[69] Free radicals can damage DNA and proteins, either through oxidation of DNA bases (primarily guanine via lipid peroxyl or alkoxyl radicals) or through covalent binding to MDA resulting in strand breaks and cross-linking.[70] ROS can also induce oxidation of critical -SH groups in proteins and DNA, which will alter cellular integrity and function with an increased susceptibility to attack by toxicants (Figure 8.1). Oxidative stress is theoretically the result of an improper balance between ROS generation and intrinsic scavenging activities. Adequate levels of superoxide dismutase (SOD), catalase, and probably glutathione (GSH) peroxidase and reductase normally maintain the free radical scavenging potential in the testes. This balance can be referred to as oxidative stress status (OSS), and its assessment may play a critical role in monitoring testicular toxicity and infertility.[9]

8.6 Assessment of Toxicity

Several methods are being evaluated for the assessment of the effects of toxicants on the male reproductive system. Essentially, any risk assessment usually has four components: (1) hazard identification, (2) dose-response

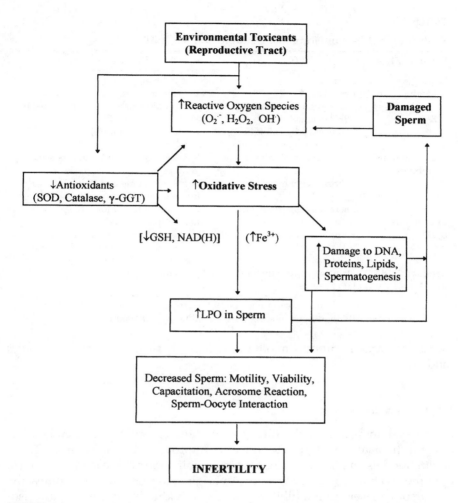

FIGURE 8.1
Scheme suggesting interacting mechanisms of environmental toxicants causing oxidative stress resulting in male infertility.

assessment, (3) human-exposure assessment, and (4) risk characterization. The hazard identification and dose-response data are developed from experimental animal studies that may be supplemented with data from *in vitro* studies. This information is then extrapolated and integrated to characterize and assess the risk to the human population.

The most common approach to evaluate the effect of cytotoxic drugs on the testis has used testicular biopsy, semen analysis, and endocrine assessment of the hypothalamic-pituitary-testicular axis (Table 8.2). Research on testicular toxicology has been advanced significantly by the introduction of *in vitro* testing systems. *In vivo* systems, however, are still essential parts of

TABLE 8.2

Evaluation of Effect of Hormonal Disruptors in the Adult Male

Potential Sites	Effects	Evaluative Tests
Testis	Necrosis	Weight, histopathology,
Leydig cells	LH/PRL	Receptor analysis, RIA
	T biosynthesis/secretion	*In vitro* production and hormone assay
Sertoli cells	FSH/inhibin/steroids	Receptor analysis, RIA
	Sertoli/Leydig cell function	*In vitro* tests (co-culture)
	Blood-testis barrier	Morphology
Seminiferous tubules	Spermatogonial mitosis	Germ cell count and % tubules without germ cells
	Spermatocyte meiosis	Spermatid counts and % tubules with luminal sperm
	Spermatid differentiation	Germ-cell culture, morphology
Epididymis	Sperm maturation	Histopathology, biochemical tests
Brain	Hypothalamic-pituitary axis	Pituitary cell-culture, hypothalamus perfusion, histopathology, hormone challenge, accessory sex-organ weights
Seminal fluid	Daily sperm production	Spermatid counts and semen evaluation
Blood	HPG-axis	Hormones/ABP assays

Note: Abbreviations: LH (luteinizing hormone); PRL (prolactin); FSH (follicle stimulating hormone); ABP (androgen binding protein); HPG (hypothalamic-pituitary-gonadal).

the risk assessment process, and they are unlikely to be eliminated by *in vitro* models.

8.6.1 *In Vitro* Systems

In vitro systems are uniquely suited to investigate specific cellular and molecular mechanisms in the testis and thus improve risk assessment.[71] These *in vitro* models can be used alone or in combination with each other to test hypotheses about testicular toxicity. An original toxicant, its metabolites, the precursors, or selective inhibitors can be individually administered to isolated cell types to evaluate specific toxicity mechanisms and to note the interaction of adjacent cell types. Numerous *in vitro* model systems are described in the literature, including Sertoli-germ-cell cocultures,[72] Sertoli-cell-enriched cultures,[73,74] germ-cell-enriched cultures,[75] Leydig-cell cultures,[33] Leydig-Sertoli-cell cocultures,[76] and peritubular and tubular cell cultures.[72,76] These *in vitro* systems are the only way to compare directly human and animal responses and to screen a class of compounds for new product development. Though these *in vitro* systems are a valuable adjunct to the *in vivo* test system, they do not replace the *in vivo* data, because they cannot provide all the facts essential for hazard assessment. Moreover, certain dynamic changes associated with spermatogenesis are difficult to model *in vitro*. For example, the release of elongated spermatids by the Sertoli cells (spermiation), which is commonly inhibited by boric acid and methyl chloride, can only be studied at present by specific *in vivo* systems.

8.6.2 *In Vivo* Systems

In vivo methods are important tools to study the integrated male reproductive system. The complete *in vivo* assessment of testicular toxicity involves multigenerational studies, now required by most regulatory agencies. These multigenerational studies have a complex design, because testicular function and spermatogenesis are very complicated processes. The spermatogenic cycle is highly organized throughout the testis. In the rat, it requires 53 d. If a toxicant affects the immature spermatogonia, the effect may not be detectable as a change in mature sperm before 7 to 8 weeks. Effects on more mature germ cells would be detected sooner. To test the sensitivity of all stages of spermatogenesis, the exposure should last the full duration of the cycle. This cannot be achieved *in vitro,* because germ cell differentiation and the physical relationship of stages within the tubules are lost in cell culture systems. The germ cells are entirely dependent upon the Sertoli cells for physical and biochemical support. Complicated endocrine and paracrine systems control Sertoli cells, Leydig cells, and germ cells. Besides the loss of paracrine interactions, the altered metabolic activity of target or adjacent cells and difficulty in isolating and testing certain spermatogenic stages are other significant limitations of *in vitro* assessment of testicular toxicity.[71] In addition, for accurate identification of stage-specific lesions of the seminiferous epithelium, critical evaluation of morphological structures is very important. Because germ cells are continuously dividing and differentiating, the staging of spermatogenesis has proven to be an extremely sensitive tool in identifying and characterizing even subtle toxicological changes.

8.6.3 Sperm Nuclear Integrity Assessment

Recent attention has been focused on assessments of sperm morphology and physiology as important endpoints in reproductive toxicology testing.[77] Structural stability of sperm nuclei varies by species, appears to be enhanced by the oxidation of protamine sulfhydryl to inter- and intramolecular disulfide bonds, and is a function of the types of protamine present. Chemicals may disrupt the structural stability of sperm nuclei, which depend upon their unique packaging either during spermatogenesis or sperm maturation. Decondensation of an isolated sperm nucleus *in vitro* can be induced by exposure to disulfide-reducing agents, and the time taken to induce extensive decondensation (assay end) is considered to be inversely proportional to the stability of the sperm nucleus. This "sperm activation assay" is also useful in the evaluation of some cases of unexplained infertility.[78] Human sperm decondenses most rapidly, followed by that of the mouse and of the hamster, while rat sperm nuclei show a slower decondensation.[79]

Other tests, called DNA stability assay or sperm chromatin structure assay (SCSA), use direct evaluation of sperm chromatin integrity and may provide information about genetic damage to sperm. A shift in DNA pattern (from double-stranded intact DNA to denatured single-stranded) can be induced by a variety of mutagenic and chemical agents and evaluated either by DNA flow cytometric analysis or by sperm chromatin structure assay.[80,81] A single cell gel electrophoresis (Comet) assay, which uses fluorescence intensity measurements by microscopy and image analysis, has also been developed recently.[78] A shift in the DNA pattern can also be evaluated by acridine orange staining, where double-stranded DNA is stained green and single-stranded DNA is stained red. Animals exposed to known mutagens demonstrate increased amounts of single-stranded DNA, indicating an increase in genetic damage.[82,83]

DNA flow cytometry is a very useful tool that permits rapid, objective assessment of a large number of cells, but it may not be readily available. Comet assay, when combined with centrifugal elutriation, can provide a useful *in vitro* model to study differences in metabolism and the susceptibility of different testicular cell types to DNA-damaging compounds. Thus, new findings through these systems should lead to greater knowledge about why a chemical or class of chemicals can cause testicular toxicity.

8.7   Scientific Debate

In the wake of media coverage dealing with possible reproductive health and cancer concerns,[84] a few toxicologists have questioned whether these adverse health effects can be attributed to environmental endocrine disruption.[63,85] Arguments for a demonstrable link between hormone-disruptive environmental agents and human reproductive health effects are supported by the fact that many pesticides and other agents with estrogenic or antiandrogenic activity operate via hormone receptor mechanisms. However, in the few studies of suspected weak estrogens, like the alkylphenols, some 1,000 to 10,000 times, or up to 10^6 more agent is required to bind 50% of the estrogen receptor than estradiol itself.[59] Of course, crucial to risk assessment is the need to know how many receptors must be occupied before activation of a response can ensue. For some hormones, such as human chorionic gonadotropin (hCG), as little as 0.5% to 5% receptor occupancy is required for full activation of response. For other hormones (those that require protein synthesis for expression of effect), higher levels of receptor occupancy are needed.

Fluctuations of hormone concentration and receptor activities, by design, absorb some environmental and physiological challenges to maintain homeostasis in adults. Only when the equilibrium control mechanisms are overwhelmed do the deleterious effects occur. An important question is whether homeostatic mechanisms are operative in the embryo and fetus.

Some investigators[86] have proposed the use of *in vitro* assays to screen for estrogenic or other hormonal activity. While steroid receptors bound to their ligand act as transcription factors for gene expression in the target tissue, simple *in vitro* screening assays based on binding to a receptor are not sufficient in themselves for measuring hormone activity. Binding of ligand to its specific receptor must be correlated with a physiologic response.

8.8 Summary

The observation that humans have experienced increased incidences of developmental, reproductive, and carcinogenic effects and the formulation of a working hypothesis that these adverse effects may be caused by environmental chemicals acting to disrupt the endocrine system that regulates these processes are supported by observations of similar effects in aquatic and wildlife species. In other words, a common theme runs through both human and wildlife reports.

In contrast, the hypothesis that the reported increased incidence of human cancers and reproductive abnormalities and infertility can be attributed to an endocrine disruption phenomenon is called into question for several reasons. First, secretion and elimination of hormones are highly regulated by the body, and mechanisms for controlling modest fluctuations of hormones are in place via negative feedback control of hormone concentrations. Therefore, minor increases of environmental hormones following dietary absorption and liver detoxification of these xenobiotics may be inconsequential in disrupting endocrine homeostasis. Second, low ambient concentrations of chemicals along with low affinity binding of purported xenobiotics to target receptors probably are insufficient to activate an adverse response in adults. Whether the fetus and the young are capable of regulating minor changes to the endocrine milieu is uncertain. Finally, the data are not available for mixtures of chemicals that may be able to affect endocrine function. At the same time, in the case of environmental estrogens as endocrine disrupters, it is known that competition for binding sites by antiestrogens in the environment may moderate estrogenic effects of some chemicals. Clearly, more research to fill data gaps and to remove the uncertainty in these unknowns is needed.

With few exceptions (e.g., DES), a causal relationship between exposure to a specific environmental agent and an adverse effect on human health operating via an endocrine disruption mechanism has not been established. Short-term screening studies could be developed and validated in an effort to elucidate mechanism. Through controlled dose-response studies, it appears that these compounds (e.g., alkyl phenol ethylates and their degradation products, chlorinated dibenzodioxins and difurans, and PCBs) can induce irreversible induction of male sex characteristics on females (imposex), which can lead to sterility and reduced reproductive performance.

In conclusion, a variety of extraneous and internal factors can induce testicular toxicity, leading to poor sperm quality and male factor infertility. Unfortunately, several of these influences (e.g., glandular infection, environmental toxicants that are mainly estrogenic chemicals, nutritional deficiencies, aging, ischemia, and oxidative stress) disrupt the hormonal milieu and have been underestimated. Partial androgen insensitivity mainly due to altered androgen-to-estrogen balance may contribute to significant oligozoospermia. The role of chronic inflammation of the reproductive organs is not completely understood because it is asymptomatic and is difficult to demonstrate objectively. There is an urgent need to characterize all the factors involved and to develop reliable animal models of testicular disease. No major advances have been made for the medical management of poor sperm quality. The application of assisted reproductive techniques, such as ICSI, to male infertility, regardless of cause, does not necessarily treat the cause and may inadvertently pass on adverse genetic consequences. Clinicians should always attempt to identify the etiology of a possible testicular toxicity, assess the degree of risk to the patients being evaluated for infertility, and initiate a plan to control and prevent exposure to others once an association between occupation/exposure and infertility has been established.

References

1. Chapin, R. E., White, R. D., Morgan, K. T., and Buss, J. S., Studies of lesions induced in the testis and epididymis of F-344 rats by inhaled methyl chloride, *Toxicol. Appl. Pharmacol.*, 76, 328, 1984.
2. Brake, A. and Krause, W., Decreasing quality of semen, *Br. Med. J.*, 305, 1498, 1992.
3. Olsen, G. W., Bodner, K. M., Ramlow, J. M., Ross, C. E., and Lipshultz, L. I., Have sperm counts been reduced 50 percent in 50 years? A statistical model revisited, *Fertil. Steril.*, 63, 887, 1995.
4. Fisch, H., Goluboff, E. T., Olson, J. H., Feldshuh, J., Broder, S. J., and Barad, D. H., Semen analyses in 1283 men from the United States over a 25-year period: no decline in quality, *Fertil. Steril.*, 65, 1009, 1996.
5. Parvinen, M., Lahdetie, J., and Parvinen, L. M., Toxic and mutagenic influences on spermatogenesis, *Arch. Toxicol.*, 7, 147, 1984.
6. Guillette, L. J., Gross, T. S., Masson, G. R., Matter, J. M., Percival, H. F., and Woodward, A. R., Developmental abnormalities of the gonad and abnormal sex hormone concentrations in juvenile alligators from contaminated and control lakes in Florida, *Environ. Health Perspect.*, 102(8), 680, 1994.
7. Kavlock, R. J. and Perreault, S. D., Multiple chemical exposure and risks of adverse reproductive function and outcome, in *Toxicology of Chemical Mixtures: From Real Life Examples to Mechanisms of Toxicology Interactions*, Yang, R. S. H., Ed., Academic Press, Orlando, FL, 1994, 245.
8. Sokol, R. Z., Hormonal effects of lead acetate in the male rat: mechanism of action, *Biol. Reprod.*, 37, 1135, 1987.
9. Sikka, S. C., Gonadotoxicity, in *Male Infertility and Sexual Dysfunction*, Hellstrom, W. J. G., Ed., Springer-Verlag, New York, 1997, 292.

10. Lamb, D. J., Hormonal disruptors and male infertility: are men at serious risk? *Reg. Toxicol. Pharmacol,* 26, 001, 1997.
11. Cheek, A. O. and McLachlan, J. A., Environmental hormones and the male reproductive system, *J. Androl.,* 19, 5, 1998.
12. Boris, A., Endocrine studies of a nonsteroid anti-androgen and progestin, *Endocrinology,* 76, 1063, 1965.
13. McLachlan, J. A. and Arnold, S. F., Environmental estrogens, *Am. Sci.,* 84, 452, 1996.
14. Colborn, T., vomSaal, F. S., and Soto, A. M., Developmental effects of endocrine-disrupting chemicals in wildlife and humans, *Environ. Health Perspect.,* 1101(5), 378, 1993.
15. Purdom, C. E., Hardiman, P. A., Bye, V. J., Eno, N. C., Tyler, C. R., and Sumpter, J. P., Estrogenic effects of effluents from sewage treatment works, *Chem. Ecol.,* 8, 275, 1994.
16. Kelce, W. R., Monosson, E., Gamcsik, M. P., Laws, S. C., and Gray, L. E., Jr., Environmental hormone disruptors: evidence that vinclozolin developmental toxicity is mediated by antiandrogenic metabolites, *Toxicol. Appl. Pharmacol.,* 126, 276, 1994.
17. Sharpe, R. M. and Skakkebaek, N. E., Are estrogens involved in falling sperm counts and disorders of the male reproductive tract? *Lancet,* 351, 1392, 1993.
18. Sokol, R. Z., Toxicants and infertility: identification and prevention, in *Management of Impotence and Infertility,* Whitehead, E. D. and Nagler, H. M., Eds., J. B. Lippincott Co., Philadelphia, 1994, 380.
19. Schrader, S. M. and Kanitz, M. H., Occupational hazards to male reproduction, in *State of the Art Reviews in Occupational Medicine: Reproductive Hazards,* Gold, E., Schenker, M., and Lesley, B., Eds., Hanley and Belfus, Pittsburgh, PA, 1994, 405.
20. Working, P. K., Male reproductive toxicity: comparison of the human to animal models, *Environ. Health Perspect.,* 77, 37, 1988.
21. Mandl, A. M., The radiosensitivity of germ cells, *Biol. Res.,* 39, 288, 1964.
22. Whorton, M. D., Krauss, R. M., Marshall, S., Infertility in male pesticide workers, *Lancet,* 2, 1259, 1977.
23. Mattison, D. R., The mechanisms of action of reproductive toxins, *Am. J. Ind. Med.,* 4, 65, 1983.
24. Potashnik, G. and Yanai-Inbar, I., Dibromochloropropane (DBCP): an 8-year reevaluation of testicular function and reproductive performance, *Fertil. Steril.,* 47, 317, 1987.
25. Chapin, R. E., Gray, T. J. B., Phelps, J. L., and Dutton, S. L., The effects of mono-(2-ethylhexyl)phthalate on rat Sertoli cell-enriched primary cultures, *Toxicol. Appl. Pharmacol.,* 96, 467, 1988.
26. Schrader, S. M., Principles of male reproductive toxicology, in *Environmental Medicine,* Brooks, S. M. and Gochfeld, M., Eds., Mosby Press, St. Louis, 1995, 95.
27. Georgellis, A., Toppari, J., Veromaa, T., Rydstrom, J., and Parvinen, M., Inhibition of meiotic divisions of rat spermatocytes *in vitro* by polycyclic aromatic hydrocarbons, *Mutat. Res.,* 231, 125, 1990.
28. Vine, M. F., Tse, C. J., Hu, P. C., and Truong, K. Y., Cigarette smoking and semen quality, *Fertil. Steril.,* 65, 835, 1996.
29. Zavos, P. M., Cigarette smoking and human reproduction: effects on female and male fecundity, *Infertility,* 12, 35, 1989.
30. Gilfillan, S. C., Lead poisoning and the fall of Rome, *J. Occup. Med.,* 7, 53, 1965.

31. Lancranjan, I., Popescu, H. I., Gavanescu, O., Klepsch, I., and Serbanescu, M., Reproductive ability of workmen occupationally exposed to lead, *Arch. Environ. Health*, 30, 396, 1975.

32. Winder, C., Reproductive and chromosomal effects of occupational exposure to lead in males, *Reprod. Toxicol.*, 3, 221, 1989.

33. Ewing, L. L., Zirkin, B. R., and Chubb, C., Assessment of testicular testosterone production and Leydig cell structure, *Environ. Health Perspect.*, 38, 19, 1981.

34. Foster, W. G., McMahon, A.,Young-Lai, E. V., Hughes, E. G., and Rice, D. C., Reproductive endocrine effects of chronic lead exposure in the male cynomolgus monkey, *Reprod. Toxicol.*, 7, 203, 1992.

35. Braunstein, G. D., Dahlgren, J., Loriaux, D. O., Hypogonadism in chronically lead poisoned men, *Infertility*, 1, 33, 1978.

36. Weir, R. J. and Fisher, R. S., Toxicological studies on borox and boric acid, *Toxicol. Appl. Pharmacol.*, 23, 251, 1972.

37. Friberg, L., Piscator, M., and Nordberg, G. F., *Cadmium in the Environment*, 2nd ed., CRC Press, Inc. Cleveland, 1974, 37.

38. King, L. M., Andrew, M. G., Sikka, S. C., and George, W. J., Murine strain differences in cadmium-induced testicular toxicity, *The Toxicologist*, 36(2), 186, 1997.

39. Snow, E. T., Metal carcinogenesis: mechanistic implications, *Pharmacol. Ther.*, 53, 31, 1992.

40. Knuth, U. A., Maniera, H., and Nieschlag, E., Anabolic steroids and semen parameters in body builders, *Fertil. Steril.*, 52, 1041, 1989.

41. Jarow, J. P. and Lipshultz, L. I., Anabolic steroid-induced hypogonadotropic hypogonadism, *Am. J. Sports Med.*, 18, 429, 1990.

42. Ericsson, R. J. and Baker, V. F., Binding of tetracycline to mammalian spermatozoa, *Nature*, 214, 403, 1967.

43. Schlegel, P. N., Chang, T. S. K., and Maeshall, F. F., Antibiotics: potential hazards to male fertility, *Fertil. Steril.*, 55, 235, 1991.

44. Shalet, S. M., Effects of cancer chemotherapy on testicular function of patients, *Canc. Treat. Rev.*, 7, 41, 1980.

45. Spitz, S., The histological effects of nitrogen mustards on human tumors and tissues, *Cancer*, 1, 383, 1948.

46. Meistrich, M. L., Quantitative correlation between testicular stem cell survival, sperm production, and fertility in mouse after treatment with different cytotoxic agents, *J. Androl.*, 3, 58, 1982.

47. Qiu, J., Hales, B. F., and Robaire, B., Adverse effects of cyclophosphamide on progeny outcome can be mediated through post-testicular mechanisms in the rat, *Biol. Reprod.*, 46, 926, 1992.

48. Trasler, J. M., Hales, B. F., and Robaire, B., A time course study of chronic paternal cyclophosphamide treatment of rats: effects on pregnancy outcome and the male reproductive and hematologic systems, *Biol. Reprod.*, 37, 317, 1987.

49. Sherins, R. J. and DeVita, V. T., Jr., Effect of drug treatment for lymphoma on male reproductive capacity, *Ann. Intern. Med.*, 79, 216, 1973.

50. Parvinen, M., Lahdetie, J., and Parvinen, L. M., Toxic and mutagenic influences on spermatogenesis, *Arch. Toxicol.*, 7, 147, 1984.

51. Oats, R. D. and Lipshultz, L. I., Fertility and testicular function in patients after chemotherapy and radiotherapy, in *Advances in Urology*, Vol. 2, Lytton B, Ed., Mosby Year Book, Chicago, 1989, 55.

52. Rowley, M. J., Leach, D. R., Warner, G. A., and Heller, C. G., Effects of graded doses of ionizing radiation on the human testis, *Radiat. Res.*, 59, 665, 1974.

53. Ogilvy-Stuart, A. L. and Shalet, S. M., Effect of radiation on the Human reproductive system, *Environ. Health Perspect.*, 101, 109, 1993.

54. Wilson, C. A., Leigh, A. J., and Chapman, A. J., Gonadotrophin glycosylation and function, *J. Endocrinol.*, 125, 3, 1990.

55. Cooper, R. L., Goldman, J. M., Rehnberg, G. L., McElroy, W. K., and Hein, J. F., Effects of metal cations on pituitary hormone secretions *in vitro, J. Biochem. Toxicol.*, 2, 241, 1987.

56. Bulger, W. H., Nuccitelli, R. M., and Kupfer, D., Studies on the *in vivo* and *in vitro* estrogenic activities of methoxychlor and its metabolites: role of hepatic monooxygenase in methoxychlor activation, *Biochem. Pharmacol.*, 27, 2417, 1978.

57. Welch, R. M., Levin, W., Kuntzman, R., Jocobson, M., and Conney, A. H., Effect of halogenated hydrocarbon insecticides on the metabolism and uterotropic actions of estrogens in rats and mice, *Toxicol. Appl. Pharmacol.*, 19, 234, 1971.

58. Mueller, G. C. and Kim, U. H., Displacement of estradiol from estrogen receptors by simple alkylphenols, *Endocrinology*, 102, 1429, 1978.

59. White, T. E., Rucci, G., Liu, Z., and Gasiewicz, T. A., Environmentally persistent alkylphenolic compounds are estrogenic, *Endocrinology*, 135, 175, 1994.

60. Kelce, W. R., Stone, C. R., Laws, S. C., Gray, L. E., Jr., Kemppainen, J. A., and Wilson, E. M., Persistent DDT metabolite p,p'-DDE is a potent androgen receptor antagonist, *Nature*, 375, 581, 1995.

61. O'Brian, C. A., Liskamp, R. M., Solomon, D. H., and Weinstein, I. B., Inhibition of protein kinase C by tamoxifen, *Canc. Res.*, 45, 2462, 1985.

62. Safe, S., Astroff, B., Harris, B., Zacharewski, T., Dickerson, R., Romkes, M., and Biegel, L., 2,3,7,8-Tetrachlorodibenzo-p-dioxin (TCDD) and related compounds as antiestrogens; characterization and mechanism of action, *Pharmacol. Toxicol.*, 69, 400, 1991.

63. Safe, S. H., Environmental and dietary estrogens and human health: is there a problem? *Environ. Health Perspect.*, 103, 346, 1995.

64. Sikka, S. C., Rajasekaran, M., and Hellstrom, W. J. G., Role of oxidative stress and antioxidants in male infertility, *J. Androl.*, 16, 464, 1995.

65. Koppenol, W. H., Moreno, J. J., Pryor, W. A., et al., Peroxynitroite, a cloaked oxidant formed by nitric oxide and superoxide, *Chem. Res. Toxicol.*, 5, 834, 1992.

66. Rosselli, M., Dubey, R. K., Imthurn, B., Macase, E., and Keller, P. J., Effects of nitric oxide on human spermatozoa: evidence that nitric oxide decreases sperm motility and induces sperm toxicity, *Hum. Reprod.*, 10, 1786, 1995.

67. Beckman, J. S., Beckman, T. W., Chen, J., Marshall, P. A., and Freeman, B. A., Apparent hydroxyl radical production by peroxynitrite: implications for endothelial injury from nitric oxide and superoxide, *Proc. Natl. Acad. Sci. U.S.A.*, 87, 1620, 1990.

68. Gagnon, C., Iwasaki, A., deLamirande, E., and Kavolski, N., Reactive oxygen species and human spermatozoa, (review) *Ann. N.Y. Acad. Sci.*, 637, 436, 1991.

69. Aitken, R. J. and Clarkson, J. S., Cellular basis of defective sperm function and its association with the genesis of reactive oxygen species by human spermatozoa, *Reprod. Fertil.*, 81, 459, 1987.

70. Alvarez, J. G., Touchstone, J. C., Blasco, L., and Storey, B. T., Spontaneous lipid peroxidation and production of hydrogen peroxide and superoxide in human spermatozoa. Superoxide dismutase as major enzyme protectant against oxygen toxicity, *J. Androl.*, 8, 338, 1987.

71. Lamb, J. C., IV, and Chapin, R. E., Testicular and germ cell toxicity: *in vitro* approaches, *Reprod. Toxicol.*, 7, 17, 1993.

72. Gray, T. J. B., Application of *in vitro* systems in male reproductive toxicology, in *Physiology and Toxicology of Male Reproduction*, Lamb, J. C., IV, and Foster, P. M. D., Eds., Academic Press, San Diego, CA, 1988, 250.

73. Chapin, R. E., Phelps, J. L., Somkuti, S. G., and Heindel, J. J., The interaction of Sertoli and Leydig cells in the testicular toxicity of tri-o-cresyl phosphate, *Toxicol. Appl. Pharmacol.*, 104, 483, 1990.

74. Steinberger, A. and Clinton, J. P., Two-compartment cultures of Sertoli cells — applications in testicular toxicology, in *Methods in Toxicology*, Part A, Male Reprod. Toxicol., Chapin, R. E. and Heindel, J. J., Eds., Academic Press, New York, 1993, 230.

75. Foster, P. M. D., Lloyd, S. C., and Prout, M. S., Toxicity and metabolism of 1,3-dinitrobenzene in rat testicular cell cultures, *Toxicol. In Vitro*, 1, 31, 1987.

76. Chapin, R. E., Phelps, J. L., Somkuti, S. G., and Heindel, J. J., The interaction of Sertoli and Leydig cells in the testicular toxicity of tri-o-cresyl phosphate, *Toxicol. Appl. Pharmacol.*, 104, 483, 1990.

77. Darney, S. P., *In vitro* assessment of gamete integrity, in *In-vitro Toxicology: Mechanisms and New Toxicology — Alternative Methods in Toxicology*, Vol. 8, Goldberg, A. M., Ed., Ann Liebert, Inc., New York, 1991, 63.

78. Brown, D. B., Hayes, E. J., Uchida, T., and Nagamani, M., Some cases of human male infertility are explained by abnormal *in vitro* human sperm activation, *Fertil. Steril.*, 64, 612, 1995.

79. Perrault, S. D., Barbee, R. R., Elstein, K. H., Zucker, R. M., and Keeler, C. L., Interspecies differences in the stability of mammalian sperm nuclei assessed *in vivo* by sperm microinjection and *in vitro* by flow cytometry, *Biol. Reprod.*, 39, 157, 1988.

80. Evenson, D. P., Flow cytometry evaluation of male germ cells, in *Flow Cytometry: Advanced Research and Clinical Applications*, Vol. 1, Yen A, Ed., CRC Press, Boca Raton, FL, 1989, 218.

81. Evenson, D. P., Baer, R. K., Jost, L. K., and Gesch, R. W., Toxicity of thiotepa on mouse spermatogenesis as determined by dual-parameter flow cytometry, *Toxicol. Appl. Pharmacol.*, 82, 151, 1986.

82. Evenson, D. P., Jost, L. K., Baer, R. K., Turner, T. W., and Schrader, S. M., Individuality of DNA denaturation patterns in human sperm as measured by the sperm chromatin structure assay, *Reprod. Toxicol.*, 5, 115, 1991.

83. Ulbrich, B. and Palmer, A. K., Detection of effects on male reproduction — a literature survey, *J. Am. Coll. Toxicol.*, 14, 293, 1995.

84. Raloff, J., The gender benders. Are environmental "hormones" emasculating wildlife? *Sci. News*, 145, 24, 1994.

85. Stone, R., Environmental estrogens stir debate, *News Comment. Sci.*, 256, 308, 1994.

86. Soto, A. M., Lin, T. M., Justicia, H., Silvia, R. M., and Sonenschein, C., An "in culture" bioassay to assess the estrogenicity of xenobiotics (E-Screen), in *Chemically Induced Alterations in Sexual and Functional Development: The Wildlife/Human Connection*, Colborn, T. and Clements, C., Princeton Scientific Publishing Co., Inc., Princeton, NJ, 1992, 295.

9

Environmental Antiandrogens as Endocrine Disruptors

William R. Kelce and L. Earl Gray, Jr.

CONTENTS

0-8493-3164-1/99/$0.00+$.50
© 1999 by CRC Press LLC

9.1   Introduction

Confirmed alterations in reproductive development in wildlife species[1,2] together with reports touting an increase in the incidence of human male reproductive tract abnormalities[3,4] and decreased adult sperm counts in some parts of the world[5-10] have increased public concern about anthropogenic chemicals with hormone activity. In an effort to differentiate these hormone-mimicking and/or -inhibiting chemicals from classical toxicants such as carcinogens, neurotoxicants, and heavy metals, the term "endocrine disrupting chemical" (EDC) has emerged. Concerns with EDCs have driven public policy to mandate, via the Food Quality Protection Act (Public Law 104-170) and the Safe Drinking Water Act (Public Law 104-182), that the Environmental Protection Agency (EPA) develop and implement a screening and testing program for environmental chemicals that produce estrogen-like effects or other effects as deemed appropriate by the EPA administrator. The development of specific EDC test protocols should improve our ability to identify and evaluate, in the context of production volume and exposure data, their potential to induce adverse effects in wildlife and human populations.

Endocrine-disrupting chemicals act to alter normal blood hormone levels or the subsequent action of those hormones, including effects on hormone production, release, transport, metabolism, and/or elimination, together with effects on cognate receptor binding and/or subsequent intracellular receptor actions. Here we focus on the effects and mechanisms of environmental chemicals that alter androgen action during fetal development, as the consequences of this disruption are especially insidious due to the crucial role of androgens in controlling transient and irreversible sex differentiation processes. Chemicals that alter androgen action typically act by inhibiting the biosynthesis of testosterone by testicular Leydig cells, by inhibiting the enzymatic activity of microsomal 5α-reductase (Type 2), which activates testosterone to the more potent androgen 5α-dihydrotesterone, or by inhibiting androgen action at the level of the androgen receptor (AR). Each of these mechanisms and their specific effects on male sex differentiation and development will be discussed where applicable. The reader is referred to a recent review[11] for a general review of environmental chemical-induced teratogenicity in rodents and humans. Due to space limitations, review articles and selected manuscripts are referenced wherever possible; no attempt has been made to cite the original literature exhaustively. Finally, as opinions vary regarding the best methods to screen for endocrine disruptor activity, ranging from using *in vitro* systems exclusively to using *in vivo* screens exclusively, we propose a comprehensive investigational strategy that identifies the chemicals/metabolites of concern but also provides information as to the mechanism responsible for the phenotypic effects. The reader is referred elsewhere for discussions of general mechanisms of environmental endocrine disruptors,[12-14] effects of environmental endocrine disruptors in wildlife,[2,15] effects of environmental estrogens in the male,[16] clinical implications of these chemicals in humans,[14,17] and proposed research needs for risk assessment.[18]

9.2 Sex Differentiation and Sensitivity to Disruption

The sex chromosomal constitution of heterogametic males (XY) and homo-gametic females (XX) is determined at fertilization in mammals. This genetic sex forms the basis for gonadal sex development, where SRY genes on the Y chromosome direct differentiation of the indifferent gonads into testes. Subsequent testicular secretions of testosterone and Müllerian inhibiting sub-stance induce differentiation of the male internal duct system and external genitalia, contributing to normal cell differentiation, normal tissue histiogen-esis, and ultimately a normal male phenotype. In the absence of testosterone, the female phenotype is expressed independent of the presence of an ovary.

In humans, testicular testosterone synthesis begins approximately 65 days after fertilization and influences differentiation of the Wolffian duct system into the epididymis, vas deferens, and seminal vesicles. The more potent androgen is the testosterone metabolite, 5α-dihydrotestosterone (DHT), which induces development of the prostate and male external genitalia. Testosterone is 5α-reduced to DHT via the enzymatic activity of 5α-reduc-tase. Both testosterone and DHT bind to the AR to initiate androgen-depen-dent gene expression; however, DHT has a higher affinity for binding, thus inducing maximal androgen agonist activity at lower concentrations than testosterone. It is thought that the Wolffian ducts receive adequate concen-trations of testosterone for development via their close proximity to the testis. The prostate and external genitalia, on the other hand, may not, thus requir-ing activation of testosterone to the more potent androgen DHT.[19] In addi-tion, the rat ventral prostate also uniquely expresses high levels of 17β-hydroxysteroid oxidoreductase during development. This enzyme metabo-lizes testosterone to the inactive androgen androstenedione; high 5α-reduc-tase activity in the developing prostate, then, may also function to shunt available testosterone to DHT, maintaining adequate concentrations of non-aromatizable, active androgens.[20] It is clear that these latter tissues are addi-tionally dependent on normal DHT formation for their proper differentiation and development. Environmental chemicals that alter growth and differen-tiation of the prostate with limited effects on Wolffian duct development (e.g., seminal vesicles) should be considered suspect 5α-reductase inhibitors. However, in rodents, even AR-mediated antiandrogens have more pro-nounced effects on the ventral prostate and external genitalia.

It appears that the same AR mediates sex differentiation in the developing fetus as well as androgen action in postnatal life, as immunoblots prepared from urogenital tract tissues of gestational day 17 male and female rats recognize the same 110 kDa protein characteristic of the adult AR.[21] The steroid-binding characteristics of AR isolated from the embryonic urogenital tract are identical to those determined from mature adult reproductive tract tissues.[21] The greater sensitivity of the developing male fetus to the antiandrogenic effects of environmental chemicals may result from reduced levels of competing endogenous androgens in the developing fetal male compared to the adult. Given the critical importance of androgen biosynthesis in the expression of the male phenotype and the importance of 5α-reductase activity and AR in mediating androgen action during sex differentiation and development, exposure to environmental antiandrogens often has unique and devastating effects on the developing male.

Chemical-induced alterations in androgen action during development warrant special concern for several reasons. First, sex development in mammals is in part an androgen-driven process, so alterations in androgen action during development induce permanent adverse effects that are likely to affect risk assessment. Second, basic mechanisms of sex development are similar among mammals, so chemicals that affect reproductive development in rodents and other test mammals are also putative human reproductive toxicants. Third, development of the reproductive system often is sensitive to low-dose chemical effects, as compensatory endocrine mechanisms (i.e., the hypothalamic-pituitary-gonadal axis) are not functional at early developmental stages. Fourth, functional alterations are often not discovered until after puberty or later in life, leading to underestimates of the effects induced by chemical treatment on reproductive development. Fifth, developmental abnormalities cannot be predicted from chemical exposures in adult animals, as adults are fully differentiated and can therefore tolerate chemical insult. That is, the same chemical at the same dose causes transient endocrine modulation in adult animals but permanent endocrine disruption in fetal animals. Sixth, the similarity in molecular size and lipophilicity of many environmental chemicals with endogenous androgens may preferentially target disruption of endocrine function at the level of this promiscuous receptor. Finally, unlike most environmental estrogens, some environmental antiandrogens, like p,p′-DDE, bioaccumulate to reach high levels. It is not unusual to see part per million levels of p,p′-DDE in animal and human tissues in contaminated areas.[22-25]

9.3   Testicular Androgen Biosynthesis: Mechanisms and Effects of Select Chemicals

9.3.1   Background

The best understood function of the Leydig cell is the synthesis and secretion of testosterone in response to stimulation by the pituitary hormone, luteinizing hormone (LH). Testosterone mediates numerous functions throughout the life cycle of the male, including the differentiation and development of the fetal male reproductive tract; the neonatal organization of androgen-dependent target tissues; masculinization of the male at puberty; growth and function of androgen-dependent organs in the adult; maintenance of spermatogenesis; permissive effects on libido; and senescent androgen-dependent changes accompanying Leydig cell dysfunction with advancing age.[26-29] As a consequence of the central role of testosterone in the male, toxicant-induced alterations in testosterone production can have a devastating impact on the development of the male reproductive system and/or its subsequent functioning in adult life.

Chemicals that affect testosterone production can exert direct effects on the Leydig cell or act indirectly through the hypothalamus-pituitary-testicular axis. In this chapter, we limit discussion to chemicals that act directly to impair Leydig cell function or to alter Leydig cell viability. We use as examples chemicals that directly alter LH-stimulated testosterone production by the rat testis *in vivo*, during *in vitro* testicular perfusion, and/or in crude testis preparations or highly purified rat Leydig cell cultures. These *in vitro* data not only corroborate *in vivo* effects but also identify putative biochemical mechanisms responsible for these effects. Lesions in the steroidogenic pathway are identified via accumulation of substrate and/or depletion of product surrounding the enzymatic step in question. Once a lesion has been identified, specific radiometric enzyme assays can be completed using various concentrations of substrate at different fixed concentrations of inhibitor to characterize further the kinetic mechanism of inhibition (e.g., competitive, noncompetitive, or uncompetitive) as well as alterations in the associated apparent rate constants.

Ex vivo assessment of Leydig cell function involves treating male rats with putative toxicants and assessing LH-stimulated hormone production by the testis *in vitro*. The major advantage of the *ex vivo* approach is the normal pharmacokinetics and metabolism of the parent chemical. In *in vitro* studies, the testes are removed from untreated rats and exposed to varying concentrations of the toxicant in the culture media, thus assessing direct effects of the toxicant on testicular steroidogenesis in the absence of other organ systems. In either case, testicular parenchyma is incubated in the presence and absence of maximally stimulating concentrations of LH/hCG for several hours, a time period when testosterone production is linear over time. Both maximum testosterone production and LH responsiveness of the Leydig cell are evaluated. The testicular parenchyma can also be incubated with specific steroid substrates to localize the enzymatic lesion. Administration of a steroid substrate that follows the enzyme defect in the steroidogenic pathway will restore normal testosterone production, while administration of a substrate that precedes the affected enzyme will not. These methods also can be used on testicular parenchyma from different-aged animals, thus assessing effects specific to one Leydig cell population or another. It often is not appreciated that Leydig cell structure and function changes throughout the life cycle of the rat, potentially rendering one population of Leydig cells either more or less susceptible to toxic insult than another. A review of the various Leydig cell populations and age-specific chemical effects has been presented in detail elsewhere.[30]

9.3.2   Chemical Effects and Mechanisms

9.3.2.1   Leydig Cell Function

Pituitary LH regulates Leydig cell volume, the volume of steroidogenic organelles such as the smooth endoplasmic reticulum and peroxisomes, the enzymatic activity of 17α-hydroxylase/$C_{17,20}$-lyase, as well as the synthesis and secretion of testosterone.[26,31,32] In this context, it is clear that chemicals that alter the synthesis and/or secretion of LH (e.g., reserpine, cyclosporin, steroid hormones) indirectly alter Leydig cell function by inhibiting the trophic effects of LH. This chapter, however, is limited to those chemicals that directly impair steroidogensis or kill rat Leydig cells. The reader is referred elsewhere for a thorough discussion of indirect (i.e., endocrine, paracrine, and autocrine) effects on Leydig cell function.[33]

9.3.2.1.1   Xenobiotic Chemicals

Toxicants that interfere with steroidogenesis typically inhibit the cytochrome P450 enzymes in the steroidogenic pathway. The fungicidal action of several major classes of fungicides (drugs and pesticides), including the imidazoles and triazoles, depends on inhibition of P450 enzymes in the sterol synthesis pathway necessary for fungal membrane formation.[34] Cytochrome P450 enzyme inhibitors tend to be nonspecific, inhibiting the activity of more than one P450 enzyme in the pathway.[35] The effects of these nonspecific inhibitors depend on which enzymes are inhibited. The types of effects vary greatly, ranging from pregnancy loss,[36] delayed parturition, demasculinization of male pups,[37] lack of normal male and female mating behavior, altered estrous cyclicity,[38] abnormal serum hormone levels, and altered reproductive organ weights.[39]

Ketoconazole is an example of a xenobiotic chemical that directly alters Leydig cell function without affecting Leydig cell viability. Ketoconazole is an imidazole antifungal drug thought to exert its toxic effects in fungi by inhibiting 14-demethylation, thereby preventing the synthesis of ergosterol, a major component of the fungal cell membrane.[40] Studies in both rats and humans demonstrate that ketoconazole administration reduces serum testosterone levels in the absence of alterations in serum LH, suggesting a direct effect on Leydig cell steroidogenesis.[40-42] The *in vivo* effects of ketoconazole on Leydig cell testosterone production have been corroborated *in vitro* using purified Leydig cell cultures from rats[43] and mice.[41,44] These studies indicate that ketoconazole directly inhibits the cytochrome-P450 activity of choles-terol side-chain cleavage and 17α-hydroxylase/$C_{17,20}$-lyase enzymes,[43-46] effects that are fully reversible following acute exposure.[40-42] The reversible effects of ketoconazole on Leydig cell steroidogenesis are consistent with studies demonstrating that ketoconazole inhibits LH-stimulated testosterone production but not Leydig cell viability, in highly purified adult rat Leydig cell cultures.[47]

Ketoconazole and other related imidazole derivatives bind directly to cyto-chrome-P450, inducing type II difference spectra.[48,49] The induction of type II difference spectra reflects ferrihemochrome formation with cytochrome-P450, thereby inhibiting enzyme activity (i.e., compounds containing amine groups bind to the ferric form of the hemoprotein to displace other potential or bound ligands from the enzyme).[50] Numerous drugs, detergents, and toxic chemicals also induce spectral changes in cytochrome-P450, suggesting their potential to impair Leydig cell function through inhibition of cytochrome-P450-depen-dent testosterone synthesis. While the direct interaction of xenobiotic chem-icals with steroidogenic cytochrome-P450 enzymes appears to be a common mechanism of chemical-induced Leydig cell dysfunction, this apparent insight may simply reflect the immense quantity of information regarding the mechanisms of cytochrome-P450. It is evident from studies using the female rat that the effects of ketaconazole are not limited to a single P450 enzyme. Administration to pregnant rats during the last third of gestation caused delayed delivery and maternal death, whereas higher doses led to pregnancy loss. These effects result from an inhibition of estradiol and proges-terone synthesis.[51] The reader is referred elsewhere for a comprehensive dis-cussion of the interactions of xenobiotic chemicals with cytochrome-P450.[50]

Several additional mechanisms by which xenobiotic chemicals are thought to directly alter Leydig cell steroidogenesis include (1) inhibition of choles-terol transport to the mitochondria by 2,3,7,8-tetrachlorodibenzo-*p*-dioxin,[52] diethylumbelliferyl phosphate,[53] and inhibitors of microtubule assembly and disassembly, such as cytochalasin B[54] and taxol;[55] (2) inhibition of calmodulin action by phenathiazines;[56,57] (3) reduced pyridine nucleotide levels by eth-anol;[58] and (4) inhibition of heme formation by cyclosporin.[59]

9.3.2.1.2 Steroid Hormones

The substrate specificity and regulatory effects of endogenous steroids on steroidogenic enzyme activity in the adrenal, ovary, testis, and placenta have been reviewed in detail.[60] Here the ability of glucocorticoids, androgens, and estrogens to alter LH-stimulated testosterone production by the testis *in vivo*, during *in vitro* testicular perfusion, and/or in highly purified Leydig cell cul-tures is examined. In all cases, the *in vitro* data not only corroborate the *in vivo* effects but also identify several unique biochemical and molecular mecha-nisms by which these compounds inhibit Leydig cell function. Environmental chemicals with similar mechanisms of action have not yet been identified, but then mechanisms beyond inhibition of steroidogenesis are often not pursued.

Glucocorticoids — The direct involvement of glucocorticoids in Leydig cell steroidogenesis was shown in adult male rats when glucocorticoid (i.e., cortisol) administration reduced the normal nocturnal rise in plasma testosterone levels without altering plasma levels of LH.[61] To determine whether the effects of glucocorticoids were specific to the testis or mediated by other organs or organ systems, *in vitro* experiments were completed with isolated testicular tissue. Direct inhibitory effects of stress levels of glucocorticoids on testicular LH receptor content and steroidogenesis were demonstrated using dispersed testicular and crude interstitial cell preparations.[62] Crude interstitial cell preparations subsequently were used to isolate the glucocorticoid-induced steroidogenic lesion to reduced cAMP production and reduced cytochrome-P450 enzyme activity.[63]

The direct effects of glucocorticoids on cytochrome-P450 enzymes intrinsic to the Leydig cell were obtained using purified mouse Leydig cell cultures.[64] These studies demonstrated that glucocorticoids, acting via the glucocorticoid receptor, negatively regulate the *de novo* synthesis and steady-state mRNA levels of cytochrome-P450 cholesterol side-chain cleavage enzyme ($P450_{SCC}$).[64] In this context, it is interesting that Leydig cells appear to have evolved a parallel enzymatic mechanism (i.e., 11β-hydroxysteroid dehydrogenase) for protection from the inhibitory effects of nonstress levels of glucocorticoids.[65] That is, 11β-hydroxysteroid dehydrogenase inactivates endogenous glucocorticoids in Leydig cells by oxidizing them to the 11-keto forms, which do not bind the glucocorticoid receptor.[65] This protective mechanism is simply overwhelmed with glucocorticoid under stress conditions resulting in inhibition of Leydig cell function. Clearly, these studies underscore the importance of considering potential confounding effects of toxicant-induced stress in whole animal studies, including those during development, on Leydig cell steroidogenesis. In the context, maternal stress levels of glucocorticoids have been demonstrated to lower serum testosterone levels in perinatal male rats.[66]

Androgens — *In vivo* studies suggest that testosterone may control its own synthesis and secretion via a short-loop negative feedback mechanism.[67,68] *In vitro* studies with the isolated-perfused rat testis suggest that when testosterone is perfused into the testis, subsequent testosterone synthesis is reduced.[69] Similar inhibitory effects of testosterone exist at the level of the purified adult rat Leydig cell, where testosterone inhibits cAMP-induced testosterone production by negatively regulating the *de novo* synthesis of 17α-hydroxylase.[70,71] This short-loop negative feedback effect of testosterone is likely mediated through the androgen receptor, as the negative effect of testosterone could be mimicked by mibolerone (an androgen receptor agonist) and blocked by hydroxyflutamide (an androgen receptor antagonist).[70]

In addition to an androgen receptor-mediated mechanism, purified cultures of adult rat[72] and mouse[73,74] Leydig cells have been used to identify a testosterone-induced oxygen-mediated increase in the rate of decay of the 17α-hydroxylase protein. The generation of reactive oxygen by this cytochrome-P450 enzyme is thought to result from the rebinding of reaction products like testosterone (i.e., a pseudosubstrate) to the enzyme active site.[75] That is, testosterone binds to the active site of the P450-dependent 17α-hydroxylase, induces electron flow and activation of molecular oxygen, but because it is no longer a substrate for hydroxylation (i.e., it already has been hydroxylated), the highly reactive oxygen attacks and destroys the enzyme.[73,76] Taken together, these studies suggest that androgens alter the synthesis and the stability of adult Leydig cell steroidogenic enzymes. Whether these mechanisms are operative in the fetal Leydig cell population is unknown, but it appears unlikely, since fetal Leydig cells are not desensitized by high concentrations of LH and continue to produce high levels of testosterone when they are repeatedly stimulated (see below).[77,78a,78b]

Estrogens — Estrogens have long been recognized to exert inhibitory effects on adult rat Leydig cell function through at least two different mechanisms, including a suppression of LH release by the pituitary and a direct effect of estrogen on testicular steroidogenesis.[79] *In vivo* experiments suggest that pharmacological levels of estrogen inhibit testosterone synthesis and secretion via inhibition of 17α-hydroxylase activity.[79,80] These *in vivo* testicular effects have been corroborated *in vitro* as estrogen appears to interact directly with the 17α-hydroxylase/$C_{17,20}$-lyase enzyme. These experiments used purified enzyme preparations to demonstrate that 17β-estradiol can bind to the enzyme and act as a noncompetitive inhibitor of 17α-hydroxylase and a competitive inhibitor of $C_{17,20}$-lyase activity.[81] The role of endogenous or environmental estrogens in the regulation of LH-stimulated testosterone production by the adult testis is not clear.

In addition to competing with substrate for binding to the catalytic site of steroidogenic enzymes, estrogens also have been implicated in the late lesion of gonadotropin-induced Leydig cell desensitization.[82] Gonadotropin-induced desensitization is defined as the diminished capacity of the testis to synthesize and secrete testosterone following a second injection of LH, i.e., compared to the capacity following the first LH injection.[81] This regulatory mechanism involves LH receptor downregulation and inhibition of steroidogenic enzyme activity via an estradiol-dependent 28 kd protein that inhibits cholesterol side-chain cleavage, 17α-hydroxylase and $C_{17,20}$-lyase.[82-85] The presence of estrogen receptors in Leydig cell nuclei is consistent with this estrogen-mediated mechanism for late-desensitization.[86-88] Perhaps most interesting, however, is the absence of this desensitization mechanism in fetal-type Leydig cells,[77,78] presumably protecting androgen-induced sexual differentiation of male fetuses from maternal estrogens.

Many different mechanisms exist to inhibit LH-stimulated testosterone production by the Leydig cell. While steroid hormones have been some of the most extensively studied to date, the recent attention attracted by environmental chemicals exhibiting endocrine disruptor activity may prompt additional mechanistic studies of environmental chemicals that impair Leydig cell function. A good example is the ability of ethanol to inhibit the enzymatic activity of 17α-hydroxylase in fetal but not immature or adult rat testes.[89,90] These studies suggest that fetal Leydig cells may be especially sensitive to the direct effects of ethanol and again emphasize the importance of comprehensively investigating the effects of chemicals on all Leydig cell populations.

9.3.2.2   Leydig Cell Viability

Although ethane-1,2-dimethanesulfonate (EDS) is not an environmental contaminant, it is included here as an example of a chemical that irreversibly alters Leydig cell function by specifically killing Leydig cells. EDS is a simple diester of methane sulfonic acid that selectively kills Leydig cells in the adult rat testis following *in vivo* administration.[91-94] The effects of EDS are specific for adult rat Leydig cells following a single ip injection (75-85 mg/kg). This dose of EDS does not affect growth of the rat,[95,96] result in the death of other interstitial or germinal cells in the adult testis,[91,94] or result in the death or elimination of Leydig cells from the fetal or immature rat testis.[97] The specificity of EDS for adult rat Leydig cells is underscored by the observation that closely related alkylating agents (e.g., butane dimethanesulfonate), which kill spermatogonia, have no effect on Leydig cells.[93]

The *in vivo* effects of EDS have been corroborated extensively *in vitro* using adult (i.e., EDS-sensitive) and immature (i.e., EDS-refractory) rats. Testes from adult and immature rats were perfused *in vitro* with EDS to determine the effects of EDS on Leydig cells maintained in their normal cytoarchitectural environment. Testosterone secretion by rat testes perfused *in vitro* with EDS was reduced significantly in adult but not immature animals, suggesting that EDS is not metabolically activated and that peripheral actions of EDS on other organs or organ systems do not mediate the toxic effects of EDS on Leydig cells.[97] The effects of EDS on the function and viability of highly purified adult and immature rat Leydig cell cultures were examined to determine whether EDS effects were intrinsic to the Leydig cell. EDS-induced alterations in Leydig cell function (LH-stimulated testosterone production) and viability (35S-methionine incorporation and reduction of MTT to formazan) were far more pronounced in adult than immature Leydig cells, as is the case *in vivo*.[97-99] These results indicate that other testicular cell types do not activate EDS to a toxic metabolite or mediate the disparate effects of EDS on androgen production by adult and immature rat Leydig cells. Taken together, Leydig cells from immature rats appear to be less sensitive intrinsically to the functional effects of EDS than Leydig cells from adult rats.

9.4   5-α-Reductase Activity: Mechanisms and Effects of Select Chemicals

9.4.1   Background

Androgen action is essential for the normal masculinization of the XY embryo during development. In fact, without androgen or the androgen receptor (e.g., androgen insensitivity syndrome), the phenotype of the fetus is female, irrespective of genetic sex.[100] Testosterone is the major circulating androgen in males; however, within certain target tissues testosterone is enzymatically reduced to the more potent androgen, 5α-dihydrotestosterone (DHT). The enzymatic activity of 5α-reductase (Type 2), the enzyme that converts testosterone to DHT in reproductive tissues, is high in the external genital anlage and urogenital sinus of rabbits, rats and humans during sex differentiation and development.[19,101,102] In contrast, 5α-reductase activity is low in the developing Wolffian ducts during their fetal development, suggesting that the external genitalia and prostate are dependent upon DHT for normal cell differentiation and histiogenesis, whereas those structures derived from the Wolffian ducts (epididymis, seminal vesicle, and vas deferens) are likely dependent on testosterone. This conclusion is supported by the findings that 5α-reductase-deficient males display ambiguous external genitalia, together with absent or nonpalpable prostates, while the development of the epididymis, seminal vesicle, and vas deferens is normal.[19,103,104]

Environmental chemicals that inhibit the activity or expression of 5α-reductase will likely induce a phenotype similar to 5α-reductase deficiency if exposure is during fetal development at the time of male reproductive tract differentiation. If 5α-reductase inhibition is suspected following developmental studies with test chemicals, their ability to directly inhibit enzyme activity is typically examined using radiometric enzyme assays that assess enzymatic conversion of radiolabeled substrate to radiolabeled product under defined conditions. To assess direct effects on enzyme activity, it is best to complete *in vitro* kinetic inhibition studies using varying concentrations of substrate at different fixed levels of test chemical.[105] These studies assess direct test chemical effects on both apparent substrate binding affinity (K_m) and the apparent number of catalytic sites (V_{max}), as well as information on the apparent affinity constant of the test chemical for its enzyme binding site (K_i). Alternatively, animals are dosed with test chemical, and the epididymis, seminal vesicle, and/or vas deferens are subsequently removed to assess the effect of chemical exposure on 5α-reductase activity (*ex vivo*). It is important to remember that these latter *ex vivo* experiments typically use near-saturating concentrations of substrate in single point assays to assess the effects of the test chemical on 5α-reductase enzyme expression. That is, they are used to determine whether chemical exposure alters the number of enzyme molecules in that tissue. Ideally, both types of experiments should be completed if inhibition of 5α-reductase activity is suspect as a mechanism for adverse reproductive effects. Recent studies by Nukui provide a good example of the use of these *in vitro* and *ex vivo* procedures in human tissues from patients being treated for prostate cancer.[106]

9.4.2   Chemical Effects and Mechanisms

9.4.2.1   Pharmacological Agents

Inhibition of 5α-reductase activity in adult males leads to reduced androgenic support for the maintenance of those tissues, such as the prostate, that are dependent on DHT. Medical conditions of uncontrolled prostate growth in humans, such as benign prostatic hyperplasia and androgen-dependent prostate cancers, have led to the development of pharmaceuticals (e.g., finasteride, etc.) that specifically inhibit the enzymatic activity of the Type 2 enzyme present in these reproductive tissues. As anticipated, administration of these pharmaceutical agents to rodents during development results in feminization of the external genitalia and underdeveloped but not absent ventral prostate tissue.[19] These latter results suggest that increased levels of testosterone may compensate for the lack of DHT at the level of the AR.[19] Obviously, the use of these drugs is contraindicated during pregnancy. A number of steroidal and nonsteroidal 5α-reductase inhibitors have been developed for pharmaceutical purposes, and the reader is referred to a recent review for additional information.[107]

9.4.2.2   Steroid Hormones and Natural Products

It has been known for some time that estrogens such as 17β-estradiol and diethylstilbestrol inhibit the enymatic activity of 5α-reductase *in vivo* and *in vitro*.[108-112] The Δ⁴-3-ketosteroid hormones competitively inhibit 5α-reductase activity, suggesting competition for binding at the level of the enzyme active site.[108,111] It is interesting that few xenobiotic chemicals have been reported to inhibit the activity of Type 2 5α-reductase,[113] while a number of natural products with this activity have been identified,[114] including gossypol, a natural product derived from cotton seeds.[115] Most of the plant extracts are not effective in inhibiting human prostate 5α-reductase activity or prostate growth compared to more potent pharmaceuticals. Permixon, however, an androgen receptor antagonist with 5α-reductase inhibitory activity, appears to be effective and currently is used clinically for the treatment of benign prostatic hyperplasia (see section 9.5.2.5 below). Presumably, environmental chemicals that inhibit 5α-reductase activity would be identified in Hershbergher type assays with castrate testosterone-implanted adult male rats where the size of the ventral prostate should be reduced with little to no effect being observed on seminal vesicle size. The paucity of information regarding environmental 5α-reductase inhibitors may simply be due to limited studies of this type or with this enzyme, or the active binding site of the 5α-reductase enzyme may not be conducive to binding by structurally diverse environmental chemicals. The Type 1 5α-reductase activity also can be inhibited by natural products, as catechins in green tea have been shown to inhibit Type 1 5α-reductase activity *in vitro*.[116]

9.5 Androgen Receptor Anatagonists: Mechanism and Effects of Select Chemicals

9.5.1 Background

The androgen testosterone produced by the Leydig cells of the testis dissociates from serum carrier proteins (e.g., albumin and sex-hormone binding globulin) to diffuse into cells, where it binds AR. In target tissues such as the prostate and epididymis, testosterone is reduced to DHT, a more potent, slower dissociating androgen.[117] Agonist-bound AR monomers undergo conformational changes, likely resulting in the loss of heat-shock proteins, and are imported into nuclei, where they dimerize[118] and bind to androgen response element DNA regulatory sequences within intron regions or flanking androgen-responsive genes, resulting in transcriptional activation.[119,120] During sex differentiation and development, androgen-induced gene products bring about androgen-dependent cell functions critical to cell differentiation, tissue histiogenesis, and normal sex differentiation and development (Figure 9.1).

Sex steroid hormone antagonists originally were thought to function as simple competitive inhibitors of natural ligand binding. However, it now is clear that these antihormones are actively involved in the process of inhibiting androgen action. Conformational differences in the AR induced by hormone or antihormone binding are readily detectable using limited proteolytic digestion techniques.[121] The altered structural conformation of the ligand binding domain most likely explains the functional ability of some antiandrogens (e.g., hydroxyflutamide) to inhibit AR dimerization and transcriptional activation. The binding of antagonists with moderate affinity for the AR also may fail to stabilize the receptor, effectively reducing the half-life of the receptor protein in target cells.[122] That is, natural ligands with high affinity for the AR slow receptor degradation by prolonging nuclear retention and thereby limiting recycling of the receptor from the nucleus to the cytosol.[122]

Binding of antihormones to AR may induce a receptor conformation that differs from that imposed by agonist binding altering its ability to activate transcription.[123-125] Proposed models of antihormone action include two mechanisms of transcriptional inhibition that reflect the ability of receptors to bind DNA. Type I antagonists bind receptors but prevent DNA binding and transcriptional activation, whereas type II antagonists promote DNA

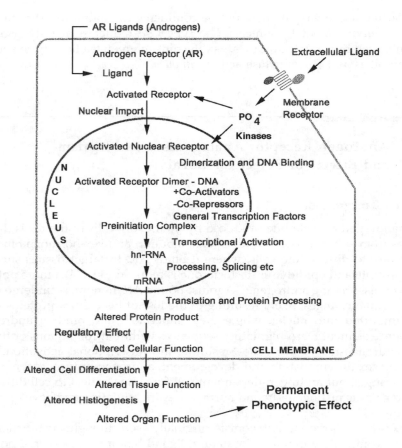

FIGURE 9.1

A simplified diagram of androgen receptor-mediated events prerequisite to normal androgen-induced cell differentiation and histiogensis of male reproductive tissues/organs that occur during sex differentiation and development. Androgens (testosterone or DHT) pass through the plasma membrane of the target cell by passive diffusion and/or active transport and bind the ligand binding domain of the intracellular androgen receptor. The activated receptor typically loses its associated heat shock proteins and imports into the nucleus from its predominantly perinuclear location in the cytosol. In some instances cell surface-acting ligands (e.g., growth factors and cytokines) bind their respective membrane receptors (these membrane receptors usually consist of an extracellular ligand binding domain, a single transmembrane region usually containing seven transmembrane spanning domains, and an intracelluar domain exhibiting kinase activity for autophosphorylation), resulting in phosphorylation of various protein substrates, which can phosphorylate either the cytosolic or the nuclear androgen receptor to modulate its transcriptional activity. The activated nuclear androgen receptor monomer then binds androgen response element DNA as a dimer and initiates formation of the preinitiation complex, whereby specific co-activators are attracted, co-repressors are released, and general transcription factors are recruited to the complex to initiate transcription. The heterogeneous nuclear RNA that is produced via transcription of the downstream androgen receptor-dependent gene is spliced to remove the introns and processed to add a poly A RNA tail characteristic of messenger RNA. The mRNA is transferred to the cytoplasm, where it is translated on ribosomes to protein, whose regulatory effect is to alter cell function to promote normal binding but nevertheless fail to initiate transcription.[126] Environmental anti-androgens identified thus far exhibit low to moderate affinity for AR and act as type I antagonists by preventing AR DNA binding.[127,128] We have previously suggested that binding of different ligands in the same receptor dimer (mixed-ligand dimer) is required for AR antagonism;[128] however, the specific mechanisms responsible for inhibition of AR DNA binding remain unknown. This mechanism could include (1) increased AR degradation via an inappropriate receptor conformation; (2) an inability of rapidly dissoci-ating ligands to stabilize AR;[117,129] (3) incompatibility of the AR dimerization interface for agonist and antagonist bound AR whereby mixed ligand dimers fail to form; and/or, (4) failure of mixed-ligand AR dimers to bind DNA due to an inappropriate dimer conformation[130] or an inability to release receptor-associated proteins requisite for subsequent DNA binding.[121,131]

9.5.2 Chemical Effects and Mechanisms

9.5.2.1 Pharmaceuticals

Several nonsteroidal pharmaceuticals (e.g., flutamide, casodex, and niluta-mide) have been developed by pharmaceutical companies to treat androgen-dependent prostate carcinoma and benign prostatic hyperplasia/hypertro-phy. Flutamide is hydroxylated *in vivo* to hydroxyflutamide, which acts as a pure AR antagonist; it binds the AR, is efficiently imported into the nucleus but, like the active vinclozolin metabolites and p,p'-DDE (see below), fails to initiate transcription.[129] ICI 176,334 (Casodex) binds to the AR and fails to induce receptor accessory protein dissociation, DNA binding, or transcrip-tional activation.[132,133] Nilutamide is a nonsteroidal antiandrogen with weak affinity for the AR; it has a long biological half-life and exhibits potent antiandrogenic activity *in vivo*, likely reflecting its inhibitory action on andro-gen synthesis in addition to inhibition of AR binding.[134] Developmental reproductive alterations induced by drugs specifically designed to inhibit androgen action have previously been described[19,135] and resemble alter-ations produced by natural mutations in the AR gene[100,136] and those induced by environmental antiandrogens.[137]

9.5.2.2 Steroid Hormones

9.5.2.2.1 Androgens

As discussed above, androgens are absolutely required for the masculiniza-tion of the reproductive tract of the fetal male. Paradoxically, exogenously administered testosterone adversely affects sex differentiation in male rats,

---

FIGURE 9.1 (continued)

cellular differentiation and, subsequently, normal histiogenesis requisite for organ formation. Alterations in this process at any level may lead to permanent effects and characterize an altered phenotype.

as males treated neonatally with high doses of testosterone exhibit small testes with hypospermatogenesis and reduced prostate, seminal vesicle, and epididymal weights.[138] The effects on the prostate and epididymis are thought to be mediated via reduced 5α- reductase activity.[139] These results indicate that while androgens are required for male reproductive development, their presence in excess is detrimental.

9.5.2.2.2   Estrogens

Antiandrogenic effects seen in male animals exposed *in utero* or neonatally to estrogens resemble those seen in human males exposed to DES during development. Male mice, given DES perinatally, develop epididymal cysts, hypospadias, phallic hypoplasia, inhibition of growth and descent of the testes, and underdevelopment or absence of the vas deferens, epididymis, and seminal vesicles.[140] *In vitro* ligand binding experiments suggest that the estrogenic chemicals estradiol, DES, and o,p′-DDT all compete with endogenous androgens for binding to the AR.[141] Once bound to the receptor, these estrogenic chemicals act as AR antagonists by inhibiting transcriptional activation. These results suggest that the demasculinizing action of estrogenic chemicals on male offspring after *in utero* exposure may result from an antagonistic interaction of the "estrogenic" compound with the androgen receptor, rather than acting exclusively through the ER. In support of this hypothesis is the report that human male external genitalia at 18-22 weeks of gestation exhibit intense positive immunohistochemical staining for the androgen, but not the estrogen, receptor.[141] The fact that ER was not detectable in human male external genitalia during development questions whether estrogenic chemicals act through the ER to influence directly the development of the male external genitalia.

9.5.2.2.3   Progestins

Depending on the dose, ligand structure, and individual tissue responsiveness, progestins interact with a functional AR to induce androgenic (mimic androgen action), synandrogenic (potentiate androgen action), and antiandrogenic (inhibit androgen action) effects.[142] In the kidney, androgens act via the AR to stimulate β-glucuronidase and ornithine decarboxylase activity.[143,144] Progestins like medroxyprogesterone acetate (MPA) but not progesterone itself also act via the AR to stimulate the activity of these enzymes.[142] As these effects are not demonstrable when the AR is mutated and nonfunctional (e.g., Tfm/y mice,[145,146] androgen-insensitive rats,[143] or humans with testicular feminization[147]), it is clear that the androgenic action of these progestins requires a functional AR.

Cyproterone acetate is a synthetic derivative of hydroxyprogesterone that exhibits antiandrogenic as well as progestational activity.[135,148,149] Exposure to cyproterone acetate during development induces antiandrogenic effects in the male mouse, rat, guinea pig, hamster, sheep, pig, and dog consistent with those induced by testicular feminization.[135] The antiandrogenic activity of cyproterone acetate results from competitive inhibition at the level of the

AR. Cyproterone acetate is not considered a true antiandrogen as it exhibits both agonist (at high concentrations) and antagonist (at lower concentrations) activity *in vivo*.[129] At high concentrations, cyproterone acetate, progesterone, and the synthetic anti-progestin RU486 not only bind the AR, but they promote nuclear transport, AR DNA binding and transcriptional activation.[129] This correlates precisely with the *in vivo* observations that at high concentrations, progestational steroids act as androgens by stimulating the growth of the male reproductive tract and virilization of the female fetus.[129]

9.5.2.3   Vinclozolin

The fungicide vinclozolin alters sex differentiation in male rats by inhibition of AR-mediated gene activation.[128,150] In male rat offspring, perinatal exposure to vinclozolin causes reduced anogenital distance, hypospadias, ectopic testes, vaginal pouch formation, agenesis of the ventral prostate, and nipple retention; females are phenotypically normal.[137] While a transient reduction in anogenital distance is the most sensitive endpoint to detect environmental chemicals with antiandrogen activity, these effects are usually accompanied by permanent alterations, such as retained nipples and permanently reduced seminal vesicle and ventral prostate weights. Dosages of 12 mg vinclozolin/kg/d or lower administered to pregnant rats result in reduced anogenital distance, retained nipples, and permanently reduced ventral prostate weights in male offspring, while 100 mg/kg/d cause hypospadias, deformity, and infertility in all males. In contrast, fertility is unaffected in male rats exposed as adults following prolonged exposure to 100 mg vinclozolin/kg/d for 25 weeks.[151] These results suggest that the developing male fetus is particularly sensitive to endocrine disruptors such as vinclozolin, which can produce malformations at dosages that have little reproductive effect in adult males.

The molecular mechanism responsible for the antiandrogenic effects of vinclozolin has been elucidated.[128,152] Vinclozolin is hydrolyzed to two ring opened metabolites, M1 and M2, which compete for AR androgen binding, induce AR nuclear import, and inhibit DHT-induced transcriptional activation by blocking AR DNA binding.[128] The parent chemical vinclozolin is a poor inhibitor of AR androgen binding and subsequent transactivation, suggesting that vinclozolin developmental toxicity is mediated via the formation of active metabolites.[152] The enhanced activity of the vinclozolin metabolites, compared to vinclozolin itself, was perhaps predictable based on the structural similarity of these metabolites with the potent antiandrogen hydroxyflutamide.

9.5.2.4   DDT Metabolites

Recently, we demonstrated both *in vivo* and *in vitro* that p,p'-DDE, the persistent metabolite of p,p'-DDT that bioaccumulates in the environment, is a potent environmental antiandrogen.[127] While o,p'-DDT is a well-known environmental estrogen, the predominant p,p'-DDT metabolite, p,p'-DDE, does not bind the estrogen receptor.[127] When administered to pregnant rats from gestational day 14-18, p,p'-DDE (100 mg/kg/d) reduces anogenital distance and causes retention of thoracic nipples in male progeny,[127] both of which are indicative of prenatal antiandrogen exposure.[19] p,p'-DDE binds AR *in vitro* with moderate affinity and inhibits DHT-induced transcriptional activation with a potency similar to that of the antiandrogenic drug, hydroxyflutamide. The mechanism responsible for transcriptional inhibition was determined using electrophoretic mobility shift and promoter interference assays to be inhibition of AR-DNA binding.[127] A similar mechanism was observed for the structurally related pesticide, methoxychlor, and its primary o-demethylated metabolite, 2,2-bis-*p*-hydroxyphenol-1,1,1-trichloroethane (manuscript submitted). The most potent environmental antiandrogens identified to date bind AR and inhibit transcription of androgen-dependent genes *in vitro* by blocking AR-DNA binding, implicating this as a common mechanism.

To determine whether these model chemicals inhibit the expression of androgen-regulated genes *in vivo*, their ability to induce a testosterone-repressed prostatic mRNA (TRPM-2) or repress a testosterone-induced prostatic mRNA (prostatein subunit C3) was assessed in adult rats. The results indicate that exposure to vinclozolin or p,p'-DDE induces testosterone-repressed TRPM-2 mRNA and represses the androgen-induced C3 mRNA compared to vehicle treated control rats, consistent with the mechanism of an antiandrogen.[150] Vinclozolin metabolites and p,p'-DDE inhibit the expression of androgen-regulated genes *in vivo* and *in vitro* at biologically relevant concentrations. These endocrine data (i.e., both mechanistic and morphological) are currently being used in the risk assessment process for vinclozolin and provide an *in vivo/in vitro* investigational strategy for the study of environmental antiandrogens.

Birth defects in humans that could result from inhibition of androgen action include alterations in the development of the male external genitalia.[153,154] Environmental chemicals with antiandrogen activity may contribute to the increasing incidence of isolated hypospadias in the human population, as this anomaly is not frequently associated with mutations in the AR coding sequence,[155,156] with steroid 5α-reductase (type 2) deficiency,[157] or with decreased levels of AR.[158] Hypospadias has been linked to fetal exposure to estrogenic chemicals during the first trimester;[159] however, the external genitalia of the human male fetus may lack estrogen receptor.[141] As estrogens bind AR with moderate affinity,[160] the increased incidence of hypospadias following developmental exposure to estrogenic chemicals may be mediated at the level of the AR. Environmental antiandrogens could induce male pseudohermaphroditism (incomplete masculinization of the male fetus) to differing degrees, depending on the time of exposure and chemical potency.[11]

9.5.2.5   Plant Products

A natural plant product has been shown to possess antiandrogenic activity. Permixon is a liposterolic extract from the fruit of the American dwarf palm tree Serenoa Repens B, native to Florida.[161] In clinical trials, this palm tree extract was found to lessen the signs and symptoms of benign prostatic hyperplasia, including dysuria, nocturia, and poor urinary flow.[162] The anti-androgenic effects of Permixon are mediated through direct action at the level of the AR (IC_{50} = 367 µg/ml) and via inhibition of 5α-reductase activity (IC_{50} = 88 µg/ml).[161] To the best of our knowledge, effects of Permixon on the development of the male or female reproductive systems have not been reported.

9.6 Screening for Environmental Antiandrogens

It has been argued that we, the public, are safeguarded from EDCs, as these chemicals would be detected in the safety assessment studies required of industry before marketing chemicals. However, many chemicals, including environmental antiandrogens, are poorly characterized in these standardized multigenerational tests due to the failure of these tests to measure the most sensitive endpoints and the lack of appreciation for the complexity of animal responses to EDCs. Standard tests have missed some of the malformations and all of the low-dose effects (e.g., reduced anogenital distance, presence of nipples on males, reduced adult sex accessory organ weights, undescended testes, vaginal pouches, and bladder stones) of chemicals like vinclozolin and procymidone, both of which were later identified in mechanistic studies to be antiandrogens. Multigenerational studies with DDT, the prototype EDC, failed to detect the estrogenic effects of o,p'-DDT or the antiandrogenic effects of p,p'-DDE in rats, mice, and beagle dogs.[163] New test guidelines implemented by the U.S. Environmental Protection Agency (US EPA) will improve antiandrogen detectability for pesticides, but these tests will not be routinely used for most chemicals (i.e., toxic substances or pharmaceuticals) and are long-term (years) and resource-intensive studies.

Some have proposed that the release of EDCs into the environment, where they either act alone or in concert with other environmental pollutants, will be identified in epidemiology studies. However, this seems very unlikely, as many of the developmental effects of EDCs are not manifest until steroid hormone levels increase with the onset of puberty. It is then difficult to associate these latent effects with a specific developmental exposure. For example, if antiandrogen exposure delayed or prevented testicular descent in humans (cryptorchidism), the associated increase in testicular cancer would not be seen until 30-40 years later.[164] Epidemiological studies are rarely conducted to search for such latent reproductive effects and are more effective at detecting increases in rare events, such as vaginal cancer associated with developmental exposure to diethylstilbestrol. Cryptorchidism occurs at a rate of about 3% in the population.[164] A doubling of this incidence in a population exposed to environmental antiandrogens may go undetected because of the large sample size of exposed individuals needed to detect events occurring against a high normal background. The absence of a national health data base, inconsistent reporting and characterization of these adverse developmental effects, and poor funding for epidemiological studies in general compound the problem of hazard identification in humans.

In response to deficiencies in current testing requirements and the growing public concern with EDCs, the U.S. Congress recently mandated via the Food Quality Protection Act (Public Law 104-170) and the Safe Drinking Water Act (Public Law 104-182) that chemicals specifically be screened for hormone activity. *In vivo* and *in vitro* testing protocols being recommended for EDC screening include cell-free and whole-cell receptor binding assays, hormone-dependent cell proliferation assays, transcriptional activation assays to distinguish agonists from antagonists, and short-term, hormone-specific *in vivo* assays (assays such as the Hershbergher or delayed male pubertal maturation assays for estrogen and androgen/antiandrogen activity).[165] The application of these protocols will certainly increase EDC identification and also will contribute to the evaluation of their potential to induce adverse effects in wildlife and human populations.

As it is doubtful that any one single *in vivo* or *in vitro* test will assess adequately endocrine disrupting activity, we also suggest combining *in vivo* and *in vitro* test strategies. *In vivo* tests identify chemicals with endocrine-disrupting activity, whereas *in vitro* tests reveal the effective chemical or metabolite and provide information regarding the biochemical mechanism. Given this information, human susceptibility and risk assessment issues can subsequently be addressed. For example, vinclozolin administered for 30 days starting at weaning delayed puberty, reduced the weights of the sex accessory glands, and increased serum testosterone and LH levels consistent with the endocrine profile of an antiandrogen. In a developmental study, vinclozolin caused alterations in male rat sex differentiation, such as reduced anogenital distance, cleft phallus, hypospadias, ectopic testes, and retained thoracic nipples in male offspring,[137] all indicative of antiandrogen activity. Subsequent *in vitro* studies demonstrated that although the parent chemical, vinclozolin, bound AR weakly, its two primary hydrolysis products were stronger androgen antagonists.[152] Maternal serum concentrations of these metabolites were at levels near the Ki for inhibition of androgen binding, suggesting that the developmental toxicity of vinclozolin was mediated by its hydrolysis products, M1 and M2.[152] Molecular studies determined that the mechanism of inhibition of androgen-induced transcriptional activation was inhibition of AR-DNA binding.[128] Within a relatively short period and with a limited number of animals, the antiandrogenic activity of vinclozolin was identified, its adverse developmental effects characterized, and the biochemical and molecular mechanism established. Thus, combining *in vivo* and *in vitro* test strategies is effective in the identification and characterization of environmental endocrine disruptors.

Some of the above testing strategy was used to identify over 25 environmental chemicals predicted to have an affinity for AR. Those structures shown biochemically to interact with AR were introduced into a computer model, together with known androgen agonists and antagonists, to develop a three-dimensional quantitative structure-activity relationship (3D-QSAR) paradigm that predicts AR binding affinity solely from chemical structure, taking into account steric and electrostatic properties.[166] The model is being used to search structural databases for potential androgen agonists and antagonists. Chemicals identified using the computer are subsequently examined empirically for AR binding activity, induction or inhibition of androgen-dependent transcriptional activity, and the potential to induce antiandrogenic *in vivo* developmental effects. Alternatively, in situations where a chemical is found to induce antiandrogenic effects *in vivo* but not *in vitro*, the computer model is useful for searching structural variations of the parent chemical for potential active metabolite(s) responsible for the antiandrogenic effects. To date, the computer model has identified several hundred chemicals with the potential to bind AR. Empirical testing has begun and already several novel androgen antagonists have been identified.[166]

References

1. Fox, G. A., Epidemiological and pathobiological evidence of contaminant-induced alterations in sexual development in free-living wildlife, in *Chemically-Induced Alterations in Sexual and Functional Development: The Wildlife/Human Connection*, Colborn. T. and Clement, C., Eds., Princeton Scientific Publishing Co., Inc, Princeton, NJ, 1992.
2. Guillette, L. J. and Crain, D. A. Endocrine-disrupting contaminants and reproductive abnormalities in reptiles, *Comm. Toxicol.*, 5, 381, 1996.
3. Jirasek, J. E., in Cohen, M. M., Ed., *Development of the Genital System and Male Pseudohermaphroditism*, Johns Hopkins Press, Baltimore, 1971.
4. Leung, T. J., Baird, P. A., and McGillivray, B., Hypospadias in British Columbia, *Am. J. Med. Genet.*, 21, 39, 1985.
5. Nelson, C. M. K. and Bunge, R. G., Semen analysis: evidence for changing parameters of male fertility potential, *Fertil. Steril.*, 25, 503, 1974.
6. Leto, S. and Frensilli, F. J., Changing parameters of donor semen, *Fertil. Steril.*, 36, 766, 1981.
7. Bostofte, E., Serup, J., and Rebbe, H., Has the fertility of Danish men declined through the years in terms of semen quality? A comparison of semen qualities between 1952 and 1972, *Int. J. Fertil.*, 28, 91, 1983.
8. Carlsen, E., Giwercman, A., Keiding, N., and Skakkebaek, N. E., Evidence for decreasing quality of semen during the past 50 years, *Br. Med. J.*, 305, 609, 1992.

This manuscript has been reviewed in accordance with the policy of the National Health and Environmental Effects Research Laboratory, U.S. Environmental Protection Agency, and approved for publication. Approval does not signify that the contents necessarily reflect the views and policies of the Agency, nor does mention of trade names or commercial products constitute endorsement or recommendation for use.

9. Skakkebaek, N. E. and Keiding, N., Changes in semen and the testis, *Br. Med. J.*, 309, 1316, 1994.
10. Auger, J., Kunstmann, J. M., Czyglik, F., and Jouannet, P., Decline in semen quality among fertile men in Paris during the past 20 years, *N. Engl. J. Med.*, 332, 281, 1995.
11. Schardein, J., Hormones and hormone antagonists, in *Chemically Induced Birth Defects*, 2nd ed., Dekker, New York, 1993, 271.
12. Kelce, W. R. and Gray, L. E., Antiandrogens as environmental endocrine disruptors, *Health Environ. Dig.*, 11, 9, 1997.
13. Peterson, R., Cooke, P., Gray, L. E., and Kelce, W. R., Endocrine disruptors, in *Reproductive and Endocrine Toxicology: Male Reproductive Toxicology*, Vol. 10, Comprehensive Toxicology, Boekelheide, K. and Chapin, R., Eds., 1997, 181.
14. Gray, L. E., Monosson, E., and Kelce, W. R., Emerging issues: the effects of endocrine disruptors on reproductive development, in *Interconnections Between Human and Ecosystem Health*, Di Giulio, R. and Monosson, E., Eds., Chapman and Hall, New York, 1996, 46.
15. Guillette, L. J., Arnold, S. F., and McLachlan, J. A. Ecoestrogens and embryos — is there a scientific basis for concern? *An. Reprod. Sci.*, 42, 13, 1996.
16. Toppari, J., Larsen, J. C., Christiansen, P., Giwercman, A., Grandjean, P., and Guillette, L. J., Male reproductive health and environmental chemicals with estrogenic effects, *Miljoprojekt nr*, 290, 1995, 1.
17. Kelce, W. R. and Wilson, E. M., Clinical, functional and molecular implications of environmental antiandrogens, *J. Mol. Med.*, 75, 198, 1997.
18. Kavlock, R. J., Daston, G. P., DeRosa, C., and Fenner-Crisp, P., Research needs for the risk assessment of health and environmental effects of endocrine disruptors: a report of the US EPA-sponsored workshop, *Environ. Health Perspect.*, 104, 715, 1996.
19. Imperato-McGinley, J., Sanchez, R. S., Spencer, J. R., Yee, B., and Vaugan, E. D., Comparision of the effects of the 5alpha-reductase inhibitor finasteride and the antiandrogen flutamide on prostate and genital differentiation: dose response studies, *Endocrinology*, 131, 1149, 1992.
20. George, F. W., Androgen metabolism in the prostate of the finasteride-treated, adult rat: a possible explanation for the differential action of testosterone and 5α-dihydrotestosterone during development of the male urogenital tract, *Endocrinology*, 138, 871, 1997.
21. Bentvelsen, F. M., McPhaul, M. J., Wilson, J. D., and George, F. W., The androgen receptor of the urogenital tract of the fetal rat is regulated by androgen, *Mol. Cell. Endocrinol.*, 105, 21, 1994.
22. Curley, A., Copeland, M. F., and Kimbrough, R. D., Chlorinated hydrocarbon insecticides in organs of stillborn and blood of newborn babies, *Arch. Environ. Health*, 19, 628, 1969.
23. Bouwman, H., Reinecke, A. J., Cooppan, R. M., and Becker, P. J., Factors affecting levels of DDT and metabolites in human breast milk from Kwazulu, *J. Toxicol. Environ. Health*, 31, 93, 1990.
24. Bouwman, H., Cooppan, R. M., Becker, P. J., and Ngxongo, S., Malaria control and levels of DDT in serum of two populations in Kwazulu, *J. Toxicol. Environ. Health*, 33, 141, 1991.
25. Simonich, S. L. and Hites, R. A., Global distribution of persistent organochlorine compounds, *Science*, 269, 1851, 1995.

26. Ewing, L. L. and Zirkin, B. R., Leydig cell structure and steroidogenic function, *Rec. Prog. Horm. Res.*, 39, 599, 1983.

27. Hall, P. F., *The Physiology of Reproduction*, Knobil, E. and Neill, J. D., Eds., Raven Press, New York, 1988, 975.

28. de Krester, D. M. and Kerr, J. B., *The Physiology of Reproduction*, Knobil, E. and Neill, J. D., Eds., Raven Press, New York, 1988, 837.

29. Dufau, M. L., The endocrine regulation and communicating functions of the Leydig cell, *Annu. Rev. Physiol.*, 50, 483, 1988.

30. Kelce, W. R., The Leydig cell: mechanisms of toxicity, in *Reproductive and Endocrine Toxicology: Male Reproductive Toxicology*, Vol. 10, Comprehensive Toxicology, Boekelheide, K. and Chapin, R., Eds., Elsevier Science, New York, 1997, 113.

31. Wing, T.-Y., Ewing, L. L., and Zirkin, B. R., Effect of LH withdrawal on Leydig cell smooth endoplasmic reticulum and steroidogenic reactions which convert pregnenolone to testosterone, *Endocrinology*, 115, 2290, 1984.

32. Mendis-Handagama, S. L. M. C., Zirkin, B. R., and Ewing, L. L., Comparision of components of the testis interstitium with testosterone secretion in hamster, rat and guinea pig testes perfused *in vitro*, *Am. J. Anat.*, 181, 12, 1988.

33. Saez, J. M., Leydig cells: endocrine, paracrine and autocrine regulation, *Endocr. Rev.*, 15, 574, 1994.

34. Taton, M., Ullmann, P., Benveniste, P., and Rahier, A., *Pest. Biochem. Physiol.*, 30, 178, 1988.

35. Murray, M. and Reidy, G., Selectivity in the inhibition of mammalian cytochromes P-450 by chemical agents, *Pharmacol. Rev.*, 42, 85, 1990.

36. Glasser, S., Northcutt, R., Chytil, F., and Strott, C., The influence of an antisteroidogenic drug (aminoglutethimide phosphate) on pregnancy maintenance, *Endocrinology*, 90, 1363, 1972.

37. Goldman, A. S., Eavey, R. D., and Baker, M. K., Production of male pseudohermaphroditism in rats by two new inhibitors of steroid 17α-hydroxylase and C17-20 lyase, *J. Endocrinol.*, 71, 289, 1976.

38. Milne, C., Hasmall, R., Russell, A., Watson, S., Vaughan, Z., and Middleton, M., Reduced estradiol production by a substituted triazole results in delayed ovulation in rats, *Toxicol. Appl. Pharmacol.*, 90, 427, 1987.

39. Tayeb, E., Salih, Y., and Pillay, A., Effects of aminoglutethimide on ovarian histology in the rat, *Acta Anat.*, 122, 212, 1985.

40. Pont, A., Williams, P. L., Azhar, S., Reitz, R. E., Bochra, C., Smith, E. R., and Stevens, D. A., Ketoconazole blocks testosterone synthesis, *Arch. Int. Med.*, 142, 2137, 1982.

41. Schurmeyer, T. and Nieschlag, E., Effect of ketoconazole and other imidazole fungicides on testosterone biosynthesis, *Acta Endocrinol.*, 105, 275, 1984.

42. Vawda, A. I. and Davies, A. G., An investigation into the effects of ketoconazole on testicular function in Wistar rats, *Acta Endocrinol.*, 111, 246, 1986.

43. Kan, P. B., Hirst, M. A., and Feldman, D., Inhibition of steroidogenic cytochrome-P450 enzymes in rat testes by ketoconazole and related imidazole antifungal drugs, *J. Steroid Biochem.*, 23, 1023, 1985.

44. Chaudhary, L. R. and Stocco, D. M., Inhibition of hCG- and cAMP-stimulated progesterone production in MA-10 Leydig tumor cells by ketoconazole, *Biochem. Inter.*, 18, 251, 1989.

45. Rajfer, J., Sikka, S. C., Xie, H. W., and Swerdloff, R. J., Effect of *in vitro* ketoconazole on steroid production in rat testis, *Steroids*, 46, 867, 1985.

46. Sikka, S. C., Swerdloff, R. S., and Reifer, J., *In vitro* inhibition of testosterone biosynthesis by ketoconazole, *Endocrinology,* 116, 1920, 1985.

47. Kelce, W. R., Zirkin, B. R., and Ewing, L. L., Leydig cell cultures can be used to identify toxicants acting to impair or kill Leydig cells, *Alt. Meth. Toxicol.,* 8, 397, 1991.

48. Higashi, Y., Yoshida, K.-I., and Oshima, H., *In vitro* inhibition by ketoconazole of human testicular steroid oxidoreductases, *J. Steroid Biochem.,* 36, 667, 1990.

49. Mason, J. I., Murray, B. A., Olcott, M., and Sheet, J. J., Imidazole antimycotics: inhibitors of steroid aromatase, *Biochem. Pharmacol.,* 34, 1087, 1985.

50. Schenkman, J., Sligar, S. G., and Cinti, D. L., Substrate interaction with cyto-chrome-P450, *Pharm. Ther.,* 12, 43, 1981.

51. Gray, L. E., Kelce, W. R., and Laskey, J. L., Pesticides affect mammalian repro-ductive development and function via multiple mechanisms of action, Wing-spread Conference on Contemporary Use Pesticides, Racine, WI, 1996.

52. Moore, R. W., Jefcoate, C. R., and Peterson, R. E., 2,3,7,8-Tetrachlorodibenzo-*p*-dioxin inhibits steroidogenesis in the rat testis by inhibiting the mobilization of cholesterol to cytochrome P-450$_{scc}$, *Toxicol. Appl. Pharmacol.,* 109, 85, 1991.

53. Gocze, P. M. and Freeman, D. A., A cholesterol ester hydrolase inhibitor blocks cholesterol translocation into the mitochondria of MA-10 Leydig tumor cells, *Endocrinology,* 131, 2972, 1992.

54. Murono, E. P., Lin, T., Osterman, J., and Nankin, H. R., The effects of cytocha-lasin B on testosterone synthesis by interstitial cells of rat testis, *Biochem. Bio-phys. Acta.,* 633, 228, 1980.

55. Rainey, W. E., Kramer, R. E., Mason, J. I., and Shay, J. W., The effects of Taxol, a microtubule stabilizing drug, on steroidogenic cells, *J. Cell Physiol.,* 123, 17, 1985.

56. Melner, M. H., Zimniski, S. J., and Puett, D., Divergent effects of phenothiazines on Leydig tumor cell steroidogenesis and adenylate activity, *J. Steroid Biochem.,* 19, 1111, 1983.

57. Sullivan, M. H. F. and Cooke, B. A., Effects of calmodulin and lipoxygenase inhibitors on LH (lutropin)- and LHRH (luliberin)-agonist-stimulated steroido-genesis in rat Leydig cells, *Biochem. J.,* 232, 55, 1985.

58. Gordon, G. G., Vittek, J., Southren, A., Munnagi, P., and Lieber, C. S., Effect of chronic alcohol ingestion on the biosynthesis of steroids in rat testicular ho-mogenate *in vitro, Endocrinology,* 106, 1880, 1980.

59. Krueger, B. A., Trakshel, G. M., Sluss, P. M., and Maines, M. D., Cyclosporin-mediated depression of luteinizing hormone receptors and heme biosynthesis in rat testes: A possible mechanism for decrease in serum testosterone, *Endo-crinology,* 129, 2647, 1991.

60. Gower, D. B. and Cooke, G. M., Regulation of steroid transforming enzymes by endogenous steroids, *J. Steroid Biochem.,* 19, 1527, 1983.

61. Doerr, P. and Pirke, K. M., Cortisol-induced suppression of plasma testosterone in normal adult males, *J. Clin. Endocrinol. Metab.,* 43, 622, 1976.

62. Bambino, T. H. and Hsueh, A. J. W., Direct inhibitory effect of glucocorticoids upon testicular luteinizing hormone receptor and steroidogenesis *in vivo* and *in vitro, Endocrinology,* 108, 2142, 1981.

63. Welsh, T. H., Bambino, T. H., and Hsueh, A. J. W., Mechanism of glucocorticoid-induced suppression of testicular androgen biosynthesis *in vitro, Biol. Reprod.,* 27, 1138, 1982.

64. Hales, D. B. and Payne, A. H., Glucocorticoid mediated repression of P450$_{SCC}$ mRNA and *de novo* synthesis in cultured Leydig cells, *Endocrinology*, 124, 2099, 1989.
65. Monder, C., Hardy, M. P., Blanchard, R. J., and Blanchard, D. C., Comparative aspects of 11B-hydroxysteroid dehydrogenase. Testicular 11B-hydroxysteroid dehydrogenase: development of a model for the mediation of Leydig cell function by corticosteroids, *Steroids*, 59, 69, 1994.
66. Ward, I. L. and Weisz, J., Maternal stress alters plasma testosterone in fetal males, *Science*, 207, 328, 1980.
67. Chen, Y.-D. I., Shaw, M. J., and Payne, A. H., Steroid and FSH action on LH receptors and LH sensitive testicular responsiveness during sexual maturation of the rat, *Mol. Cell. Endocrinol.*, 8, 291, 1977.
68. Purvis, K., Clausen, O. P. F., and Hansson, V., Androgen effects on rat Leydig cells, *Biol. Reprod.*, 20, 304, 1979.
69. Darney, K. J. and Ewing, L. L., Autoregulation of testosterone secretion in perfused rat testes, *Endocrinology*, 109, 993, 1981.
70. Hales, D. B., Sha, L., and Payne, A. H., Testosterone inhibits cAMP-induced *de novo* synthesis of Leydig cell cytochrome P450$_{17}$α by an androgen receptor-mediated mechanism, *J. Biol. Chem.*, 262, 11200, 1987.
71. Payne, A. H., Youngblood, G. L., Burgos-Trinidad, M., and Hammond, S. H., Hormonal regulation of steroidogenic enzyme gene expression in Leydig cells, *J. Steroid Biochem. Mol. Biol.*, 43, 895, 1992.
72. Georgiou, M. G., Perkins, L. M., and Payne, A. H., Steroid synthesis-dependent, oxygen-mediated damage of mitochondrial and microsomal cytochrome P450 enzymes in rat Leydig cell cultures, *Endocrinology*, 121, 1390, 1987.
73. Quinn, P. G. and Payne, A. H., Steroid product-induced, oxygen-mediated damage of microsomal cytochrome P450 enzymes in Leydig cell cultures. Relationship to desensitization, *J. Biol. Chem.*, 260, 2092, 1985.
74. Perkins, L. M., Hall, P. F., and Payne, A. H., Testosterone-enhanced oxygen-mediated degradation of P450$_{17}$α in mouse Leydig cell cultures, *Endocrinology*, 122, 2257, 1988.
75. Hornsby, P. J., Regulation of cytochrome P-450 supported 11β-hydroxylation of deoxycortisol by steroids, oxygen, and antioxidants in adrenalcortical cell cultures, *J. Biol. Chem.*, 255, 4020, 1980.
76. Quinn, P. G. and Payne, A. H., Oxygen-mediated damage of microsomal cytochrome P450 enzymes in cultured Leydig cells. Role in steroidogenic desensitization, *J. Biol. Chem.*, 259, 4130, 1984.
77. Huhtaniemi, I. T., Nozu, K., Warren, D. W., Dufau, M. L., and Catt, K. J., Acquisition of regulatory mechanisms for gonadotropin receptors and steroidogenesis in the maturing rat testis, *Endocrinology*, 111, 1711, 1982.
78a. Brinkman, A. O., Leemborg, F. G., Roodnat, E. M., De Jong, F. H., and van der Molen, H. J., A specific action of estradiol on enzymes involved in steroidogenesis, *Biol. Reprod.*, 23, 801, 1980.
78b. Warren, D. W., Dufau, M. L., and Catt, K. J., Hormonal regulation of gonadotropin receptors and steroidogenesis in cultured fetal rat testes, *Science*, 218, 375, 1982.
79. Kalla, N. R., Nisula, B. C., Menard, R., and Loriaux, D. L., The effect of estradiol on testicular testosterone biosynthesis, *Endocrinology*, 106, 35, 1980.

80. Brinkman, A. O., Leemborg, F. G., Roodnat, E. M., De Jong, F. H., and van der Molen, H. J., A specific action of estradiol on enzymes involved in steroidogenesis, *Biol. Reprod.*, 23, 801, 1980.

81. Onoda, M. and Hall, P. F., Inhibition of testicular microsomal cytochrome P-450 (17α-hydroxylase/$C_{17,20}$-lyase) by estrogens, *Endocrinology*, 109, 763, 1981.

82. Dufau, M. L., Winters, C. A., Hattori, M., Aquilano, D., Baranao, J. L. S., Nozu, K., Bauka, A., and Catt, K. J., Hormonal regulation of androgen production by the Leydig cell, *J. Steroid Biochem.*, 20, 161, 1984.

83. Nozu, K., Dufau, M. L., and Catt, K. J., Estradiol receptor-mediated regulation of steroidogenesis in gonadotropin-desensitized Leydig cells, *J. Biol. Chem.*, 256, 1915, 1981.

84. Ciocca, D. R., Winters, C. A., and Dufau, M. L., Expression of an estrogen-regulated protein in rat testis Leydig cells, *J. Steroid Biochem.*, 24, 219, 1986.

85. Nishihara, M., Winters, C. A., Buczko, E., Waterman, M. R., and Dufau, M. L., Hormonal regulation of rat Leydig cell cytochrome $P450_{17}\alpha$ mRNA levels and characterization of a partial length rat $P450_{17}\alpha$ cDNA, *Biochem. Biophys. Res. Commun.*, 154, 151, 1988.

86. Brinkman, A. O., Mulder, E., Lamers-Stahlhofen, J. G. M., Mechielsen, M. J., and van der Molen, H. J., An estradiol receptor in rat testis interstitial tissue, *FEBS Lett.*, 26, 301, 1972.

87. Mulder, E., Brinkman, A. O., Lamers-Stahlhofen, J. G. M., and van der Molen, H. J., Binding of estradiol by the nuclear fraction of rat testis interstitial tissue, *FEBS Lett.*, 31, 131, 1973.

88. van Beurden-Lamers, W. M. O., Brinkman, A. O., Mulder, E., and van der Molen, H. J., High-affinity binding of oestradiol-17β by cytosols from testis interstitial tissue, pituitary, adrenal, liver, and accessory sex glands of the male rat, *Biochem. J.*, 140, 495, 1974.

89. Kelce, W. R., Rudeen, P. K., and Ganjam, V. K., Prenatal ethanol exposure alters steroidogenic enzyme activity in newborn rat testes, *Alcoholism: Clin. Exp. Res.*, 13, 617, 1989.

90. Kelce, W. R., Ganjam, V. K., and Rudeen, P. K., Inhibition of testicular steroidogenesis in the neonatal rat following acute ethanol exposure, *Alcohol*, 7, 75, 1990.

91. Bartlett, J. M. S., Kerr, J. B., and Sharpe, R. M., The effect of selective destruction and regeneration of rat Leydig cells on the intratesticular distribution of testosterone and morphology of the seminiferous epithelium, *J. Androl.*, 7, 240, 1986.

92. Kerr, J. B., Donachie, K., and Rommerts, F. F. G., Selective destruction and regeneration of rat Leydig cells *in vivo*, *Cell Tissue Res.*, 242, 145, 1985.

93. Molenaar, R., de Rooij, D. G., Rommerts, F. F. G., Reuvers, P. J., and van der Molen, H. J., Specific destruction of Leydig cells in mature rats after *in vivo* administration of ethane dimethyl sulfonate, *Biol. Reprod.*, 33, 1213, 1985.

94. Morris, I. D., Phillips, D. M., and Bardin, C. W., Ethylene dimethanesulfonate destroys Leydig cells in the rat testis, *Endocrinology*, 118, 709, 1986.

95. Morris, I. D., Leydig cell resistance to the cytotoxic effect of ethylene dimethanesulphonate in the adult rat testis, *J. Endocrinol.*, 105, 311, 1985.

96. Zaidi, A., Lendon, R. G., Dixon, J. S., and Morris, I. D., Abnormal development of the testis after administration of the Leydig cell cytotoxic ethylene-1,2-dimethanesulphonate to the immature rat, *J. Reprod. Fertil.*, 82, 381, 1988.

97. Kelce, W. R., Zirkin, B. R., and Ewing, L. L., Immature rat Leydig cells are intrinsically less sensitive than adult Leydig cells to ethane dimethanesulfonate, *Toxicol. Appl. Pharmacol.*, 111, 189, 1991.

98. Kelce, W. R. and Zirkin, B. R., Mechanism by which ethane dimethanesulfonate kills adult rat Leydig cells: involvement of intracellular glutathione, *Toxicol. Appl. Pharmacol.*, 120, 80, 1993.

99. Kelce, W. R., Buthionine sulfoximine protects the viability of adult rat Leydig cells exposed to ethane dimethanesulfonate, *Toxicol. Appl. Pharmacol.*, 125, 237, 1994.

100. French, F. S., Lubahn, D. B., Brown, T. R., Simental, J. A., Quigley, C. A., Yarbrough, W. G., Tan, J., Sar, M., Joseph, D. R., Evans, B. A. J., Hughes, I. A., Migeon, C. J., and Wilson, E. M., Molecular basis of androgen insensitivity, *Rec. Prog. Horm. Res.*, 46, 1, 1990.

101. Wilson, J. D. and Lasnitski, I., Dihydrotestosterone formation in fetal tissues of the rabbit and rat, *Endocrinology*, 89, 659, 1971.

102. Siiteri, P. and Wilson, J. D., Testosterone formation and metabolism during male sexual differentiation in the human embryo, *J. Clin. Endocrinol. Metab.*, 38, 113, 1973.

103. Imperato-McGinley, J., Guerrero L., Gautier, T., and Peterson, R. E., Steroid 5α-reductase deficiency in man: an inherited form of male pseudohermaphroditism, *Science*, 186, 1213, 1974.

104. Imperato-McGinley, J., Peterson, R. E., Gautier, T., and Sturla, E., Male pseudohermaphroditism secondary to 5α-reductase deficiency — a model for the role of androgens in both the development of the male phenotype and evolution of a male gender identity, *J. Steroid Biochem.*, 11, 637, 1979.

105. Segel, I. H., *Enzyme Kinetics*, John Wiley and Sons, New York, 1975, chap. 3.

106. Nukui, F., Effects of chlormadinone acetate and ethinylestradiol treatment on epididymal 5α- reductase activities in patients with prostate cancer, *Endocrine J.*, 44, 127, 1997.

107. Li, X., Chen, C., Singh, S. M., and Labire, F., The enzyme and inhibitors of 4-ene-3-oxosteroid 5α-oxidoreductase, *Steroids*, 60, 430, 1995.

108. Nozu, K. and Tamaoki, B.-I., Characteristics of the nuclear and microsomal steroid 4-ene-5α-hydrogenase of the rat prostate, *ACTA Endocrinol.*, 76, 608, 1974.

109. Koninchx, P., Verhoeven, G., Heyns, W., and De Moor, P., Biochemical characterization of the NADPH:4-ene-3-ketosteroid 5α-oxidoreductase in rat ovarian suspension cultures, *J. Steroid Biochem.*, 10, 325, 1979.

110. Cheng, Y.-J. and Karavolas, H. J., Properties and subcellular distribution of 4-ene-steroid (progesterone) 5α-reductase in rat anterior pituitary, *Steroids*, 26, 57, 1975.

111. Kinoshita, Y., Studies on the human epididymis: partial characterization of 3α- and 3β-hydroxysteroid dehydrogenase, regional distribution of 5α-reductase and inhibitory effect of 4-ene-3-oxosteroids on 5α-reductase, *Endocrinol. Jpn.*, 28, 499, 1981.

112. Makela, S., Santti, R., Martikainen, P., Nienstedt, W., and Paranko, J., The influence of steroidal and nonsteroidal estrogens on the 5α-reduction of testosterone by the ventral prostate of the rat, *J. Steroid Biochem.*, 35, 249, 1990.

113. Lee, P. C., Patra, S. C., and Struve, M., Modulation of rat hepatic CYP3A by nonylphenol, *Xenobiotica*, 26, 831, 1996.

114. Rhodes, L., Primka, R. L., Berman, C., Vergult, G., Gabriel, M., Pierre-Malice, M., and Gibelin, B., Comparision of finasteride (Proscar), a 5α-reductase inhibitor, and various commercial plant extracts in *in vitro* and *in vivo* 5α-reductase inhibition, *Prostate*, 22, 43, 1993.

115. Moh, P. P., Chang, G. C. J., Brueggemeier, R. W., and Lin, Y. C., Effect of gossypol on 5α-reductase and 3α-hydroxysteroid dehydrogenase activities in adult rat testes, *Res. Commun. Chem. Pathol. Pharmacol.*, 82, 12, 1993.

116. Liao, S. and Hiipakka, R. A., Selective inhibition of steroid 5α-reductase isozymes by tea epicatechin-3-gallate and epigallocatechin-3-gallate, *Biochem. Biophys. Res. Commun.*, 214, 833, 1995.

117. Zhou, Z.-X., Lane, M. V., Kemppainen, J. A., French, F. S., and Wilson, E. M., Specificity of ligand-dependent androgen receptor stabilization: receptor domain interactions influence ligand dissociation and receptor stability, *Mol. Endocrinol.*, 9, 208, 1995.

118. Wong, C. I., Zhou, Z. X., Sar, M., and Wilson, E. M., Steroid requirement for androgen receptor dimerization and DNA binding: modulation by intramolecular interactions between the NH2-terminal and steroid binding domains, *J. Biol. Chem.*, 268, 19004, 1995.

119. Tan, J. A., Marschke, K. B., Ho, K. C., Perry, S. T., Wilson, E. M., and French, F. S., Response elements of the androgen regulated C3 gene, *J. Biol. Chem.* 267, 4456, 1992.

120. Ho, K. C., Marschke, K. B., Tan, J. A., Power, S. G. A., Wilson, E. M., and French, F. S., A complex response element in intron 1 of the androgen regulated 20 kDa protein gene displays cell-type dependent androgen receptor specificity, *J. Biol. Chem.*, 268, 27226, 1993.

121. Kuil, C. W. and Mulder, E., Mechanism of antiandrogen action: conformational changes of the receptor, *Mol. Cell. Endocrinol.*, 102, R1, 1994.

122. Zhou, Z. X., Wong, C.-I., Sar, M., and Wilson, E. M., The androgen receptor: an overview, *Rec. Prog. Horm. Res.*, 49, 249, 1994.

123. Eckert, R. L. and Katzenellenbogen, B. S., Physical properties of estrogen receptor complexes in MCF-7 human breast cancer cells, *J. Biol. Chem.* 257, 8840, 1982.

124. Hansen, J. C. and Gorski, J., Conformational transitions of the estrogen receptor monomer, *J. Biol. Chem.*, 261, 13990, 1986.

125. Martin, P. M., Berthois, Y., and Jensen, E. V., Binding of antiestrogens exposes an occult antigenic determinant in the human estrogen receptor, *Proc. Natl. Acad. Sci. U.S.A.* 85, 2533, 1988.

126. Truss, M., Bartsch, J., and Beato, M., Antiprogestins prevent progesterone receptor binding to hormone responsive elements *in vivo*, *Proc. Natl. Acad. Sci. U.S.A.*, 91, 11333, 1994.

127. Kelce, W. R., Stone, C. S., Laws, S. C., Gray, L. E., Kemppainen, J. A., and Wilson, E. M., Persistent DDT metabolite, p,p'-DDE is a potent androgen receptor antagonist, *Nature*, 375, 581, 1995.

128. Wong, C. I., Kelce, W. R., Sar, M., and Wilson, E. M., Androgen receptor antagonist vs. agonist activities of the fungicide vinclozolin relative to hydroxyflutamide, *J. Biol. Chem.*, 270, 19998, 1995.

129. Kemppainen, J. A., Lane, M. V., Sar, M., and Wilson, E. M., Androgen receptor phosphorylation, turnover, nuclear transport, and transcriptional activation, *J. Biol. Chem.*, 267, 968, 1992.

130. Langley, E., Zhou, Z.-X., and Wilson, E. M., Evidence for an anti-parallel orientation of the ligand-activated human androgen receptor dimer, *J. Biol. Chem.*, 270, 29983, 1995.

131. Kuil, C. W., Berrevoets, C. A., and Mulder, E., Ligand-induced conformational alterations of the androgen receptor analyzed by limited trypsinization, *J. Biol. Chem.*, 270, 27569, 1995.

132. Wakeling, A. E., Steroid antagonists as nuclear receptor blockers, *Canc. Surv.*, 14, 71, 1992.

133. Freeman, S. N., Mainwaring, W. I. P., and Furr, B. J. A., A possible explanation for the peripheral selectivity of a novel non-steroidal pure antiandrogen, Casodex (ICI 176 334), *Br. J. Canc.*, 60, 664, 1989.

134. Harris, M. G., Coleman, S. G., Faulds, D., and Chrisp, P., Nilutamide: a review of its pharmacodynamic and pharmacokinetic properties and therapeutic efficacy in prostate cancer, *Drugs Aging*, 3, 9, 1993.

135. Neumann, F., Pharmacology and potential use of cyproterone acetate, *Horm. Metab. Res.*, 9, 1, 1977.

136. Polani, P. E., Abnormal sex development in man. 1. Anomalies of sex determining mechanisms, in *Mechanisms of Sex Differentiation in Animals and Man*, Austin, R. and Edwards, R. G., Eds., Academic Press, Inc, New York, 1981, 465.

137. Gray, L. E., Ostby, J. S., and Kelce, W. R., Developmental effects of an environmental antiandrogen: the fungicide vinclozolin alters sex differentiation of the male rat, *Toxicol. Appl. Pharmacol.*, 129, 46, 1994.

138. Wilson, J. G. and Wilson, H. C., Reproductive capacity in adult rats treated prepubertally with androgenic hormone, *Endocrinology*, 33, 353, 1943.

139. Baranao, J. L. S., Chemes, H. E., Tesone, M., Chiauzzi, E. H., Scacchi, P., Calvo, J. C., Faigon, M. R., Moguilevsky, J. A., Charreau, E. H., and Calandra, R. S., Effects of androgen treatment of the neonate on the rat testis and the sex accessory organs, *Biol. Reprod.*, 25, 851, 1981.

140. McLachlan, J. A., Rodent models for perinatal exposure to diethylstilbestrol and their relation to human disease in the male, in *Developmental Effects of Diethylstilbestrol in Pregnancy*, Herbst, A. L. and Bern, H. A., Eds., Thieme-Stratton, Inc., New York, 1981, 48.

141. Kalloo, N. B., Gearhart, J. P., and Barrack, E. R., Sexually dimorphic expression of estrogen receptors, but not of androgen receptors in human fetal external genitalia, *J. Clin. Endocrinol. Metab.*, 77, 692, 1993.

142. Jänne, O. A. and Bardin, C. W., Steroid receptors and hormone action: physiological and synthetic androgens and progestins can mediate inappropriate biological effects, *Pharmacol. Rev.*, 36, 35S, 1984.

143. Bardin, C. W., Bullock, L. P., Sherins, R., Mowszowicz, I., and Blackburn, W. R., Androgen metabolism and mechanism of action in male pseudohermaphroditism: a study of testicular feminization, *Rec. Prog. Horm. Res.*, 29, 65, 1973.

144. Pajunen, A. E., Isomaa, V. V., Janne, A. O., and Bardin, C. W., Androgenic regulation of ornithine decarboxylase activity in mouse kidney and its relationship to changes in cytosol and nuclear androgen receptor concentrations, *J. Biol. Chem.*, 257, 8190, 1982.

145. Bullock, L. P., Barthe, P. L., Mowszowicz, I., Orth, D. N., and Bardin, C. W., The effect of progestins on submaxillary gland epidermal growth factor: demonstration of androgenic, synandrogenic and antiandrogenic actions, *Endocrinology*, 97, 189, 1975.

146. Mowszowicz, I., Bieber, D. E., Chung, K. W., Bullock, L. P., and Bardin, C. W., Synandrogenic and antiandrogenic effect of progestins: comparision with non-progestational antiandrogens, *Endocrinology*, 95, 1589, 1974.

147. Perez-Palacios, G., Chavez, B., Escobar, N., Vilchis, F., Larrea, F., Lince, M., and Perez, A. E., Mechanism of action of contraceptive synthetic progestins, *J. Steroid Biochem.*, 15, 125, 1981.

148. Brinkmann, A. O., Lindh, L. M., Breedveld, D. I., Mulder, E., and Van Der Molen, H. J., Cyproterone acetate prevents translocation of the androgen receptor in the rat prostate, *Mol. Cell. Endocrinol.*, 32, 117, 1983.

149. Huang, J. K., Bartsch, W., and Voigt, K. D., Interactions of an antiandrogen (cyproterone acetate) with the androgen receptor system and its biological action in the rat ventral prostate, *ACTA Endocrinol.*, 109, 569, 1985.

150. Kelce, W. R., Lambright, C. S., Gray, L. E., and Roberts, K. P., Vinclozolin and p,p'-DDE alter androgen dependent gene expression: *in vivo* confirmation of and androgen receptor mediated mechanism, *Toxicol. Appl. Pharmacol.*, 142, 192, 1997.

151. Fail, P. A., Pearce, S. W., Anderson, S. A., Tyl, R. W., and Gray, L. E., Endocrine and reproductive toxicity of vinclozolin (vin) in male Long-Evans Hooded rats, *Fund. Appl. Toxicol.*, 15, 293, 1995.

152. Kelce, W. R., Monosson, E., Gamcsik, M. P., Laws, S. C., and Gray, L. E., Environmental hormone disruptors: evidence that vinclozolin developmental toxicity is mediated by antiandrogenic metabolites, *Toxicol. Appl. Pharmacol.*, 126, 276, 1994.

153. Sweet, R. A., Schrott, H. G., Kurland, R., Culp, O. S., Study of the incidence of hypospadias in Rochester, Minn., 1940-1970, and a case-control comparision of possible etiologic factors, *Mayo Clin. Proc.*, 49, 52, 1974.

154. Paulozzi, L. J., Erickson, J. D., and Jackson, R. J., Hypospadias trends in two US surveillance systems, *Pediatrics*, 100, 831, 1997.

155. Allera, A., Herbst, M. A., Griffin, J. E., Wilson, J. D., Schweikert, H. -U., and McPhaul, M. J., Mutations of the androgen receptor coding sequence are infrequent in patients with isolated hypospadias, *J. Clin. Endocrinol. Metab.*, 80, 2697, 1995.

156. Hiort, O., Klauber, G., Cendron, M., Sinnecker, G. G. H., Keim, L., Schwinger, E., Wolfe, H. J., and Yandell, D. W., Molecular characterization of the androgen receptor gene in boys with hypospadias, *Eur. J. Pediatr.*, 153, 317, 1994.

157. Wilson, J. D., Griffin, J. E., and Russell, D. W., Steroid 5α-reductase 2 deficiency, *Endocr. Rev.*, 14, 577, 1993.

158. Bentvelsen, F. M., Brinkmann, A. O., van der Linden, J. E. T. M., Schroder, F. H., and Nijman, J. M., Decreased immunoreactive androgen receptor levels are not the cause of isolated hypospadias, *Br. J. Urol.*, 76, 384, 1995.

159. Henderson, B. E., Benton, B., Cogsgrove, M., Baptista, J., Aldrich, J., Townsend, D., Hart, W., and Mack, T. M., Urogenital tract abnormalities in sons of women treated with diethylstilbestrol, *Pediatrics*, 58, 505, 1976.

160. Wilson, E. M. and French, F. S., Binding properties of androgen receptors. Evidence for identical receptors in rat testis, epididymis and prostate, *J. Biol. Chem.*, 25, 5620, 1976.

161. Carilla, E., Briley, M., Fauran, F., Sultan, C. H., and Duvilliers, C., Binding of Permixon, a new treatment for prostatic benign hyperplasia, to the cytosolic androgen receptor in the rat prostate, *J. Steroid Biochem. Mol. Biol.*, 20, 521, 1984.

162. Champault, G., Patel, J. C., and Bonnard, A. M., A double-blind trial of an extract of the plant Serenoa repens in benign prostatic hyperplasia, *Br. J. Clin. Pharmacol.*, 18, 461, 1984.

163. Ware, G. W., Effects of DDT on reproduction in higher animals, *Residue Rev.*, 59, 119, 1975.

164. Giwercman, A., Carlsen, E., Keiding, S., and Skakkebaek, N. E., Evidence for increasing incidence of abnormalities of the human testis: a review, *Environ. Health Perspect. (suppl.)*, 101, 65, 1993.

165. Gray, L. E., Kelce, W. R., Wiese, T., Tyl, R., Gaido, K., Cook, J., Klinefelter, G., Desaulniers, D., Wilson, E., Zacharewski, T., Waller, C., Foster, P., Laskey, J., Reel, J., Giesy, J., Breslin, W., Cooper, R., Di Giulio, R., Welshons, W., Miller, R., Safe, S., McLachlan, J., McMaster, S., and Colborn, T., Endocrine screening methods workshop: Detection of estrogenic and androgenic hormonal and antihormonal activity for chemicals that act via receptor or steroidogenic enzyme mechanisms, *Reprod. Toxicol.*, 11, 719, 1997.

166. Waller, C. L., Juma, B. W., Gray, L. E., and Kelce, W. R., Three-dimensional quantitative structure activity relationships for androgen receptor ligands, *Toxicol. Appl. Pharmacol.*, 137, 219, 1996.

10

Endocrine Disruptors and Sexual Dysfunction

Suresh C. Sikka and Rajesh K. Naz

CONTENTS

0-8493-3164-1/99/$0.00+$.50
© 1999 by CRC Press LLC

10.1   Introduction

Male sexual dysfunction, in general, can be defined as the inability of a man to obtain penile rigidity sufficient to permit coitus of adequate duration to satisfy himself and his partner. It is estimated that 20 to 30 million Americans suffer from erectile dysfunction.[1] However, with the recent availability of oral medication for impotence, the so-called "magic pill" (Viagra), it has become difficult to accurately estimate the true prevalence of impotence in the general population. The onset of impotence is mostly very gradual, interrupted by seemingly partial recoveries. The Massachusetts Male Aging Study (MMAS) reported that 52% of men aged 40-70 experienced some degree of erectile dysfunction and that with advancing age there is a progressive decline in libido, frequency of nocturnal or morning erections, and intercourse.[2] However, sexual satisfaction did not decline, suggesting that men accommodate for age-related changes in sexual capacity by altering expectations. The decline in libido with age has been associated with a similar decrease in the male hormone testosterone. This association between low libido, declining androgen, and the onset of impotence is not clear at present. In order to understand the complexity of this process and the role of hormonal disruptors, it is important first to focus on what is currently known about male sexual function, with the penis being the most important target organ.

Many widely used synthetic chemicals and sometimes their more harmful breakdown products are found in soil, water, plants, and animals all over the world. These are carried to other places by air, water, and animals. Animals, including humans, can and do accumulate some of these chemicals in their fat and often pass them along to offspring and predators as part of the food chain. These foreign substances have been associated with health, development, and reproductive problems in wildlife, domestic and laboratory animals, and humans. For example, environmental estrogens can mimic or act like estrogens, the hormones that control female characteristics; antiestrogens or antiandrogens can both mimic and/or block hormone actions; and environmental disruptors or modulators can alter biosynthesis, metabolism, and the action of natural hormones and their protein receptors.[3] Fetuses and embryos, whose growth and development are highly controlled by the endocrine system, seem especially vulnerable to such toxic exposure. Mothers can pass contaminants to their offspring prenatally in eggs (amphibians, reptiles, birds) or through the womb (mammals) or after birth by breastfeeding newborns.[4] So, even though adult animals exposed to contaminants may not show any ill effects, their offspring may have distinct lifelong health and reproductive abnormalities, including reduced fertility, altered sexual behavior, lowered immunity, and even cancer.

10.2 Background

The idea that manmade chemicals could mimic estrogens, disrupt endocrine balance, and have adverse health effects is not entirely new.[5] For instance, male fish living near municipal sewage outlets in England had both male and female sex characteristics, and their livers produced vitellogenin, a female egg-yolk protein not normally found in males. The fish living close to the sewage outlet had severe abnormalities, while the fish living farther downstream had less severe symptoms. Several different chemicals, especially the alkylphenols, the breakdown products of chemicals found in detergents and plastics, are suspected of causing these feminizing effects.[6]

Alligators living in Florida's Lake Apopka were exposed to the estrogenic pollutants dicofol, DDT, and its metabolites (DDD, DDE, and chloro-DDT), when a nearby chemical plant had an extensive spill in 1980. Researchers trying to find out why alligator populations were dropping in the lake found higher than normal mortality among eggs and newborn alligators. They also found that adolescent females had severe ovarian abnormalities and blood estrogen levels two times higher than normal. The male juvenile alligators were feminized, with smaller than normal penises, abnormal testes, higher estrogen levels, and lower testosterone levels in their blood than normal males of the same age.[7] The researchers concluded that chemicals from the spill not only killed developing eggs outright but also altered the embryos' endocrine systems (hormone levels and sexual development), which severely limited the alligators' ability to reproduce.

Furthermore, there is ample evidence that the pesticide DDT and its potent metabolite dichlorodiphenyl-dichloroethylene (DDE) caused a dwindling Western gulls population in Southern California in the 1960s, due to testicular feminization of male embryos, leading to abnormal sex ratios.[8] Sons born to mothers who took the synthetic estrogen DES (diethylstilbestrol) during pregnancy to prevent miscarriage had higher rates of malformed or small penises, undescended testicles, and abnormal sperm.[4] However, a recent study found no evidence of reduced fertility in DES sons.[9] Daughters of these mothers had higher rates of reproductive problems, reproductive cancer (vagina, cervix), and malformed reproductive organs (uterus, cervix). DES is not only a potent estrogen, similar in strength to the natural estrogen estradiol, but it also has the unique ability to concentrate in target tissues, such as the reproductive tracts of birds, reptiles, and other animals, during development and cause abnormalities.[10] This drug serves as an example of what potent estrogenic compounds can do and may illustrate the health effects that other environmental estrogens can produce.

Considerable controversy surrounds a study that found the sperm counts in men were falling worldwide, that rates of testicular cancer were increasing, and that environmental estrogens may be responsible for these trends.[11] Other studies do not support all of these findings and suggest that lower sperm counts and decreased fertility may only occur in certain human populations.[12]

Because many of these synthetic chemicals are suspected of acting like natural estrogens, the most likely health problems would be related to sexual development, reproduction, and breast and reproductive cancers. In females, estrogens, mainly the hormone estradiol, foster development of female characteristics (breasts, no facial hair, reproductive cycles, and behavior). In males, estrogens play a secondary role to testosterone, which defines male characteristics and aids sperm production. But, when the ratio of estrogen to testosterone is increased, feminization can occur. This may lead to poor semen quality, altered sexual behavior, testicular cancer, malformed reproductive tissue (undescended testes, small testes and penis size), prostate disease, and other recognized abnormalities of male reproductive tissues. As with any potential health risk, many factors such as length of exposure, dose, age, and individual differences will influence the kinds and severity of health problems experienced. That is, one person may experience many problems while another may experience none.

These studies have (1) helped identify and restrict use of the most harmful chemicals, (2) aided in deciphering how these substances can interfere with hormones and lead to health problems, and (3) broadened the definition of toxic chemical exposure, measured for so long by cancer, to include reproductive and developmental health problems. In response to this research, some of the most dangerous chemicals, such as DDT and PCBs, have been banned in the U.S. and Europe. Chemical manufacturers continue to replace the more persistent chemicals with shorter-lived ones that will not accumulate in soil, wildlife, or our bodies. However, at high doses, some of these chemicals can affect the endocrine and reproductive systems, especially during critical developmental stages. In addition to the developmental and reproductive health problems, these hormonal disruptors are likely to affect the sexuality and sexual function, resulting in impotence-related problems in the male, an area poorly evaluated until recently.

10.3   What is Impotence or Erectile Dysfunction?

The word impotence is derived from the Latin impotentias, meaning lack of power, and was first used to describe loss of sexual power in 1655 in a treatise entitled 'Church History of Britain' by Thomas Fuller. Impotence is usually defined as a man's failure to achieve or maintain an erection until the completion of the "satisfactory" sexual act. Because the failure may be partial or complete, persistent or recurrent, impotence in the true medical sense is now referred to as erectile dysfunction. Certain impotence-related conditions that may be mistaken for erectile dysfunction are premature/delayed ejaculation, low level of sexual desire, and prolonged refractory period (time taken for repeat ejaculation). The penis in the male is the major target site for understanding the pathophysiology of erectile dysfunction and the role of environmental disruptors.

10.3.1   Anatomy and Physiology of the Penis

The human penis is a tubular appendage consisting of three distinct cylindrical compartments, each one of which is encased by connective tissue. The ventral compartment is the corpus spongiosum, containing the bulbar and penile urethra. The paired dorsal compartments are the corpora cavernosa, or erectile bodies of the penis. The corpora cavernosa are covered by a thick fascial layer, called the tunica albuginea. The tunica albuginea in the midline septum is permeable to blood flow, which allows free exchange of nutrients and pharmacological agents between the corpora cavernosa. Penile blood supply originates in the internal pudendal artery, which divides into the paired dorsal penile arteries and the paired cavernosal arteries. The dorsal penile arteries supply the corpus spongiosum through the circumflex arteries, while the cavernosal arteries supply the corpora cavernosa through the helical arteries.

Penile erection is a result of passive dilation of the lacunar spaces and relaxation of the smooth musculature of the cavernosal arteriovenous bed and trabecular network.[13] Three neuroeffector pathways coordinate the smooth muscle tone in the corpora cavernosa. These are the adrenergic, cholinergic, and nonadrenergic/noncholinergic (NANC) pathways.[14] Penile flaccidity is maintained by the adrenergic-mediated sympathetic tone of the cavernosal smooth muscle. Erection is triggered by stimulation of a dual-innervated neuronal pathway involving both cholinergic and NANC mediators. The primary mediator of penile erections is nitric oxide, originating from NANC neurons, cavernosal smooth muscle cells, and cholinergic-stimulated endothelial cells.[14] Nitric oxide synthase (NOS) generates nitric oxide (NO) from its precursor, L-arginine. Nitric oxide acts on the enzyme guanylate cyclase to increase cGMP levels. Cyclic GMP is the active second messenger responsible for smooth muscle relaxation that initiates this first phase of erection.[15] This is followed by the emissary veins and subtunical venules compression against the fibroelastic tunica albuginea, leading to the "steady-state," where arterial inflow and venous outflow both decrease. The contraction of the bulbocavernosus and ischiocavernosus muscles results in the rigidity of the erection.[16] Finally, a sympathetic stimulation leads to seminal emission, ejaculation, and contraction of the lacunar space, followed by detumescence and return of the basal adrenergic-mediated cavernosal smooth muscle tone. Other neurotransmitters have also been postulated to play some role in penile tumescence/detumescence.[17] Any agent, including hormonal disruptors, causing imbalances between a vasoconstrictive mediator (e.g., endothelin-1) and cavernosal smooth muscle relaxation, especially in an aging male, may therefore play a significant role in erectile dysfunction.

10.3.2   Aging and Impotence

While it is undeniable that aging brings changes to every man's sexual life, it is equally undeniable that plenty of men enjoy a healthy, active sex life through their fifties, sixties, seventies, and even into their eighties! In spite of continuing good health, all men have to accept some loss in their sensitivity to touch and in the tone of their penile smooth muscle. As early as 1948, Kinsey[18] reported that by age 75 about 25 percent of men become impotent and that the incidence of impotence increases with age, but later studies (e.g., the Baltimore Longitudinal Study of Aging and the Charleston Heart Study Cohort) increased this number to 55 percent. As men get older, it usually takes longer for them to achieve an erection. Older men also have longer refractory periods. The number of failures to achieve functional erection can be indicative of trouble along the following lines:

10% of encounters = little reason for immediate concern

25% of encounters = strong possibility of chronic impotence

50% of encounters = strong evidence that chronic impotence exists

Going from a 1-in-10 to a 1-in-2 failure rate may take from 2 to 5 years. Some early warning signs of sexual dysfunction include the following:

1. Fewer morning erections,
2. Fewer spontaneous erections,
3. Increasing inability to induce an erection,
4. Increasing inability to maintain an erection,
5. Increasing inability to assume sexual positions.

Cellular senescence results in increased deposition of a less compliant collagen subtype in the corpora cavernosa and tunica albuginea. This can lead to veno-occlusive dysfunction and decreased neuronal transmission to the cavernosal smooth muscle.[15] Aging also is believed to result in altered endothelial function, which manifests in decreased basal nitric oxide release and increased basal endothelin-1.[19,20] There is evidence for upregulation of endothelin-1 mRNA with aging.[20] Correlations have been demonstrated between androgen levels and mRNA levels for nitric oxide synthase.[21] Thus, any hormonal control of this balance between NO and endothelin may play a significant role in the onset of impotence in the aging male.

10.4 Endocrinology of Sexual Function

10.4.1 Testosterone as the Sex Hormone

Testosterone is the main sex hormone in men. Low testosterone levels have a strong correlation with decreased libido, which suggests a major role for androgens in sexual function.[22] With advancing age, bioavailable testosterone shows a typical pattern (Figure 10.1). Testosterone levels have been shown to correlate significantly with nocturnal penile tumescence.[23] Studies have demonstrated a significant decline in penile NOS activity in castrated animals that can be reversed by androgen supplementation, especially with dihydrotestosterone (DHT). Increases in NOS mRNA have been demonstrated with androgen supplementation.[24] These studies suggest active biochemical pathways for the influence of androgens on erectile function and dysfunction. However, the clinical use of androgens for the treatment of erectile response not resulting from hypogonadism is controversial. The effects of testosterone can be grouped into the following categories.

10.4.1.1 Effects on the Reproductive System Before Birth

Before birth, testosterone secretion by the fetal testes is responsible for masculinizing the reproductive tract and external genitalia and for promoting

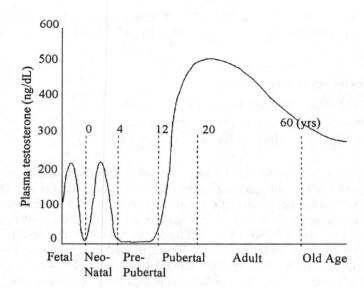

FIGURE 10.1
Note that, unlike the female sex hormone estrogen, testosterone does not peak and fall in a monthly cycle.

descent of the testes into the scrotum. After birth, testosterone secretion ceases, and the testes and the balance of the reproductive system remain small and nonfunctional until puberty. Environmental chemicals acting as antiandrogens can disrupt this normal sexual development during fetal life.[25]

10.4.1.2   Effects on Sex-Specific Tissues After Birth

At the onset of puberty, the Leydig cells once again start secreting testosterone, and spermatogenesis is initiated in the seminiferous tubules for the first time. Testosterone is responsible for the growth and maturation of the entire male reproductive system. Ongoing testosterone secretion is essential for spermatogenesis and for maintaining a mature male reproductive tract throughout adulthood. Potent hormonal disruptors in the environment can impair normal development of these organs of the male reproductive system and can affect sperm production.[26]

10.4.1.3   Other Related Effects

Other effects of testosterone include development of libido at puberty, maintenance of the adult male sex drive, control of the secretion of luteinizing hormone (LH) by the anterior pituitary via feedback mechanisms, development and maintenance of male secondary sexual characteristics, and general protein anabolic effects, including bone growth and induction of aggressive behavior. How environmental toxicants alter these effects in the male is not clear.

10.5   Erectile Dysfunction

There are four major causes of erectile dysfunction, (1) hormonal, (2) neurological, (3) psychological, and (4) vascular. Normal erection and sexual function require complex multiple interactions, which make it difficult to understand the etiology of impotence due to hormonal disruptors.

10.5.1   Hormonal Causes of Male Sexual Dysfunction

10.5.1.1   *Primary Hypogonadism*

For thousands of years, it was known that castration decreased sexual interest and activity, revealing the essential role of the testicles. A fascinating fact is that men with nonfunctioning testicles and low testosterone may sometimes continue to have normal desire and erections. In most cases, however, reduced libido and sexual performance accompany a decrease in testosterone.[27] The extent to which less-than-optimal testosterone impairs sexual function is influenced by the state of penile blood flow and nerve conduction. A younger man in good health except for diminished testosterone may often continue to have good erections, but for an older man whose penile blood flow is beginning to be reduced by arteriosclerosis or whose nerve conduction is diminished by diabetes or other neuropathy, even a moderate decrease in testosterone may interfere with erections, with improvement following supplementation.[28] Different studies estimate that up to 30% of men with sexual dysfunction have hormonal causes, with the majority having hypogonadism.[29] The most frequent cause of hypogonadism is age-related primary testicular failure.

While many studies have documented the restoration of serum testosterone levels with androgen supplementation (using injection, patch, implant, or oral routes), few have evaluated its efficacy in the management of erectile dysfunction.[30] One study reported significant improvements in frequency, duration, and rigidity of nocturnal penile tumescence with testosterone supplementation.[24] Sexual desire and arousal were also improved significantly. However, only 35-60% of men can expect a measurable improvement in sexual performance with restoration of normal serum testosterone levels.[31,32]

10.5.1.2   *Secondary Hypogonadism*

Low testosterone not accompanied by elevated gonadotropins suggests defective pituitary or hypothalamic function, also known as secondary hypogonadism. The most frequent cause of secondary hypogonadism in the population of impotent men is idiopathic LH deficiency, probably resulting from hypothalamic dysfunction.[33] A hypothalamic cause is suggested and a pituitary cause made less likely by observing LH rise after stimulation testing with GnRH.[27,29]

10.5.1.3   Role of Estrogen Excess in the Male

Estrogens belong to a family of steroid hormones that regulate and sustain female sexual development and reproductive function and stimulate tissue growth by (1) promoting cell proliferation (DNA synthesis and cell division) in female sex organs (breasts, uterus); (2) promoting hypertrophy in female breast and male muscle during puberty; and (3) initiating the synthesis of specific proteins.[34] Under these guidelines, any natural steroid, plant compound, or synthetic chemical that elicits these responses in laboratory tests is considered estrogenic. Estrogen excess causes LH suppression with resulting diminished testosterone production which is most often seen in obese men.[35] This is probably a result of adipose tissue conversion of testosterone to estrogen. Chronic liver disease can also produce estrogen excess, both because of hepatic aromatization of testosterone to estrogen and because of increased sex hormone binding globulin, which can result in a reduced amount of active testosterone in the circulation.[36]

A rarer cause of estrogen excess during occupational exposure is production of an adrenal androgen, DHEA, which is also converted to estrogen in the liver and adipose tissue. These men may have gynecomastia and feminine fat distribution, and blood tests reveal low testosterone and LH, accompanied by elevated total estrogen (estrone + estradiol).[37] Measurement of estradiol alone is not sufficient, since much of the estrogen in men is in the form of estrone. Hormonal ablation therapy using LHRH agonists or estrogens to reduce circulating testosterone to castrate levels is the mainstay of therapy for metastatic prostate cancer. However, this leads to a decrease in libido and erectile dysfunction.

10.5.2   Neurological Causes of Male Sexual Dysfunction

Agents that affect the central or peripheral nervous system or alter the pituitary-hypothalamic-gonadal axis may directly impair sexual function by altering endocrine function.[33,34] GnRH release from the hypothalamus is suppressed by stress-induced increases in catecholamines, prolactin, corticotropin-releasing factor, and opiates. Cranial irradiation may lead to irradiation-induced hypothalamic dysfunction, with hyperprolactinemia resulting in impotence.[38] Hyperprolactinemia decreases the secretion of GnRH, resulting in low testosterone levels.[27] Erectile dysfunction (88%) and decreased libido (80%) are the most common presenting symptoms of hyperprolactinemia.[38] Oral bromocriptine can normalize prolactin levels and restore normal erections.

10.6   Endocrine Disruptors and Erectile Dysfunction

An environmental hormone disruptor, in general, may be defined as an exogenous agent that interferes with the synthesis, secretion, transport, binding, action, or elimination of natural hormones that are responsible for the maintenance of homeostasis, reproduction, development, and/or behavior in the body. Endocrine disruptors are usually either natural products or synthetic chemicals that mimic, enhance (an agonist), or inhibit (an antagonist) the action of biological hormones. Dose, duration, and timing of exposure at critical periods of life are important considerations for assessing the adverse effects of endocrine disruptors. Effects may be reversible or irreversible, immediate (acute) or latent, and not expressed for a period of time.

10.6.1 Selected Endocrine-Disrupting Chemicals

Recent reports suggest that many chemicals released into the environment can affect normal endocrine function.[39] Some deleterious effects observed in animals have been attributed to persistent organic chemicals, such as polychlorinated biphenyls (PCBs), DDT, dioxin, and some pesticides.[25] These chemicals existing in the environment even in minute quantities, if ingested, may mimic natural hormones and disrupt bodily functions. Convincing evidence exists that chemical exposures in rodents have led to increased estrogenic activity and reduced androgen levels or otherwise have interfered with the action of androgen during development, causing male reproductive system abnormalities.[40] Results obtained from the observation of men exposed to DES *in utero* demonstrate that environmental agents may alter neuroendocrine function both during development and in the sexually mature organism.[41] Testing for the endocrine-disrupting potential of environmental chemicals should include the ability to detect antiandrogenic activity as well as estrogenic activity. Testing also should be able to detect alteration in androgen receptor and all receptor function as reflected in genome expression.[42]

10.6.1.1 *Organochlorines*

PCBs are a group of commercially produced organic chemicals, used since the 1940s in industrial applications and throughout the nuclear weapons complex. PCBs are found in many of the gaskets and large electrical transformers, as well as in the capacitors in gaseous diffusion plants. Many studies and reviews have found PCBs to be toxic to both humans and laboratory animals.[25,39,41,43]

10.6.1.2 *Pesticides*

Vinclozolin, a fungicide used on grapes, and p,p'-DDE, the major persistent metabolite of DDT, have been shown to feminize the reproductive systems of male [rat] pups born in a multigenerational study.[44,45] These pups had a very small anal-genital distance, which is an androgen-dependent measure, and the external genitalia of older animals had female characteristics, suggesting that these agents inhibited the action of androgens. For the male reproductive tract to develop, a number of proteins have to be synthesized, and that synthesis depends on androgens secreted by the testes during development. These chemicals interfere with androgens by binding to the androgen receptor and preventing the transcription of DNA. On the other hand, testicular cancer, undescended testis, and urethral abnormalities can arise during fetal development in the mother. These medical conditions may be due to altered exposure to estrogens during pregnancy and not due to androgen interference. Whereas androgens normally act like keys that open doors to reproductive development, certain androgenic toxicants may act like keys that jam the locks. In spite of the wave of publicity about endocrine disruptors in the past year, most men are still unaware that their reproductive health is under scrutiny.

In addition to chemical exposure, many drugs and medications, disease states, and environmental factors are likely to disturb the endocrine profile, resulting in decreased sexual performance (Table 10.1).

10.6.2   Drugs and Impotence

Many prescription and nonprescription drugs directly or indirectly act as hormonal disruptors and can affect sexual functioning in both men and women. In men, loss of libido (sexual desire), impotence, delayed (or absent) orgasm, failure of ejaculation, and priapism (prolonged painful erection) are common consequences of many drugs.[46,47] Women are often less affected but can experience loss of libido, inhibition of orgasm, or lack of orgasm from medicines. Unfortunately, many patients blame old age and low hormonal activity for diminishing sexual abilities, when, in truth, the problem may be the direct consequence of a drug.

10.6.2.1   Antihypertensives

About one-third of men who take thiazide diuretics (hydrochlorothiazide, chlorthalidone, beneroflumethiaide) as therapy for high blood pressure have problems with libido, erection, and ejaculation, but the mechanism is not known.[48] Spironolactone (Aldactone) at high doses blocks androgen receptors and lowers the sex drive, leading to impotence and gynecomastia.[49] Digoxin, a cardiac drug similar in structure to sex steroids, decreases testosterone and increases estrogen and is associated with erectile failure and gynecomastia.[50] Methyldopa (Aldomet), a synthetic relative of the neurotransmitter dopamine, is a well-documented cause of erectile problems.[48] Guanethidine and clonidine, which oppose the action of the sympathetic nervous system, also cause impotence. Clonidine (Catapress), an α_2-agonist, impairs erectile function and decreases libido in up to 40% of patients. β-blockers are used for many cardiovascular problems as well as for high blood pressure. Men taking propranolol (Inderal), the most common β-blocker, complained of loss of libido and erection. When a β-blocker causes problems, a drug of a different class should immediately replace it. Although loss of libido can be attributed to hypogonadism, reduced perfusion pressure

TABLE 10.1

Hormonal Disruption and Male Sexual Dysfunction

Class	Agent/Condition	Effects
(A) Pharmacological		
Antiandrogen	Cimetidine, cyproterone, spironolactone ketoconazole, finasteride, flutamide, progestins, anabolic steroids	↓DHT, altered HPG-axis, ↓Libido Impotence
Estrogen	Estradiol, estriol, DES	↓T; gynecomastia
Phytoestrogens	Flavonoids, lignans, alkaloids	↓Libido, delayed orgasm, gynecomastia
Antihypertensives	Calcium channel blockers, thiazides, β-blockers, methyldopa, digoxin	Impotence, libido
Antidepressants	Trazodone, Prozac, lithium, sertraline	Delayed ejaculation, priapism, ↓orgasm
(B) Environmental		
Chemicals	DBCP, DDT, PCBs, dioxins, methyl chloride, vinclozolin	↓HPG-axis, ↓T, ↓libido, deformities of sex-organs
Heavy metals	Lead, mercury, cadmium, cobalt, lithium	Central, gonadal, ↓HPG-axis
Radiations	∝-and β-rays; X-and ∝-rays	Nerve damage, impotence, low ejaculatory volume
(C) Recreational	Alcohol, nicotine, marijuana valium, cocaine, morphine	Depression, impotence
(D) Physiological	Cardiac/hepatic/pulmonary/renal failure; genitourinary conditions	↓Libido, impotence
(E) Disease States		
Hypertension/diabetes	Nerve/vascular/muscular damage	Organic impotence
Depression	Sickness, death, emotional stress	Psychogenic impotence, ↓libido
Other endocrine disorders	Testicular feminization, hyperthyroidism, hyperprolactinemia, hypogonadism, pituitary tumor	↓T, ↓libido, impotence altered HPG-axis

Note: Abbreviations: DBCP (dibromochloropropane); DDT (dichlorodiphenyl-trichloroethane); DHT (dihydrotestosterone); DES (diethyl stilbestrol); PCBs (polychlorinated biphenyls); T (testosterone).

of the lacunar spaces after antihypertensive therapy is probably the main cause of reduced penile rigidity.

10.6.2.2 Depression and Related Drugs

Depression itself is associated with impaired sexual function in terms of lost desire and performance. However, most antidepressant drugs, such as serotonin reuptake inhibitors, clomipramine, lithium carbonate, and monoamine oxidase inhibitors are associated with higher rates of impotence than other antidepressant classes.[51] Ejaculation and orgasmic difficulties, as well as alterations in libido, arousal, and erectile function, are prominent adverse effects of taking these medications.[51,52] The new antidepressant, selective serotonin reuptake inhibitor (Prozac), has negative effects on men's potency but has been found to be useful in delaying premature ejaculation.

10.6.2.3   Other Brand-Name Drugs

Over extended periods of usage, these drugs can cause impotence, possibly due to altered hormone synthesis and/or action. Some of these listed drugs are included in the table.[48]

Alcoholism drugs — Antabuse

Antifungal drugs — Ketoconazole

Arthritis drugs — Indocin

Bleeding drugs — Amicar

Epilepsy drugs — Dilantin

Gastrointestinal drugs — Antrocol, Arco-Lase, Butabell, Pro-Banthene, Probocon, Regian, Tagamet, Uretron, Zantac

Glaucoma drugs — Diamox

Headache drugs — Sansert

Infection drugs — Flagyl, Satiric

Muscle spasm drugs — Flexural, Norflex, Norgesic, X-Otag

Parkinson's disease drugs — Akineton, Artane, Cogentin, Kemadrin, Pagitane

Prostate drugs — Estrace, Eulexin, Lupron, Proscar, Zoladex

Tuberculosis drugs — Trecator-SC[48]

10.6.3   Recreational Agents

Many recreational agents in our daily environment directly or indirectly affect hormonal profile and can cause partial or complete impotence.

10.6.3.1   Marijuana

Cannabinoids are psychoactive chemicals found in marijuana. In a frequent marijuana user, THC (tetrahydrocannabinol) and other cannabinoids are stored in body fat and released slowly over time. This slow release could disturb hormonal profile, leading to decreased fertility and sexual function. Marijuana use also decreases blood testosterone levels.[48] The National Institute on Drug Abuse reports that new cultivation and breeding techniques produce plants many times more potent than the pot smoked three decades ago. The extent of the actual damage caused by these drugs is still unclear, but there is the belief that the damage is irreversible.

10.6.3.2 Smoking

Smoking in itself does not appear to be a direct cause of impotence, but chemical substances (nicotine) in tobacco smoke and its metabolite cotinine cause arterial constriction that may lead to impotence.[53] Men with treated heart disease who smoke are almost three times more likely to be completely impotent than those who do not. Similarly, men with treated high blood pressure and untreated arthritis who smoke are more than twice as likely to be completely impotent as those who do not. However, such interactions and the role of altered hormonal profiles leading to decreased libido or sexual performance in smokers is not clearly understood.

10.6.3.3 Alcohol

Nominal alcohol consumption often leads to changes in sexual behavior for a majority of people. Alcohol use is likely to increase subjective sexual desire, arousal, and pleasure, while lowering physiological arousal. Alcohol provokes the desire, but it takes away the performance. After drinking even moderate amounts of alcohol, many men find it difficult to achieve or maintain an erection. Alcohol abuse can cause hypogonadism and increased risk of sexual dysfunction.[43,47] Experimental rats given a large dose of ethyl alcohol are almost incapable of having an erection. High estrogen and low testosterone levels are often found in alcoholic men.

10.6.3.4 Street Drugs

Heroin, morphine, methadone, cocaine, LSD, marijuana, amphetamines, and barbiturates are widely known to affect a man's sexual performance.[48,54] To what extent these may have any direct or indirect interactions with hormone secretion causing sexual impairment needs to be investigated. Street drugs in relatively small quantities are considered to act as aphrodisiacs for some men within a few hours of ingestion, either through their own action or through a placebo effect.

10.6.4 Sexual Stimulants

Many men and women have chosen to go back to nature in search of sexual well-being. Recently some more new herbal products have emerged, claiming to help control hormonal imbalance and increase sexual potency. Herbal products are commonly used to improve health and prevent disease. Garlic, ginseng, and Ginkgo biloba are some of the most commonly ingested herbs. Though some studies suggest their effectiveness for improving libido and sexual performance in humans, actual scientific data established in a controlled environment are lacking.

10.6.4.1 Herbal

"Ginseng" in traditional Chinese medicine and "Shilajeet" in the Indian Ayurvedic system have been used for centuries to enhance stamina, capacity, and androgenicity to cope with fatigue and physical stress. These are thought to improve libido and sexual function. However, their mechanism of action is unclear. Recent studies have suggested that the antioxidant potential of vitamin E, especially in diabetics[55] and the organ-protective actions of ginseng[56] may help prevent the onset of impotence. Enhanced NO synthesis thus could contribute to ginseng-associated vasodilatation and perhaps also to an aphrodisiac action of this root. Further controlled scientific studies are needed to confirm or refute these claims.

10.6.4.2   Phytoproducts

Dietary phytoestrogens and their interactions in the body at the endocrine level may significantly affect various functions.[57,58] A unique combination of rainforest botanicals has recently become available as a natural sexual stimulant for men. It is referred to as "Rainforce Touchfire." It has a long documented history of use by the rainforest Indians. It is formulated to support male sexual function and desire nutritionally. It includes several herbal male tonics combined with nettle root which has been documented recently to increase bioavailable testosterone levels in the bloodstream by as much as ten times. Another powerful natural product designed to enhance sexual desire in men is extract of Muira puma, also known as potency wood. Muira puma has recently been the subject of clinical research (unpublished data). In two recent clinical trials performed at the Institute of Sexology in Paris, France, an herbal extract of Muira puma was shown very effective. It is likely that more clinical trials will be needed to test the effects of herbal substances on human sexuality.

Proanthocyanidins occur naturally in many fruits and vegetables and in high concentrations in both pine bark and grape seeds. Pycnogenols, another phytoproduct, constitute the most potent antioxidants known to man, up to 50 times more potent than vitamin E and 20 times more than vitamin C. These are considered to strengthen the immune system, help protect against the damage of free radicals, support collagen, and serve as natural protectors against aging. Because of their association in the maintenance of a healthy body, they may play an important role in human sexuality, possibly via increased hormonal output.

Jatoba tea is a unique treasure of the Amazon rainforest. Different tribes in the Amazon have been drinking this herbal tea for hundreds of years as an energizer to help them feel strong and vigorous. It has been used for the treatment of fatigue and as a tonic for the respiratory and urinary systems to fight fungus and yeast-like candida albicans. Its wonderful health-producing benefits have been associated with increased sexual desire and potency.

10.6.4.3   Pheromones

The richness of olfactosexual behavior has been recognized throughout human experience, even in cultures that found the idea embarrassing.[59] All releaser effects of odors in man tend to be more variable than in lower mammals because of the large variety of human signal systems and the size of the override from learned or conditioned behavior. This is almost certainly in part genetic, but psychoanalytic writers have documented the possibility of a special role for odor in psychosexual development. The known candidates for pheromonal roles are those self-selected by man and used in perfumery (muskone, civet one, castoreum, and synthetics such as exaltolide); those derived from steroids and observed incidentally, such as boar paint; and a few special cases (*cis*-4-hydroxydodeca-6-enoic acid lactone) in deer tarsal gland odor. The substances of initial choice as probable releasers and possible sexual primers in man are all musk odors (steroids, large-ring cycloketones, and lactones). The part played by 6-, 8-, and 10-carbon acids and lactones is unknown. Odors fixed from a partner might also have a playback function as hormonal releasers.

10.6.5 Environment and Impotence

Our daily environment plays a significant role in supporting or undermining normal sexual performance. Physical and mental illness due to many disease states, divorce, death in the family, depression, anxiety, stress, etc., all can disturb the hormonal status and contribute to impaired sexual performance.

10.6.5.1 Physical Condition

Physically ill men, especially cigarette smokers, are six times more likely to be impotent than healthy men. The medical conditions most often associated with impotence, according to the MMAS, are cardiovascular disease, diabetes, hypertension, untreated ulcer, arthritis, and allergy.[2] It is usually hard to tell whether the medical condition itself is the most important risk factor or the medication being taken for it or a combination of the two. Men who have had coronary bypass surgery or who suffer from myocardial infarction (stroke) or peripheral blood disease most likely have problems with the supply of arterial blood to the penis. Radiation therapy of the pelvic area frequently causes scarring that results in the penile arteries losing their ability to dilate. With age and the ingestion of toxic agents, neurotransmitter levels may be lower, and the sense of touch decreases. The most frequent neurologic disorders associated with impotence are prostate surgery, spinal cord injury, multiple sclerosis, and peripheral neuropathy.[2] Also in an obese man, the body elastin is progressively replaced by less elastic collagen. This may affect the framework of the smooth muscle in the penis, although the MMAS found no correlation between obesity and impotence. Thus, most of these conditions do alter the endocrine system.

10.6.5.2 Endocrine Status

Male hormones certainly affect sexual desire and behavior, but their role in the erection mechanism is uncertain.[29] Their deficiencies lead to loss of libido rather than erectile dysfunction. Men with testosterone levels close to castration can have erections as potent as men with normal levels. Of the 17 hormones measured in the MMAS, only dehydroepiandrosterone sulfate (DHEAS) was found to have a major correlation with impotence.[2] This hormone, made by the adrenal gland, decreases more rapidly with age than many other male hormones. High plasma prolactin (PRL) levels are also associated with decreased libido and impotence.[60] Because testosterone is also usually low in these cases, the effect of hyperprolactinemia per se in causing impotence is not clear. Men with hypothyroidism may be impotent, while men with hyperthyroidism are more likely to have diminished sexual desire but are less likely to be impotent. Unless a deficiency exists, administration of testosterone will not affect libido or sexual function and thus should be avoided.[61]

10.6.5.3 Male Menopause?

Since men begin to undergo a drop in levels of the male hormone testosterone in their late forties and early fifties, some questions naturally arise. Is there a male menopause at midlife in which sexual potency is, to some extent, lost? And if there is a male menopause, would testosterone therapy reverse these symptoms? The answer to the existence of male menopause is yes and no — no, because men do not usually experience the sudden drop in hormone levels that women do, and yes, because many men do have a gradual decline in testosterone levels.[62] But even when men have almost zero levels of testosterone, they can still have erections and normal sex.[63] Researchers have not been able to link testosterone directly with impotence problems. While men do not have a hormone-driven change of life like women, this does not mean that they do not have a midlife crisis.[63] As the body ages physically, it no longer has the vigor and fast recovery time of youth. Testosterone levels begin to decrease before middle age, and fibrous tissue in the intertubular spaces of the testes and penis increases. Low male hormone levels usually result in lower sexual desire. Testosterone replacement in hypogonadal men often results in improved libido and self-esteem, not necessarily erection.[64,65]

10.6.5.4 Psychological or Emotional Risk Factors

More than 80 percent of all cases of persistent impotence can be traced to one or more physical causes. The remaining 20 percent are caused by unknown physical or psychological factors.[62] However, even when the cause is wholly psychological or emotional, it is expressed in physical terms. That is, some message does not travel along a nerve or a specific hormone is not secreted into the bloodstream. Psychiatrists divide sexual dysfunction into sexual desire disorders, sexual arousal disorders, orgasm disorders, sexual pain disorders, and a miscellaneous category.[18,63] Many men occasionally pass through a phase of low interest in sex. It is natural that a man should wonder if his impotence problem has a physical or psychological cause.

10.7 Mechanism of Action of Hormonal Disruptors

Natural sex hormones (estrogens or androgens) travel in the bloodstream searching out compatible receptor sites located in the nucleus of specific cells. The hormones enter the cell, lock onto a specific receptor, and turn on specific genes. The genes tell the cell to make new proteins or other substances that can change cell functions (grow, divide, or make more enzyme). Unlike some hormones that act in seconds or minutes, this process may take hours to complete.

Although natural steroid hormones generally function by binding to specific receptor sites, synthetic environmental estrogens can affect the hormonal system in a number of different ways.

1. They bind to specific receptor sites inside the nucleus of a cell, which mimic or evoke a proper hormone response.
2. They block or inhibit a normal hormone response.
3. They mimic and block hormones (PCBs do both).
4. They elicit a weaker or a stronger hormone response or make a totally new response.
5. They bind to other receptors and create a novel reaction or interfere indirectly with normal hormonal action.
6. They alter production and breakdown of hormone receptors and natural hormones, which changes hormonal blood concentrations and endocrine responses.

Thus, several normal and abnormal responses can occur when any imposter binds with specific hormone receptors.

10.7.1 Effect on Specific Receptors

The action of androgen, mediated via androgen receptors (AR), is essential for normal development of the mammalian male reproductive system. Under normal physiological conditions, testosterone and DHT are the primary androgens that activate the AR. Three classes of chemicals, when administered during the developmental period, that influence androgen levels are: (1) those that have antagonistic properties with the AR (antiandrogens); (2) those that interact with the estrogen receptor; and (3) those that interact with the aromatic hydrocarbon (Ah) receptor.

10.7.1.1 Antiandrogens

Chemicals that can bind to the AR without activating it and simultaneously prevent binding of true androgens are called antiandrogens. Examples of antiandrogens include hydroxyflutamide, the pesticides procymidone[66] and vinclozolin,[67] and the DDT metabolite p,p'-DDE.[45] O,p'-DDT has weak estrogenic activity. Estradiol and DES have some affinity for the AR.[10,45] Therefore, the mechanism by which estrogenic chemicals impair development of the male reproductive system may be via antiandrogenic properties rather than or in addition to activity related to estrogen receptor activation.

Failure to activate the AR due to low androgen levels or antiandrogen activity (e.g., due to fungicide vinclozolin) would produce results similar to the less severe alterations seen in individuals with defective ARs. The range of those effects is seen clearly in human 45,XY genetic males who have defects in the AR (androgen insensitivity syndrome).[68] Similar effects have been observed in genotypic males exposed prenatally to DES. Gray et al. (1994) administered DES to pregnant rats from gestation day 14 to postnatal day 3. Male offspring had a variety of reproductive effects that are characteristic of interference with AR action, including reduction of ano-genital distance to that characteristic of females, impaired penis development, existence of vaginal pouches, prostate gland agenesis, delayed preputial separation, and reduced or absent sperm production as judged by seminiferous tubule atrophy.[67]

10.7.1.2   Estrogen Receptor Interactions

Exposure *in utero* to exogenous chemicals (octyphenol, octyphenol phenoxylate, and butyl benzyl phthalate, as well as DES) with estrogenic activity can reduce sperm production and can cause improper development of the penis, cryptorchidism, and testicular tumors.[69,70] Male offspring exposed to DES *in utero* had increased incidence of genital malformations, including epididymal cysts (nonmalignant; 21% vs. 5% for controls) and testicular abnormalities (11% vs. 3%), including small (hypoplastic) testes and microphallus.[4,71] In considering these results, it is important to note that DES is a potent synthetic estrogen that also has antiandrogen properties. With exposure *in utero* to relatively high levels of a potent exogenous estrogen, about one-third of the men who were recontacted have clinically detectable reproductive system effects. The types of effects that were observed are consistent with those that would be predicted from studies with rodents, but men appear to be less sensitive.

10.7.1.3   Aryl hydrocarbon (Ah) Receptor Agonists

Dioxin (2,3,7,8-TCDD) and other halogenated Ah that cause male reproductive system abnormalities can activate the Ah receptor.[72,73] The effects seen during development appear to result from the ability of dioxin to impair testosterone biosynthesis and normal sexual differentiation. The low androgen level is not accompanied by increased LH levels, indicating impairment of the feedback mechanism for control of LH synthesis and release. Observed effects include decreased anogenital distance, delayed testis descent, impaired spermatogenic function, decreased accessory sex gland weights, and feminization of male sexual behavior.

10.7.2 Effect on Receptor Gene Expression

Abnormality in the expression of the genome or interference with the action of gene products, as well as acceleration of the rate of cell division, can be induced in male reproductive organs by chemicals having endocrine activity. Because the male reproductive endocrine system involves components from the hypothalamus and pituitary (affecting gonadotropin production), as well as the testes (affecting testosterone production), opportunities for disruption exist at multiple levels and with a variety of types of endocrine action.[73,74] Thus, chemicals with estrogenic, antiandrogenic, or aryl hydrocarbon receptor binding activity are primary disruptor suspects, as are chemicals that influence the synthesis or release of follicle stimulating hormone (FSH), luteinizing hormone (LH), or prolactin.[74]

Although disruption of the endocrine balance will adversely affect the adult male reproductive system, the developing male reproductive system pre- and postnatally appears to be particularly susceptible and uniquely sensitive. In mammals, including humans, development of the male phenotype requires activation of the SRY gene on the Y chromosome. In the absence of expression of that gene, the female phenotype develops. The mechanisms of action of the SRY gene and the cascade of events that follows have not been elucidated fully. However, any interference with Müllerian ducts to regress will result in the presence of rudimentary components of the female reproductive tract in general. Depending on the extent and the timing of that interference, the consequences would be complete or partial failure of the development of the male reproductive system, which could limit androgen production, delay or prevent onset of puberty, and affect sexual behavior in adults.[74]

10.7.3 Effect on Ion Channels

The research currently undertaken using cavernosal smooth muscle cells in primary culture has shown the importance of ion channels on the surface of penile smooth muscle cells (Sikka et al., unpublished data). Two ion channels of particular significance are calcium and potassium. Simply speaking, calcium ion is responsible for smooth muscle contraction (i.e., penile flaccidity), and potassium ion is responsible for smooth muscle relaxation (i.e., erection). Alteration of those two ion channels by hormonal disruptors and other toxic agents represents important venues of future research.

10.7.4 How Do Environmental Estrogens Differ from Natural Hormones?

Environmental estrogens are a diverse group of synthetic chemicals and natural plant compounds that may act like estrogen hormones in animals and humans. Although most are weaker than natural estrogens, some have been associated with reproductive and developmental problems in wildlife and laboratory animals. Natural hormones and phytoestrogens are short lived, do not accumulate in tissue, and are easily broken down by our bodies.

Most natural estrogens stay in the bloodstream only minutes or at most a few hours.[75] Although opinions vary about their benefits, the health effects associated with phytoestrogens are influenced by the age of the individual during exposure (for instance, fetus, child, or adult) and the length and concentration of exposure. The estrogenic drugs, such as ethynylestradiol, are more stable and remain in the body longer than natural estrogens, like estradiol. However, pesticides and other environmental estrogens are not easily or readily broken down and are more persistent and long-lived, remaining intact in the environment and in living organisms for many years.[75]

In most cases, the chemical structures of natural hormones and the synthetic environmental estrogens are strikingly different. Chains of carbon rings form the backbone of the sex steroid hormones (estrogens, androgens, progestins). Each hormone differs only in the location and number of attachments to the main stem. Environmental estrogens (e.g., PCBs), on the other hand, come in all shapes and sizes. Many of the compounds have carbon rings stacked in various ways (polycyclic or many rings). Some have chlorine atoms or other side chains extending off the main structure. Still others contain no rings or chlorine. These structural differences between natural hormones and environmental estrogens may lead to functional difference.[75]

10.8   Evaluation for Hormonal Causes of Impotence

10.8.1   Assessment of Endocrine Profile

A complete history and physical examination should be done, with careful evaluation of hair and fat distribution, skin texture, thyroid size and consistency, gynecomastia, central and distal pulses, reflexes and vibration sensation, penis and testicles, and prostate size and consistency. Laboratory evaluation, in addition to routine urinalysis, CBC, and chemistries, should include free T4 index, TSH, testosterone, LH, FSH, and prolactin. Random glucose may not reveal diabetes and in a diabetic patient would not reveal the degree of control, so a test for glycosylated hemoglobin, which is a measure of the average glucose for the prior few months, should be done.[74] This battery of tests, plus others if suggested by the history and physical, is essential to look for a hormonal disorder that may be readily reversible with medication, and would certainly be easier to correct than vascular disease or neuropathy.

10.8.2   Assessment of Impotence

With the recent approval of Viagra, an oral medication for treating erectile dysfunction, more sophisticated studies usually practiced may not be required for the goal-directed therapy of the impotent man. Additional studies should be reserved for those select patients for whom primary therapies are unsuccessful and for those patients who choose surgical intervention. Nocturnal penile tumescence (NPT) usually shows REM-sleep-associated erections and normal tumescence. This test is useful in differentiating organic from psychogenic impotence.[76] Duplex ultrasonography can be conducted to measure peak flow velocity rates (25 cm/sec or more) in the cavernosal arteries. Duplex ultrasonography can differentiate between arterial insufficiency, veno-occlusive dysfunction, or mixed vascular disease.[77] Penile angiography and dynamic infusion cavernosography are invasive tests that should be reserved for those patients who are considering vascular surgery for arterial or venous disease, respectively. Intracavernosal vasodilators and visual sexual stimulation can be used to augment ultrasonographic or radiographic evaluation of inflow and outflow.

10.9 Conclusions

The endocrine disruptor story gets more and more complicated as new research findings are revealed. One of the biggest and probably most complex mysteries is how substances with different shapes and structures produce similar physiological results. Certain substances can mimic hormones by binding to specific hormone receptors inside cells (e.g., DDT, some PCBs, and many phytoestrogens bind to estrogen receptors). Not all endocrine disruptors alter hormonal action by binding to hormone receptors, however. Some relay molecular messages through a complex array of cellular proteins, hormone, and nonhormone response elements that indirectly turn genes on and alter cell growth and division. DDT, at or below levels found in human breast fat tissue, can bypass the estrogen receptor and stimulate a complex mixture of cell-signaling proteins (growth factor receptors) and processes that eventually will lead to cell division. DDT can also bind to the androgen receptor and inhibit androgen binding. Thus, a chemical can influence the endocrine system in more than one way. If understood, these complex modes of action of endocrine disruptors offer answers to the questions of how different molecules impact the endocrine system and other functions, especially the least understood sexual dysfunction.

References

1. Furlow, W. L., Prevalence of impotence in the United States, *Med. Ann. Hum. Sex.*, 19, 13, 1985.
2. Feldman, H. A., Goldstein, I., Hatzichristou, D. G., Krane, R. J., and McKinlay, J. B., Impotence and its medical and psychosocial correlates: results of the Massachusetts male aging study, *J. Urol.*, 151, 54, 1994.

3. McLachlan, J. A. and Korach, K. S., Symposium on estrogens in the environment, III, *Environ. Health Perspect.*, 103, 3, 1995.
4. Gill, W. B., Schumacher, G. F. B, and Bibbo, M., Structural and functional abnormalities in the sex organs of male offspring of mothers treated with diethylstilbestrol (DES), *J. Reprod. Med.*, 16, 147, 1976.
5. McLachlan, J. A., *Estrogens in the Environment*, Elsevier Press, Holland, 1980.
6. White, R., Jobling, S., Hoare, S. A., Sumpter, J. P., and Parker, M. G., Environmentally persistent alkylphenolic compounds are estrogenic, *Endocrinology*, 135, 175, 1994.
7. Guillette, L. J., Gross, T. S., Masson, G. R., Matter, J. M., Percival, H. F., and Woodward, A. R., Developmental abnormalities of the gonad and abnormal sex hormone concentrations in juvenile alligators from contaminated and control lakes in Florida, *Environ. Health Perspect.*, 102(8), 680, 1994.
8. Fry, D. M. and Toone, C. K., DDT-induced feminization of gull embryos, *Science*, 213, 922, 1981.
9. Raloff, J., DES sons face no fertility problems, *Sci. News*, 147, 324, 1995.
10. Newbold, R. R. and McLachlan, J. A., Diethylstilbestrol associated defects in murine genital tract development, in *Estrogens in the Environment*, McLachlan, J. A., Ed., Elsevier Science, Holland, 1985, 288.
11. Carlsen, E., Giwereman, A., Keiding, N., and Skakkebaek, N. E., Evidence for decreasing quality of semen during the past 50 years, *Br. Med. J.*, 305, 609, 1992.
12. Fisch, H. and Goluboff, E. T., Geographic variations in sperm counts: a potential cause of bias in studies of semen quality, *Fertil. Steril.*, 65(5), 1044, 1996.
13. Newman, H. F., Northrup, I. D., and Devlin, J., Mechanism of human penile erection, *Invest. Urol.*, 1, 350, 1964.
14. Rajfer, J., Aronson, W. J., Bush, P. A., Dorey, F. J., and Ignarro, L. J., Nitric oxide as a mediator of relaxation of the corpus cavernosum in response to nonadrenergic, noncholinergic neurotransmission, *N. Engl. J. Med.*, 326, 90, 1992.
15. Gonzalez-Cadavid, N. F. and Rajfer, J., Nitric oxide and other neurotransmitters of the corpus cavernosum, in *Infertility and Sexual Dysfunction*, Hellstrom, W. J. G., Ed., Springer-Verlag, New York, 1997, 425.
16. Wagner, G., Vascular mechanisms involved in erection and erectile disorders, *Clin. Endocrinol. Metab.*, 11, 717, 1983.
17. Saenz deTejada, I., Commentary on mechanisms for the regulation of the penile smooth muscle contractility, *J. Urol.*, 153, 1762, 1995.
18. Kinsey, A. C., Pomeroy, W. B., and Martin, C. E., Sexual behavior in the human male, W. B. Saunders, Philadelphia, 236, 1948.
19. Garban, H., Vernet, D., Freedman, A., Rajfer, J., and Gonzalez-Cadavid, N., Effect of aging on nitric oxide-mediated penile erection in the rat, *Am. J. Physiol.*, 268, H467, 1995.
20. Saenz deTejada, I., Carson, M., Morenas, A., Goldstein, I., and Traish, A. M., Endothelin: localization, synthesis, activity, and receptor types in human penile corpus cavernosum, *Am. J. Physiol.*, 261, H1078, 1991.
21. Lugg, J., Rajfer, J., and Gonzalez-Cadavid, N. F., Dihydrotestosterone is the active androgen in the maintenance of nitric oxide mediated penile erection in the rat, *Endocrinology*, 136, 1495, 1995.
22. Tsitouras, P. D., Martin, C. E., and Harman, S. M., Relationship of serum testosterone to sexual activity in healthy elderly men, *J. Gerontol.*, 37, 288, 1982.
23. Schiavi, R. C., White, D., Mandeli, J., and Schreiner-Engel, P., Hormones and nocturnal tumescence in healthy aging men, *Arch. Sex Behav.*, 22, 207, 1993.

24. Morales, A., Johnston, B., Heaton, J. P. W., and Lundie, M., Testosterone supplementation for hypogonadal impotence: assessment of biochemical measures and therapeutic outcomes, *J. Urol.*, 157, 849, 1997.

25. Cheek, A. O. and McLachlan, J. A., Environmental hormones and the male reproductive system, *J. Androl.*, 19, 5, 1998.

26. Thomas, K. B. and Coloran, T., Organochlorine endocrine disruptors in human tissue, in *Chemically-Induced Alterations in Sexual and Functional Development: The Wildlife/Human Connection*, Colborn, T. and Clement, C., Eds., Princeton Scientific Publishing Co., Inc., New Jersey, 1992, 365.

27. Pogach, L. M. and Vaitukaitis, J. L., Endocrine disorders associated with erectile dysfunction, in *Male Sexual Dysfunction*, Krane, R. J., et al., Ed., Little Brown, Boston, 1983, 63.

28. Tenover, J. S., Effects of testosterone supplementation in the aging male, *J. Clin. Endocr. Metab.*, 75, 1092, 1992.

29. Schürmeyer, T. H. and Hesch, R. D., Endocrinology of impotence, in *Erectile Dysfunction*, Jonas, U., Springer-Verlag, Berlin, 1991, 78.

30. Eardley, I., New oral therapies for the treatment of erectile dysfunction, *Br. J. Urol.*, 181, 122, 1998.

31. Ben-Galim, E., Hillman, R. E., and Weldon, V. V., Topically applied testosterone and phallic growth, *Am. J. Dis. Child*, 134, 296, 1980.

32. Findlay, J. C., Place, V., and Synder, P. J., Treatment of primary hypogonadism in men by the transdermal administration of testosterone, *J. Clin. Endocrinol. Metab.*, 68, 369, 1989.

33. Guay, A. T., Bansal, S., and Hodge, M. B., Possible hypothalamic impotence: male counterpart to hypothalamic amenorrhea, *Urology*, 38, 317, 1991.

34. Marcus, R. and Korenman, S. G., Estrogens and the human male, *Annu. Rev. Med.*, 27, 357, 1976.

35. Wortsman, J., Hamidinia, A., and Winters, S. J., Hypogonadism following long-term treatment with diethylstilbestrol, *Am. J. Med. Sci.*, 297, 364, 1989.

36. Adlercreutz, H., Hepatic metabolism of estrogens in health and disease, *N. Engl. J. Med.*, 290, 1081, 1974.

37. Willems, H., Occupational exposure to estrogens and screening for health effects, *J. Occup. Med.*, 23, 813, 1981.

38. Leonard, M. P., Nickel, C. J., and Morales, A., Hyperprolactinemia and impotence: why, when, and how to investigate, *J. Urol.*, 142, 992, 1989.

39. Roa, K. S. and Schwetz, B. A., Reproductive toxicity of environmental agents, *Annu. Rev. Publ. Health*, 3, 1, 1982.

40. Kavlock, R. J. and Perreault, S. D., Multiple chemical exposure and risks of adverse reproductive function and outcome, in Toxicological of *Chemical Mixtures: From Real Life Examples to Mechanisms of Toxicology Interactions*, Yang, R. S. H., Ed., Academic Press, Orlando, FL, 1994, 245.

41. Zaebst, D. D., Tanaka, S., and Haring, M., Occupational exposure to estrogens — problems and approaches, in *Estrogens in the Environment*, McLachlan, M. J. A., Ed., Elsevier/North-Holland, New York, 1980, 377.

42. Soto, A. M., Lin, T. M., Justicia, H., Silvia, R. M., and Sonenschein, C., An "in culture" bioassay to assess the estrogenicity of xenobiotics (E-Screen), in *Chemically Induced Alterations in Sexual and Functional Development: The Wildlife/Human Connection*, Colborn, T. and Clements, C., Princeton Scientific Publishing Co., Princeton, NJ, 1992, 295.

43. Sikka, S. C., Gonadotoxicity, in *Male Infertility and Sexual Dysfunction*, Hellstrom, W. J. G., Ed., Springer-Verlag, New York, 1997, 292.

44. Kelce, W. R., Monosson, E., Gamcsik, M. P., Laws, S. C., and Gray, L. E., Jr., Environmental hormone disruptors: evidence that vinclozolin developmental toxicity is mediated by antiandrogenic metabolites, *Toxicol. Appl. Pharm.*, 126, 1392, 1993.

45. Kelce, W. R., Stone, C. R., Laws, S. C., Gray, L. E., Jr., Kemppainen, J. A., and Wilson, E. M., Persistent DDT metabolite Pp-DDE is a potent androgen receptor antagonist, *Nature*, 375, 581, 1995.

46. Mills, L. C., Drug-induced impotence, *Clin. Pharmacol.*, 12, 104, 1975.

47. Horowitz, I. D. and Goble, A. J., Drugs and impaired male sexual function, *Drugs*, 18, 206, 1979.

48. Drugs that cause sexual dysfunction: An update, in *The Medical Letter on Drugs and Therapeutics*, Vol. 34, Abramowicz, M., Ed., The Medical Letter, Inc., New Rochelle, NY, 1992, 73.

49. Greenblatt, D. J. and Koch-Weser, J., Gynecomastia and impotence: complications of spironolactone therapy, *JAMA*, 223, 82, 1973.

50. Neri, A., The effect of long-term administration of digoxin on plasma androgens and sexual dysfunction, *J. Sex Marital Ther.*, 13, 58, 1987.

51. Mitchell, J. E. and Popkin, M. K., Antipsychotic drug therapy and sexual dysfunction in men, *Am. J. Psych.*, 139, 633, 1982.

52. Blay, S. L., Ferraz, M. P., and Calill, H. M., Lithium-induced male sexual impairment: two case reports, *J. Clin. Psych.*, 43, 497, 1982.

53. Xie, Y., Garban, H., Ng, C., Rajfer, J., and Gonzalez-Cadavid, N. F., Effect of long term passive smoking on erectile function and penile nitric oxide synthase in the rat, *J. Urol.*, 157(3), 1121, 1997.

54. Mattson, R. H., Cramer, J. A., Collins, J. F., Smith, D. B., Delgado-Escueta, A. V., Browne, T. R., Williamson, P. D., Treiman, D. M., McNamara, J. O., and McCutchen, C. B., Comparison of carbamazepine, phenobarbital, phenytoin and primidone in partial and secondarily generalized atonic-clonic seizures, *N. Engl. J. Med.*, 313(3), 145, 1985.

55. Sikka, S. C., Rajasekaran, M., Hellstrom, W. J. G., and Jain, S. K., Role of vitamin E and oxidative stress in the pathophysiology of diabetic impotence, *J. Urol.*, 155(5), 623, 1996.

56. Chen, X. and Lee, T. J., Ginsenosides-induced nitric oxide-mediated relaxation of the rabbit corpus cavernosum, *Br. J. Pharm.*, 115, 15, 1995.

57. Hughes, C. L., Phytochemical mimicry of reproductive hormones and modulation of herbivore fertility by phytoestrogens, *Environ. Health Prespect.*, 78, 171, 1988.

58. Chapin, R. E., Stevens, J. T., Hughes, C. L., Kelce, W. R., Hess, R. A., and Daston, G. P., Endocrine modulation of reproduction, *Fund. Appl. Toxicol.*, 29, 1, 1996.

59. Morris, N. M. and Udry, J. R., Pheromonal influences on human sexual behavior: an experimental search, *J. Biosoc. Sci.*, 10, 147, 1978.

60. Leonard, M. P., Nickel, C. J., and Morales, A., Hyperprolactinemia and impotence: why, when, and how to investigate, *J. Urol.*, 142(4), 992, 1989.

61. Buvat, J. and Lemaire, A., Endocrine screening in 1022 men with erectile dysfunction: clinical significance and cost-effective strategy, *J. Urol.*, 158, 1764, 1997.

62. Carroll, J. L., Ellis, D. J., and Bagley, D. H., Age-related change in hormones in impotent men, *Urology*, 36, 42, 1990.

63. Ryan, G., Reclaiming male sexuality, in *A Guide to Potency, Vitality and Prowess* (with Foreword by Arnold Melman), M. Evans and Co., Inc., New York, 1997.

64. Davidson, J. M., Kwan, M., and Greenleaf, W., Hormonal replacement and sexuality in men, *Clin Endocrinol. Metab*, 11, 599, 1982.

65. Davidson, J. M., Camargo, C. A., and Smith, E. R., Effects of androgen on sexual behavior in hypogonadal men, *J. Clin. Endocrinol. Metab.*, 45, 955, 1979.

66. Hosokawa, S., Murakami, M., Ineyama, M., Yamada, T., Yoshitake, A., Yamada, H., and Miyamoto, J., The affinity of procymidone to androgen receptor in rats and mice, *J. Toxicol. Sci.*, 18, 111, 1993.

67. Gray, L. E., Jr., Ostby, J. S., and Kelce, W. R., Developmental effects of an environmental antiandrogen: the fungicide vinclozolin alters sex differentiation of the male rat, *Toxicol. Appl. Pharmacol.*, 129, 46, 1994.

68. Quigley, C. A., De Bellis, A., Marschke, K. B., El-Awady, M. K., Wilson, E. M., and French, F. S., Androgen receptor defects: historical, clinical and molecular perspectives, *Endocr. Rev.*, 16, 271, 1995.

69. Sharpe, R. M., Commentary. Declining sperm counts in men — is there an endocrine cause? *J. Endocrinol.*, 136, 357, 1993.

70. Sharpe, R. M. and Skakkebaek, N. E., Are oestrogens involved in falling sperm counts and disorders of the male reproductive tract? *Lancet,* 341, 1392, 1993.

71. Gill, W. B., Schumacher, F. B., Bibbo, M. , Straus, F. H., and Schoenberg, H. W., Association of diethylstilbestrol exposure *in utero* with cryptorchidism, testicular hypoplasia and semen abnormalities, *J. Urol.*, 122, 36, 1979.

72. Whitlock, J. P., The aromatic hydrocarbon receptor, dioxin action, and endocrine homeostasis, *Trends Endocrinol. Metab.*, 5, 183, 1994.

73. Safe, S., Astroff, B., Harris, B., Zacharewski, T., Dickerson, R., Romkes, M., and Biegel, L., 2,3,7,8-Tetrachlorodibenzo-p-dioxin (TCDD) and related compounds as antiestrogens; characterization and mechanism of action, *Pharmacol. Toxicol.*, 69, 400, 1991.

74. Klyde, B. J., Hormonal causes of male sexual dysfunction, in *Management of Impotence and Infertility,* Whitehead, E. D. and Nagler, H. M., J. B. Lippincott Co., Philadelphia, 1994, 115.

75. Lieberman, S., Are the differences between estradiol and other estrogens, naturally occurring or synthetic, merely semantical? *J. Clin. Endocr. Metab.*, 81, 850, 1996.

76. Hirshkowitz, M., Karacan, I., Howell, J. W., Arcasoy, M. O., and Williams, R. L., Nocturnal penile tumescence in cigarette smokers with erectile dysfunction, *Urology*, 39, 101, 1992.

77. Lee, B., Sikka, S. C., Randrup, E. R., Villemarette, P., Baum, N., Hower, J. F., and Hellstrom, W. J., Standardization of penile blood flow parameters in normal men using intracavernous prostaglandin E1 and visual sexual stimulation, *J. Urol.*, 149, 49, 1993.

11

The Role of Natural and Manmade Estrogens in Prostate Development

Frederick S. vom Saal and Barry G. Timms

CONTENTS

0-8493-3164-1/99/$0.00+$.50
© 1999 by CRC Press LLC

11.1 Introduction

There has been speculation for some time that estrogen plays a role in the normal development as well as subsequent disease of the prostate.[1,2] One basis for this speculation is that embryologists recognized that the region of the developing urogenital sinus just caudal to the bladder, from which the prostatic ducts emerge during fetal life, is the homologous embryonic anlage of a portion of the vagina in females. It thus seemed reasonable to speculate that, since the vagina is an estrogen-responsive organ, portions of the prostate might also be responsive to estrogen, and that estrogen might play a role in regulating prostate development and subsequent function, as well as diseases associated with aging.

In contrast to the above prediction that estrogen might play a role in normal prostate development, there are numerous reports that prenatal or neonatal exposure to high, pharmacological doses of diethylstilbestrol (DES) and other natural and synthetic estrogens dramatically interferes with prostate development in mice and rats. Prostate development in mice begins during late fetal life and continues through adolescence.[3] These findings have led to confusion concerning the role of endogenous estrogen in normal prostate development. Many questions have been raised regarding the potential for environmental chemicals with estrogenic activity to alter prostate development at concentrations encountered in the environment (referred to as environmentally relevant doses of chemicals). What has not been recognized with regard to prostate development is that a very high dose of DES can produce an opposite effect (inhibition) on prostate development in comparison to a much lower dose. This is especially important when the dose is within a physiological range of estrogenic activity and can produce a stimulatory effect on development of the prostate.[4] The view that dose is important is not a new concept in endocrinology, toxicology, or pharmacology. However, prior to recent findings based on manipulating estrogen levels within a physiological range in fetal mice, low, physiologically relevant doses of estrogen had not been examined. One reason for this was the difficulty associated with measuring estradiol in very small volumes of serum in rodents in which levels of lipids are very high, thus causing interference with the assays.[5]

This chapter reviews recent studies showing that very small differences in circulating estradiol during fetal life in male mice can lead to differences in prostate differentiation that persist into adulthood. In some of these studies we have used the technique of computer-assisted three-dimensional reconstruction of the developing prostate to visualize and quantitate prostate morphogenesis. Because the prostate is the most prone to disease during aging of any organ in humans, the potential for endogenous estrogens, and thus also low, environmentally relevant concentrations of environmental estrogens, to impact prostate pathogenesis is of immense importance as a public health issue. Benign prostatic hyperplasia (BPH) is the most common pathological condition of aging in humans (70% of men experience BPH by age 70), while as many as 40% of men are found to have prostate cancer when examined at autopsy. The detection of cancer in living men (0.14% incidence) and mortality rates (0.03%) are, however, much lower than what would be predicted based on autopsy data. Whether the cancers detected at autopsy would have progressed if these men had lived longer remains unknown.[6]

We will begin by discussing the history of our knowledge of the prostate, after which the focus will be on research examining the effects of natural and manmade estrogens on prostate development.

11.2 Historical Overview of the Prostate

Pathology of the prostate was attributed in 1685 by Samuel Collins to "indulgence in venery" (the pursuit of sexual pleasure). Collins recognized that prostate enlargement was important with regard to urethral obstruction; this was also discussed in 1769 by Giambattista Morgagni.[1,2] Franks[2] noted that Morgagni identified the site of origin of hyperplasia within the prostate and also examined the prevalence of this disease in old men.

John Hunter observed in 1786 that the prostate (and other accessory reproductive organs) underwent involution following castration. Zuckerman[1] comments on the remarkable fact that even though the implication of this observation would suggest that castration might serve as a treatment to relieve the effects of prostatic enlargement on urethral obstruction, which results in death due to uremic poisoning if untreated, the implication of this observation was not grasped until almost a hundred years later. Castration as a treatment for enlargement of the prostate was finally proposed in 1893, after which it became the method of treating this disease. However, this approach was soon abandoned, because at that time, mortality associated with surgery was unacceptably high. In addition, although it might seem surprising today, at the end of the nineteenth century there was still considerable controversy concerning the role of the testes in accessory reproductive organ function. This controversy is interesting in that it had been reported in the middle of the nineteenth century that testicular grafts reversed the effects of castration in cockerels, which led to attempts to reverse impotence in aging men by means of grafting animal testicular tissue. At this time it was believed that any effects of the testes on organs such as the prostate were probably mediated by nerves, not secreted substances. However, in 1927, methods for extracting gonadal steroids were described, and testosterone was finally identified as the most potent of the testicular hormones in 1935. Prostate growth in castrated rats was being routinely used as a bioassay for potency of testicular hormones by this time.[7,8]

Our current understanding of prostate development and anatomy appears to have progressed steadily during the past 60 years but has been partially hindered by reliance on old anatomical descriptions.[9-11] Recent advancements in computer technology now allow organ structure to be visualized by three-dimensional reconstruction from digitized serial sections, which provides a powerful tool for examining prostate anatomy. This technique has been useful particularly in understanding the complex pattern of ductal morphogenesis, a feature that is extremely difficult to grasp when viewing two-dimensional histological sections in a microscope.[11,12] Three-dimensional reconstructions are accomplished using computer-assisted analysis of histological serial sections. This requires tracing, digitizing, and axial alignment of identified objects (anatomical structures) within each section. The main advantage of the computer-generated three-dimensional image data is that the digitized information used to reconstruct the prostate provides the basis for making quantitative comparisons. These data can be used to study the effects on the developing prostate of experimental manipulations.[4,12]

Descriptive anatomy prior to computer assisted three-dimensional reconstruction was aided by the use of wax modeling. Lowsley[13] made a wax reconstruction of serial histological sections from a fetal and newborn human male prostate, and generated considerable subsequent controversy due to his interpretation of the anatomy. Lowsley's description of prostatic lobes has been replaced by the now widely accepted concept that the human prostate is better described as consisting of zones.[14]

11.3   Prostate Development

11.3.1   Testosterone and 5α-Dihydrotestosterone

At about the eighth week of gestation in humans and at gestation day 12 in mice, Leydig cells in the developing testes begin production of androgen, with testosterone being the major androgen secreted throughout sexual differentiation.[15-17] Testosterone mediates differentiation of the Wolffian (mesonephric) duct system (Figure 11.1[18]). Secretion of Müllerian-inhibiting hormone (MIH) by the Sertoli cells, which line the seminiferous tubules, suppresses the development of the Müllerian (paramesonephric) ducts; estrogen antagonizes the action of MIH, while testosterone facilitates the action of MIH.[19]

For normal masculinization of the urogenital sinus and perineal tissue (external genitalia) in males to occur, mesenchymal tissue associated with the urogenital sinus must express the enzyme 5α-reductase, which converts testosterone to 5α-dihydrotestosterone. This relates to the dose of androgen required to induce masculinization. 5α-dihydrotestosterone has a higher affinity for androgen receptors relative to testosterone, thus enabling it to

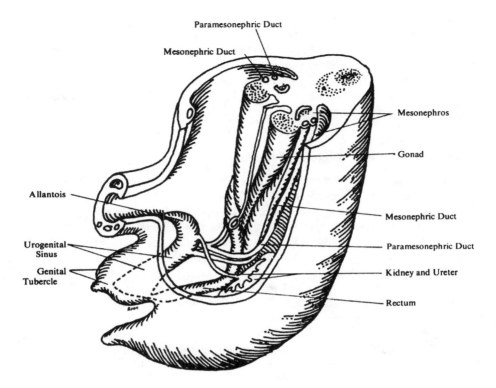

FIGURE 11.1
Genital ducts prior to differentiation. Drawing of a human embryo at about 42 d of age with
the upper half and left body wall cut away to demonstrate the gonad, mesonephros, and
associated ducts, and urogenital sinus. The gut and its mesentery have also been removed.
(From Allan, F. D., *Essentials of Human Embryology,* Oxford University Press, New York, 1960,
119. With permission.)

induce the same response as testosterone at a lower concentration, and the
concentration of testosterone in the systemic circulation is not sufficient to
result in normal prostate development. This is revealed by studies in which
testosterone levels in the fetal blood are in a normal range and androgen
receptor numbers in fetal tissues are normal, but 5α-reductase activity is
inhibited by administration of drugs. If there is a deficiency in the capacity
to normally produce 5α-dihydrotestosterone due to a genetic defect, normal
development of the prostate and external genitalia does not occur.[19,20]

5α-dihydrotestosterone binds to androgen receptors expressed in urogenital sinus mesenchyme, which induces outgrowths (glandular buds) of the
adjacent urothelium of the urogenital sinus. The epithelial buds show little
capacity to bind androgen; they form the anlage of the prostate at about
10 weeks of gestation in humans and gestation day 17 in mice.[21-23] These
outgrowths begin as solid epithelial buds, which later branch extensively
during late fetal life in humans, forming a compound tubulo-alveolar gland

structure. In mice, birth occurs within 2 d of the beginning of prostate differentiation, and extensive ductal branching occurs throughout infancy and adolescence, with the adult structure not achieved until approximately postnatal day 50.[3] In humans, the pubertal reawakening of androgen secretion by the testes results in the prostatic glandular ducts forming patent lumens within the terminal acini, and the epithelial lining becomes highly differentiated and begins secretory activity.

11.3.2   Anatomic Regions of the Prostate

The ejaculatory ducts form from the embryonic Wolffian ducts. The ejaculatory ducts enter the prostatic urethra caudal and lateral to the site of the utricle, which is the remnant of the Müllerian ducts as they merge and enter the posterior urogenital sinus (Figure 11.1). The utricle becomes enclosed in the central zone of the human prostate. Each ejaculatory duct (vas deferens) merges with the ipsilateral seminal vesicle duct, which differentiates during the thirteenth week of embryonic life in humans. The ejaculatory ducts lead into the prostatic urethra next to an enlarged portion of the urethral crest, the verumontanum (also referred to as the colliculus seminalis), in the posterior wall of the urethra (Figure 11.2).

In its passage through the prostate, the urethra is divided into a proximal segment (from bladder neck to verumontanum) and a distal segment (from verumontanum to external sphincter), forming a 35-40° angle at the verumontanum. The proximal urethra is surrounded by circular smooth muscle, which is referred to as the preprostatic sphincter and functions to stop retrograde ejaculation into the bladder. In the proximal portion of the urethra in humans, prostatic glands that mingle with sphincteric stroma have been proposed as the potential site for pathogenesis of BPH.[24] The prostatic ducts from this zone exit laterally from the urethra, but these ducts are quite short in comparison to the ducts leading to the peripheral zone. Hypertrophy of the short ducts during development of BPH impinges on the urethra, which can lead to obstruction. Carcinoma is found predominantly in glands originating from the distal segment which comprise the peripheral zone of the prostate in men. McNeal introduced the hypothesis of a reawakening of embryonic inductive interactions to describe the inappropriate new ductal budding that occurs in BPH. This was thought to result from nonprostatic stroma (the proximal urethral sphincter) inducing adjacent transition zone ducts to begin new ductal formation in areas of stromal proliferation. The significance of this stromal-epithelial interaction in prostate development has been the subject of many reviews.[25-29]

The prostate in mice contributes proteins involved in coagulation and various ions to seminal fluid. In male mice, removal of this organ reduces fertility.[30] The morphology of the mouse prostate, which is divided into dorsolateral and ventral lobes, has been described in a series of papers by Sugimura.[3,31,32] Individual prostatic glandular ducts extend from the urethra

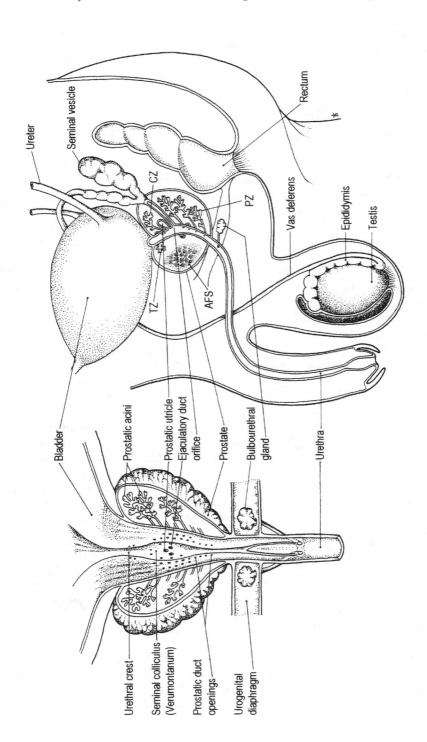

FIGURE 11.2

Diagrams of frontal and sagittal sections of the male urogenital complex showing the anatomical position of the adult prostate and associated structures. The prostatic zones are: central zone (CZ), peripheral zone (PZ) and transition zone (TZ). The anterior fibromuscular stroma (AFS) is also shown. (From Timms, B. G., Anatomical perspectives of prostate development, in *Prostate: Basic and Clinical Aspects*, Naz, R. K., Ed., CRC Press, New York, 1997, 36. With permission.)

and branch into three to six terminal ducts and are lined with pseudostrat-ified columnar epithelium with interspersed basal cells. The ducts are surrounded by a layer of smooth muscle cells.

11.4 Homology: The Basis of Comparative Biology and Pathology

It has been proposed that the variety of interspecies differences observed in the structure of the adult prostate gland reflects a diversity that makes it difficult to find a suitable animal model for the study of human prostatic disease.[24] Homology, which is based on structural and functional similarities in embryonic development rather than in adult appearance or even use of an organ, has been the basis for comparing the evolutionary relatedness of organs in different species for the past 150 years.[33,34] A well-known example is the hand in humans and the fin in a whale, which share a common embryonic development and are homologous structures, but which appear in the adult quite different on superficial examination. Thus, attempting to elucidate the appropriateness of animal models for studying human prostate pathogenesis requires comparing humans and animals during prostate development, and not simply comparing the adult appearance of the organ.

Using a computer-assisted three-dimensional approach to visualize the microanatomy of prostate development, Timms[12] has compared the ductal budding patterns during prostate morphogenesis in rat, mouse, and human (Figure 11.3). The three-dimensional reconstruction procedure revealed marked similarities between rodents and human prostate gland genesis, leading Timms to propose that the site of opening of the prostatic glandular ducts into the urethra provides a basis for assessing homologous regions of the prostate in rodents and humans. Prostatic ducts that originate from similar regions of the urogenital sinus in different species are proposed to be homologous in that they share a common structural and functional developmental pattern. This finding is significant in that Price[35] observed that the relationship of prostate ductal openings into the urethra persists in the adult in the same relative position as in the fetus. That the overall appearance of the prostate and the organization of the terminal regions of the glands (as opposed to their origin at the urethra) differ in the adult makes it appear as if the prostate in the mouse and human are quite different. In contrast, the budding patterns of the glandular ducts from the urogenital sinus in mice and humans during fetal development are remarkably similar, as described for the human hand and whale's fin. There is now no question that the formation of the fetal prostatic ducts in humans and rodents occurs from the ventral, lateral, and dorsal aspect of the urogenital sinus.[12] The question that remains to be answered relates to the grouping of these ducts into recognizable

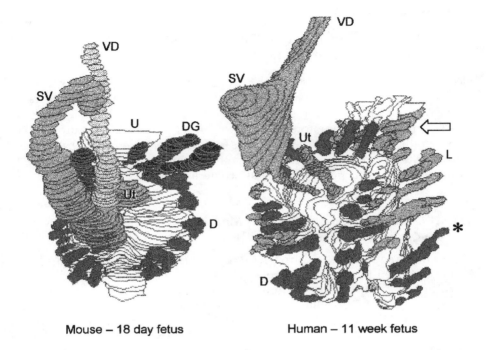

Mouse – 18 day fetus   **Human – 11 week fetus**

FIGURE 11.3

Computer-assisted serial section reconstructions from a fetal mouse (gestation day 18, left) and human prostate (70 mm CR length/11 weeks, right). The seminal vesicle (SV) and vas deferens (VD) on the right side of each reconstruction have been omitted to facilitate viewing of the prostatic budding patterns. In the mouse, dorsal prostatic bud outgrowths (D) are associated with the prostatic furrows of the urogenital sinus along the caudal-cranial axis. The dorsocranial gland (DG) exhibits three pairs of outgrowths and is associated with the dorsocranial aspect of the urogenital sinus. The human fetal prostate shows dorsal outgrowths (D) that form a horse-shoe-shaped pattern around the ejaculatory ducts and prostatic utricle (Ut). A parallel line of buds grows from the lateral wall of the urogenital sinus (L). The most caudal of these buds exhibit an anterior direction of growth (*). Several small periurethral outgrowths are evident in the proximal portion of the dorsocranial urethra (arrow). The seminal vesicle appears as a dorsal swelling on the vas deferens. Both views are from a superior right dorso-lateral perspective. At these stages of fetal growth, the mouse and human prostate budding patterns demonstrate striking similarities. Proximal urethra (U).

lobes or zones and whether these can be identified with histological, biochemical, or pathological distinctions.

Dogs and cats have homogenous prostate tissue similar to the peripheral zone in humans, while the seminal vesicles and the central zone of the prostate are absent.[36] The glandular ducts that lead from the urethra to the zones of the prostate that are prone to BPH in men, the transition and central zones,[24,27,37] are thus absent in dogs.

11.5   Estrogen and Prostate Development, Adult Function and Pathology

There is considerable evidence for estrogen responsiveness of the prostate in rodents and other mammals.[26,38-40] Our findings show that during prostate development in fetal rats (on gestation day 20), stroma strongly expresses mRNA for estrogen receptors, while estrogen receptor mRNA in urogenital sinus epithelium is at background levels (unpublished observation). A necessity for morphogenetic processes appears to be living stromal cells, through which trophic induction of epithelial proliferation is mediated.

11.5.1   The Dog and Noble Rat as Models for Human Prostate Disease

Exposure to supplemental estrogen (in combination with androgen) in adulthood has been related to hyperplasia of the prostate in dogs[41] and Noble rats. In Noble rats, neoplastic tumors can be induced to form in the dorsolateral prostatic lobes, while Sprague-Dawley rats typically do not develop tumors.[42-45] Although fewer than 1% of Noble rats spontaneously develop adenocarcinoma of the prostate, treatment with a combination of low doses of testosterone and estradiol-17β (via Silastic capsules) for 4 months leads to multifocal epithelial dysplasia,[45,46] and longer treatment (about 10 months) results in the transition from dysplasia to neoplastic tumors in about 20% of treated males. Histological examination of prostate tumors in Noble rats treated with androgen and estrogen showed that they primarily involved glandular epithelium, and metastases after transplantation into hosts revealed differentiated epithelial components.[42] Neoplastic development occurs in specific regions of the peripheral zone of the human prostate gland.[47] Dysplasia in the dorsolateral lobe of testosterone and estradiol treated Noble rats is almost identical to the premalignant lesions described in the human gland.

11.5.2   The Intrauterine Position Phenomenon: Correlation Between Estradiol and Prostate Development in Fetal Mice

Our interest in the relationship between estrogen and prostate development began with an observation that, at first, appeared to contrast with the accepted view that exposure to an increase in estrogen inhibited normal prostate development in rodents.[48] We had observed that there were higher serum concentrations of estradiol in female relative to male mouse fetuses, and higher serum testosterone levels in male relative to female mouse fetuses.[17,49,50] There is transport of both estradiol and testosterone between adjacent fetuses within a uterine horn, which serves as a source of variation in these steroids during fetal life. We refer to this as the intrauterine position phenomenon, which is mediated by steroid transport between fetuses across the placental membranes via the amniotic fluid.[51] As a consequence of steroid transport between fetuses, male mice that develop *in utero* between two female fetuses (2F males) are exposed to higher blood concentrations of estradiol (about 35% difference) and lower blood concentrations of testosterone (about 30% difference) than are male fetuses that develop between two male fetuses, referred to as 2M males.[17] There is a wide range of traits that differ as a function of random intrauterine placement in comparisons of both males and females.[17] With regard to the prostate and other reproductive organs, however, the logical prediction was that 2M males would have enlarged reproductive organs relative to 2F males. As predicted, adult 2M males were found to have larger seminal vesicles relative to 2F males,[52,53] which was associated with higher levels of 5α-reductase activity in the seminal vesicles of 2M relative to 2F males (unpublished observation). In contrast, the prostate in 2F males was found to be significantly larger (by about 30%) than that in 2M males. The enlarged prostate in 2F males was associated with a three-fold greater number of prostatic androgen receptors in 2F relative to 2M males.[53]

In dogs, estradiol synergizes with dihydrotestosterone to increase androgen binding in prostatic cells and thus increases prostate growth.[54] Studies have also shown that estradiol influences hypothalamic androgen receptors in adult male rats.[55] In addition, estradiol regulates the expression of receptors for a number of hormones, such as uterine oxytocin receptors and both uterine and brain progesterone receptors.[56,57] Taken together, these findings show that the physiological effects of exposure to estrogen can include changes in the functioning of a variety of tissues due to changes in the receptors for other hormones that regulate these tissues. Importantly, when exposure to estrogen occurs during critical periods in development, effects on tissue function are permanent.

11.5.3   Stimulating Effects on Prostate Development of an Experimental Increase in Estradiol in Male Mouse Fetuses

We examined the hypothesis that an increase in estradiol within a physiological range during fetal life would permanently increase prostate size. We experimentally increased serum estradiol levels in male mouse fetuses during the time of fetal prostate development by implanting pregnant females with a Silastic capsule containing estradiol.[4] The dose of estradiol that we chose to administer via Silastic capsule resulted in a 50% increase in free serum estradiol in male mouse fetuses from 0.2 pg/ml (in controls) to 0.3 pg/ml; the free (unbound) fraction of estradiol (and other steroids) is the biologically active fraction of total circulating steroid. This 0.1 pg/ml increase in free serum estradiol was associated with an increase in total serum estradiol of 52 pg/ml (from 94 pg/ml in controls to 146 pg/ml; the percent free

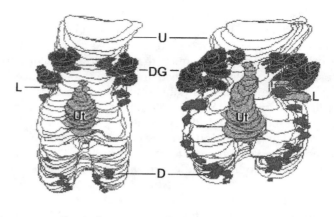

Control   Estradiol-treated mouse fetus

FIGURE 11.4

These computer-assisted serial section reconstructions show the dorsal portion of the prostate from two mouse fetuses. The prostate from an untreated male with 0.21 pg/ml free serum estradiol is shown on the left. The prostate on the right is reconstructed from a male fetus exposed to 0.32 pg/ml free serum estradiol via a maternal Silastic implant containing estradiol. Glandular buds that form the dorsal (D), lateral (L), and dorsocranial (DG) glands in the adult prostate can be seen as outgrowths of the fetal urogenital sinus (ventral buds are not visible). The prostatic utricle (Ut) is the remnant of the regressing embryonic female reproductive tract (Müllerian ducts). Compared to controls, estradiol significantly increased the number and size of the prostatic glandular buds. In contrast, estradiol caused a reduction in the size of the lumen of the urethra (U), which passes through the prostate.

estradiol in fetal mouse serum is 0.2%). This increase in estradiol was chosen since it produced a mean value for serum estradiol in all treated male fetuses that was at the high end of the normal range of estradiol values measured in the serum of 2F males, and thus represented an increase is estradiol that was within the normal physiological range.

The 0.1 pg/ml increase in free serum estradiol increased the number of developing prostate glands (by 40%) based on three-dimensional reconstruction of the prostate collected from male fetuses on gestation day 18, 1 day after initiation of fetal prostate development (Figure 11.4). The developing prostatic glandular ducts in the dorsal region of the urogenital sinus were also enlarged in estrogen-treated males relative to control males. This effect on the prostate was permanent. In adulthood, males exposed to the 50% increase in estradiol during fetal life had enlarged, hyperplastic prostates (by 40%) that showed a six-fold increase in prostatic androgen receptors relative to prenatally untreated males. The same permanent stimulation of prostate growth in male mice occurred with maternal ingestion of 0.02, 0.2, or 2 ng of the manmade estrogen, DES per gram body weight per day from gestation day 11 through 17. Males exposed during fetal life to these low doses of DES had significantly enlarged prostates in adulthood relative to control males.[4]

An interesting additional observation is that the 50% increase in serum estradiol also resulted in a significant decrease in the size of the urethra and a significant enlargement of the utriculus in male fetuses. It is well known that elevated levels of estrogen inhibit regression of the Müllerian ducts. For example, treatment of pregnant females with DES interferes with the action of Müllerian inhibiting hormone on Müllerian duct regression in mice[48] and humans.[58] The utriculus is the Müllerian duct remnant that persists within the central zone of the human prostate,[59] and the size of this area of the prostate in men may thus correlate with fetal estradiol exposure; this portion of the Müllerian duct differentiates into the dorsocranial portion of the vagina in females.[19] A critical aspect of these findings with regard to the role of estrogen in prostate differentiation, as well as effects on other reproductive organs, is that in no other *in vivo* experimental studies in rodents has the administered dose of estrogen been determined to be within a physiological range.

11.5.4   Inhibition of Prostate Development with High, Pharmacological Doses of Estrogens

An extensive literature relating to the effects of exposure to synthetic estrogens during differentiation of the prostate and other accessory reproductive organs in rodents consistently shows inhibitory effects of estrogen on prostate function. The research concerning the effects of estrogen during early life on accessory reproductive organs in male rodents has involved the use of high doses of synthetic estrogens, such as DES, and exposure to a high dose of DES (or other synthetic estrogens) causes abnormal development and lesions throughout the reproductive system in males.[60-69] Administration of high, nonphysiological levels of androgen during sexual differentiation has similar effects.[70] For example, squamous metaplasia of prostatic and coagulating gland (dorsocranial prostate) ductal epithelium in male mice and rats has been reported after exposure to exogenous estrogen during early life.[48,58,71] Similar effects of estrogen on rat prostatic cells in culture have been reported.[72] Damage to reproductive organs in females is also seen with developmental exposure to high doses of synthetic estrogens.[69,73-77]

11.5.5   Opposite Effects of High and Low Doses of Estrogen during Prostate Development

We found that a small increase in estradiol, within a physiological range, led to an increase in prostate size, associated with an increase in prostatic androgen receptors, while numerous prior studies showed exactly the opposite effect of much higher doses of manmade estrogen.[67] We thus administered increasing doses of both estradiol (via Silastic capsule) and DES (via feeding) to pregnant female mice and examined the prostate in male offspring in adulthood. Following fetal exposure to both estradiol and DES, we found an inverted-U dose-response relationship for adult prostate weight. Specifically, as serum estradiol concentrations were increased in male mouse fetuses via maternal Silastic implants from 50-800% relative to controls, first an increase and then a decrease in adult prostate weight was observed in male offspring. Similarly, while maternal doses of 0.02, 0.2, and 2 ng/g body weight per day increased prostate weight in male offspring, a DES dose of 20 ng/g led to prostate weight that did not differ significantly from control males, while 200 ng DES per gram significantly decreased adult prostate weight.[4] Taken together, the above findings provide evidence that with regard to prostate development, effects seen in response to high, pharmacological/toxicological doses of natural or manmade estrogens are opposite to effects seen with low doses within the normal physiological range of estrogenic activity.

11.5.6   Environmental Endocrine-Disrupting Chemicals that Mimic Estrogen Alter Prostate Development

Studies now identify that many chemicals have the capacity to disrupt the functioning of the endocrine system, either by binding to endogenous hormone receptors, interfering with enzyme activity, or via other mechanisms, such as interfering with plasma transport of hormones.[78,79] There are thus chemicals being used in common household products that, prior to being used to manufacture these products, were not tested for the possibility that they might be able to bind to receptors for natural steroids, such as estrogen and androgen. Because development of all organs is coordinated by endocrine signals, the disruption of endocrine signals during critical periods in organ development can lead to permanent effects on organ function. Functional effects might not be noticed based only on examination for gross malformations, which, along with cancer, has been the focus of toxicological testing.

We recently examined the effects of fetal exposure to bisphenol A, an estrogen-mimicking chemical. Bisphenol A is used to make polycarbonate plastic (for example, baby-feeding bottles are made from polycarbonate). Bisphenol A is also a component of the resin lining of food and beverage cans, in dental sealants, and many other plastic products. Approximately 2,000,000,000 pounds of bisphenol A are used per year, and another 100,000,000 pounds of brominated bisphenol A are used as flame retardants in a wide variety of products.

We used a screening assay involving human breast cancer cells (MCF-7) to assess the estrogenic potency of bisphenol A.[80] Our findings suggested that developing mouse fetuses would respond to doses of bisphenol A within the range of human exposure to this chemical through the use of polycarbonate to store food, eating canned products, and having dental sealant applied to protect teeth. Based on predictions from our *in vitro* assay, we fed pregnant mice 2 or 20 billionths of a gram of bisphenol A per gram body weight per day (2 or 20 ng/g/day) for 7 d from gestation day 11-17, prior to and during the initial period of prostate development. We observed numerous effects in male offspring, including abnormal body growth, permanent enlargement of the prostate and preputial glands, a decrease in testicular sperm production, and a decrease in seminal vesicle and epididymidal size.[80,81] In female offspring, we observed abnormal body growth and an early onset of puberty.[82] Other estrogenic effects of bisphenol A on the breast and pituitary gland have been reported recently in studies with rats.[83,84]

The Wolffian ducts and urogenital sinus express estrogen receptors during prenatal development in the mouse.[40,85] Therefore, these organs potentially can be directly affected by compounds that bind to estrogen receptors, such as bisphenol A. The decrease in the size of the epididymis and seminal vesicles suggests that bisphenol A interfered with the normal development of the Wolffian ducts as well as the testes. In contrast, bisphenol A significantly increased the size of the preputial glands and prostate relative to untreated males.

The finding that an elevation in an estrogenic chemical during fetal life decreased seminal vesicle size in adulthood is consistent with our prior findings. Specifically, male mice that developed *in utero* between two female fetuses (2F males), and were thus exposed to elevated estradiol via diffusion from the adjacent females, had smaller seminal vesicles in adulthood than their siblings who developed *in utero* between two male fetuses (2M males).[53] Subsequent studies have suggested that this effect was mediated by a permanent "imprinted" decrease in seminal vesicle 5α-reductase activity in 2F males relative to 2M males (unpublished observation). However, the larger seminal vesicles found in 2M male mice were initially thought to be due solely to the supplement in testosterone that 2M males received due to being positioned *in utero* between male fetuses. The finding that a low dose of an estrogenic chemical during fetal life can permanently decrease seminal vesicle and epididymidal size suggests that the elevated estradiol in 2F males may have contributed to the development of small seminal vesicles in these males. It has been reported that estrogen exerts an inhibitory effect on 5α-reductase activity in accessory reproductive organs.[86,87]

In contrast to findings regarding organs that differentiate from Wolffian ducts, adult 2F male mice, as well as male mice exposed experimentally as fetuses to a 50% increase in serum estradiol, exhibited enlargement of the prostate that was associated with a permanent increase in prostatic androgen receptors.[4,53] As mentioned above, the prostate develops from the urogenital sinus, while seminal vesicles develop from a different embryonic tissue, the Wolffian ducts, under different hormonal control. Taken together, these findings provide evidence that during fetal life, the specific genes influenced by estrogen are different in the Wolffian ducts and urogenital sinus. Thus, what appeared initially as contradictory findings, with some organs increasing in size and others decreasing in size associated with a small increase in serum estradiol during fetal life, now has proven to be a consistent outcome following administration of estrogenic chemicals during fetal life.

The recent discovery of two types of estrogen receptor (ER-α and ER-β), and their differential localization in prostatic epithelium and stroma has led to speculation about different biological effects.[88] This is particularly relevant when comparing effects of natural and environmental estrogens. For example, bisphenol A shows a higher binding affinity for ER-β relative to ER-α, which should result in organs, such as the prostate, which express ER-β having a greater responsiveness to bisphenol A than organs that only express ER-α.[89]

11.6   Summary

There is no information concerning whether prostate enlargement in men might be related to exposure during fetal life to estrogenic chemicals. However, there has been a doubling of the incidence of abnormal penis development in male babies over the past 20 years in the U.S., suggesting that an environmental factor is involved.[90] There is historical evidence that sperm count in men has declined by 50% over the past 50 years, while the incidence of testicular and prostate cancer has increased; there are regional differences in sperm count as well as prostate and testicular cancer rates, which suggests that environmental factors are mediating these effects.[6,91,92] Prospective studies in humans designed to examine the relationship of exposure to estrogenic chemicals during fetal life (via the mother) and health effects, such as incidence of or age of onset of prostate disease, are warranted based on findings from animal studies.

References

1. Zuckerman, S., The endocrine control of the prostate, *Proc. R. Soc. Med.*, 29, 1557, 1936.
2. Franks, L. M., Benign nodular hyperplasia of the prostate: a review, *Ann. R. Coll. Surg. Engl.*, 14, 92, 1954.
3. Sugimura, Y., Cunha, G. R., and Donjacour, A.A., Morphogenesis of ductal networks in the mouse prostate, *Biol. Reprod.*, 34, 961, 1986.
4. vom Saal, F. S., Timms, B. G., Montano, M. M., Palanza, P., Thayer, K. A., Nagel, S. C., Dhar, M. D., Ganjam, V. K., Parmigiani, S., and Welshons, W. V., Prostate enlargement in mice due to fetal exposure to low doses of estradiol or diethylstilbestrol and opposite effects at high doses, *Proc. Natl. Acad. Sci. U.S.A.*, 94, 2056, 1997.

5. vom Saal, F. S., Quadagno, D. M., Even, M. D., Keisler, L. W., Keisler, D. H., and Khan, S., Paradoxical effects of maternal stress on fetal steroid and post-natal reproductive traits in female mice from different intrauterine positions., *Biol. Reprod.*, 43, 751, 1990.

6. Hass, G. P. and Sakr, W. A., Epidemiology of prostate cancer, *CA Canc. J. Clin.*, 47, 273, 1997.

7. Burstein, S. R., The historical background of gerontology. III, The quest for rejuvenation, *Geriatrics*, 10, 536, 1955.

8. Medvei, V. C., *A History of Endocrinology*, MTP Press, Lancaster, PA, Pages, 1982.

9. Tisell, L.-E. and Salander, H., The lobes of the human prostate, *Scand. J. Urol. Nephrol.*, 9, 185, 1975.

10. McNeal, J. E., Anatomy of the prostate: An historical survey of divergent views, *The Prostrate*, 1, 3, 1980.

11. Timms, B. G., Anatomical perspectives of prostate development, in *Prostate: Basic and Clinical Aspects*, Naz, R. K., Ed., CRC Press, New York, 1997.

12. Timms, B. G., Mohs, T. J., and Didio, J. A., Ductal budding and branching patterns in the developing prostate, *J. Urol.*, 151, 1427, 1994.

13. Lowsley, O. S., The development of the human prostate gland with reference to the development of other structures at the neck of the urinary bladder, *Am. J. Anat.*, 13, 299, 1912.

14. McNeal, J. E., The prostate gland: morphology and pathobiology, *Monogr. Urol.*, 4, 1, 1983.

15. Block, E., Lew, M., and Klein, M., Studies on the inhibition of fetal androgen formation: testosterone synthesis by fetal and newborn mouse testes *in vitro*, *Endocrinology*, 88, 41, 1971.

16. Wilson, J. D., George, F. W., and Griffin, J. E., The hormonal control of sexual development, *Science*, 211, 1278, 1981.

17. vom Saal, F., Sexual differentiation in litter bearing mammals: influence of sex of adjacent fetuses *in utero*, *J. Anim. Sci.*, 67, 1824, 1989.

18. Allan, F. D., *Essentials of Human Embryology*, Oxford University Press, New York, 1960.

19. vom Saal, F. S., Montano, M. M., and Wang, H. S., Sexual differentiation in mammals, *Chemically-Induced Alterations in Sexual and Functional Development: The Wildlife/Human Connection*, Colborn, T. and Clement, C., Eds., Princeton Scientific Publishing, Princeton, NJ, 1992, 17.

20. Bardin, C. W. and Catterall, J. F., Testosterone: a major determinant of extragenital sexual dimorphism, *Science*, 211, 1285, 1981.

21. Shannon, J. M. and Cunha, G. R., Autoradiographic localization of androgen binding in the developing mouse prostate, *Prostate*, 4, 367, 1983.

22. Takeda, H., Lasnitzki, I., and Mizuno, T., Analysis of prostatic bud induction by brief androgen treatment in the fetal rat urogenital sinus, *J. Endocrinol.*, 110, 467, 1986.

23. Takeda, H., Nakamoto, T., Kokontis, J., Chodak, G., and Chang, C., Autoregulation of androgen receptor expression in rodent prostate: immunohistochemical and *in situ* hybridization analysis, *Biochem. Biophys. Res. Commun.*, 177, 488, 1991.

24. McNeal, J., Pathology of benign prostatic hyperplasia. Insight into etiology, *Urol. Clin. N. Am.*, 17, 477, 1990.

25. Tenniswood, M., Role of epithelial-stroma interactions in the control of gene expression in the prostate: an hypothesis., *Prostate*, 9, 375, 1986.

26. Cunha, G. R., Donjacour, A., Cooke, P., Mee, S., Bigsby, R., Higgins, S., and Sugimura, Y., The endocrinology and developmental biology of the prostate, *Endocr. Rev.,* 8, 338, 1987.

27. Aumüller, G., Morphologic and regulatory aspects of prostatic function, *Anat. Embryol.,* 179, 519, 1989.

28. Shapiro, E., Embryological development of the prostate, *Urol. Clin. N. Am.,* 17, 487, 1990.

29. Timms, B. G., Lee, C. W., Aumuller, G., and Seitz, J., Instructive induction of prostate growth and differentiation by a defined urogenital sinus mesenchyme, *Microsc. Res Technol.,* 30, 319, 1995.

30. Pang, S., Chow, P., and Wong, T., The role of the seminal vesicles, coagulating glands and prostate on the fertility and fecundity of mice, *J. Reprod. Fertil.,* 56, 129, 1979.

31. Sugimura, Y., Cunha, G. R., Donjacour, A. A., Bigsby, R. M., and Brody, J. R., Whole-mount autoradiography study of DNA synthetic activity during post-natal development and androgen-induced regeneration in the mouse prostate, *Biol. Reprod.,* 34, 985, 1986.

32. Sugimura, Y., Cunha, G. R., and Donjacour, A. A., Morphological and histolog-ical study of castration-induced degeneration and androgen-induced regener-ation in the mouse prostate, *Biol. Reprod.,* 34, 973, 1986.

33. Hall, B. K., Ed, *Homology: The Hierarchical Basis of Comparative Biology,* Academic Press, New York, 1994.

34. Gilbert, S. E. A., Resynthesizing evolutionary and developmental biology, *Develop. Biol.,* 173, 357, 1996.

35. Price, D., Comparative aspects of development and structure in the prostate, *Natl. Canc. Inst. Monogr.,* 12, 1, 1963.

36. McNeal, J. E., The anatomic heterogeneity of the prostate, in *Models of Prostate Cancer,* Coffey, D., Merchant, D., and Murphy, G., Eds., Liss, New York, 1980, 149.

37. Hiraoka, Y. and Akimoto, M., Anatomy of the prostate from fetus to adult — origin of benign prostatic hyperplasia, *Urol. Res.,* 177, 1987.

38. Mawhinney, M. and Neubauer, B., Actions of estrogen in the male, *Invest. Urol.,* 16, 409, 1979.

39. Jung-Testas, I., Groyer, M.-T., Bruner-Lorand, J., Hechter, O., Baulieu, E. E., and Robel, P., Androgen and estrogen receptors in rat ventral prostate epithelium and stroma, *Endocrinology,* 109, 1287, 1981.

40. Cooke, P. S., Young, P., Hess, R. A., and Cunha, G. R., Estrogen receptor ex-pression in developing epididymis, efferent ductules, and other male repro-ductive organs, *Endocrinology,* 128, 2874, 1992.

41. DeKlerk, D. P., Coffey, D. S., Ewing, L. L., McDermott, I. R., Reiner, W. G., Robinson, C. H., Scott, W. W., Standberg, J. D., Talalay, P., Walsh, P. C., Wheaton, L. G., and Zirkin, B. R., Comparison of spontaneous and experimentally in-duced canine prostatic hyperplasia, *J. Clin. Invest.,* 64, 842, 1979.

42. Noble, R. L., Prostate carcinoma of the Nb rat in relation to hormones, 23, 113, 1982.

43. Leav, I., Ho, S.-M., Ofner, P., Merk, F. B., Kwan, P. W. L., and Damassa, D., Biochemical alterations in sex hormone-induced hyperplasia and dysplasia of the dorsolateral prostates of Noble rats, 80, 1045, 1988.

44. Leav, I., Merk, F. B., Kwan, P. W. L., and Ho, S.-M., Androgen-supported estrogen enhancement of epithelial proliferation in the prostate of intact Noble rats, *The Prostrate,* 15, 23, 1989.

45. Ofner, P., Bosland, M., and Vena, R. L., Differential effects of diethystilbestrol and estradiol-17β in combination with testosterone on rat prostate lobes, *Toxicol. Appl. Pharmacol.*, 112, 300, 1992.
46. Ho, S.-M., Yu, M., Leav, I., and Viccione, T., The conjoint actions of androgens and estrogens in the induction of proliferative lesions in the rat prostate, in *Hormonal Carcinogenesis*, Li, J. J., Li, S. A., and Nandi, S., Eds., Springer-Verlag, New York, 1992.
47. McNeal, J. E. and Bostwich, D. G., Intraductal dysplasia: a premalignant lesion of the prostate, 17, 64, 1986.
48. McLachlan, J., Newbold, R., and Bullock, B., Reproductive tract lesions in male mice exposed prenatally to diethylstilbestrol, *Science*, 190, 991, 1975.
49. vom Saal, F. S. and Bronson, F. H., Sexual characteristics of adult female mice are correlated with their blood testosterone levels during prenatal development, *Science*, 208, 597, 1980.
50. vom Saal, F. S., Grant, W., McMullen, C., and Laves, K., High fetal estrogen concentrations: correlation with increased adult sexual activity and decreased aggression in male mice, *Science*, 220, 1306, 1983.
51. Even, M. D., Dhar, M., and vom Saal, F. S., Transport of steroids between fetuses via amniotic fluid mediates the intrauterine position phenomenon in rats, *J. Reprod. Fertil.*, 96, 709, 1992.
52. vom Saal, F. S., Grant, W., McMullen, C., and Laves, K., High fetal estrogen concentrations: correlation with increased adult sexual activity and decreased aggression in male mice, *Science*, 220, 1306, 1983.
53. Nonneman, D., Ganjam, V., Welshons, W., and vom Saal, F., Intrauterine position effects on steroid metabolism and steroid receptors of reproductive organs in male mice., *Biol. Reprod.*, 47, 723, 1992.
54. Trachtenberg, J., Hicks, L. L., and Walsh, P. C., Androgen- and estrogen-receptor content in spontaneous and experimentally induced canine prostatic hyperplasia, *J. Clin. Invest.*, 65, 1051, 1980.
55. Roselli, C. E. and Fasasi, T. A., Estradiol increases the duration of nuclear receptor occupation in the preoptic area of the male rat treated with testosterone, *J. Steroid Biochem. Mol. Biol.*, 42, 161, 1992.
56. Challis, J. R. G. and Lye, S. J., Parturition, in *Physiology of Reproduction*, Knobil, E., Neill, J., and Pfaff, D., Eds., Raven Press, New York, 1994, 985.
57. Clark, J. H. and Mani, S. K., Actions of ovarian steroid hormones, in *Physiology of Reproduction*, Knobil, E., Neill, J., and Pfaff, D., Eds., Raven Press, New York, 1994, 1011.
58. Driscoll, S. and Taylor, S., Effects of prenatal maternal estrogen on the male urogenital system, *Obstet. Gynecol.*, 56, 537, 1980.
59. Blacklock, N. J., The development and morphology of the prostate, *The Endocrinology of Prostate Tumours*, Ghanadian, R, Eds., MTP Press, Lancaster, England, 1983, 1.
60. Kincl, F., Pi, A., and Lasso, L., Effects of estradiol benzoate treatment in the newborn male rat, *Endocrinology*, 72, 966, 1963.
61. Arai, Y., Nature of metaplasia in rat coagulating glands induced by neonatal treatment with estrogen, *Endocrinology*, 86, 918, 1970.
62. Rajfer, J. and Coffey, D. S., Sex steroid imprinting of the immature prostate, *Invest. Urol.*, 16, 186, 1978.
63. Rajfer, J. and Coffey, D., Effects of neonatal steroids on male sex tissues, *Invest. Urol.*, 17, 3, 1979.

64. Vannier, B. and Raynaud, J. P., Long-term effects of prenatal oestrogen treatment on genital morphology and reproductive function in the rat, *J. Reprod. Fertil.*, 59, 43, 1980.

65. Lung, B. and Cunha, G. R., Development of seminal vesicles and coagulating glands in neonatal mice. I. The morphogenetic effects of various hormonal conditions, *Anat. Rec.*, 199, 73, 1981.

66. Prins, G. S., Neonatal estrogen exposure induces lobe-specific alterations in adult rat prostate androgen receptor expression, *Endocrinology*, 130, 2401, 1992.

67. Prins, G. S., Woodham, C., Lepinske, M., and Birch, L., Effects of neonatal estrogen exposure on prostatic secretory genes and their correlation with androgen receptor expression in the separate prostate lobes of the adult rat, *Endocrinology*, 132, 2387, 1993.

68. Santti, R., Newbold, R. R., Makela, S., Pylkkanen, L., and McLachlan, J. A., Developmental estrogenization and prostatic neoplasia, *Prostate*, 24, 67, 1994.

69. Newbold, R., Cellular and molecular effects of developmental exposure to diethylstilbestrol: implications for other environmental estrogens, *Environ. Health Perspect.*, 103, 83, 1995.

70. Baranao, J., Chemes, H., Tesone, M., Chauzzi, V., Scacchi, P., Calvo, J., Faugon, M., Moguilevsky, J., Charreau, E., and Calandra, R., Effects of androgen treatment of the neonate on rat testis and sex accessory organs, *Biol. Reprod.*, 25, 851, 1981.

71. Arai, Y., Chen, C.-Y., and Nishizuka, Y., Cancer development in male reproductive tract in rats given diethylstilbestrol at neonatal age, *Jpn. J. Canc. Res.*, 69, 861, 1978.

72. Martikainen, P., Makela, S., Santti, R., Harkonen, P., and Souminen, J., Interaction of male and female sex hormones in cultured rat prostate, *Prostate*, 11, 291, 1987.

73. Herbst, A. L. and Bern, H. A., Ed., *Developmental Effects of Diethylstilbestrol (DES) in Pregnancy*, Thieme-Stratton, New York, 1981.

74. Bern, H., Diethylstilbestrol (DES) syndrome: present status of animal and human studies, *Hormonal Carcinogenesis*, Li, J., Li, S. A., and Nandi, S., Eds., Springer-Verlag, New York, 1992, 1.

75. Bern, H. A., The fragile fetus, *Chemically-Induced Alterations in Sexual and Functional Development: The Wildlife/Human Connection*, Colborn, T. and Clement, C., Eds., Princeton Scientific Publishing, Princeton, NJ, 1992, 9.

76. Greco, T. L., Duello, T. M., and Gorski, J., Estrogen receptors, estradiol, and diethylstilbestrol in early development: the mouse as a model for the study of estrogen receptors and estrogen sensitivity in embryonic development of male and female reproductive tracts, *Endocr. Rev.*, 14, 59, 1993.

77. Mittendorf, R., Teratogen update: carcinogenesis and teratogenesis associated with exposure to diethylstilbestrol (DES) *in utero*, *Teratology*, 51, 435, 1995.

78. Colborn, T., vom Saal, F. S., and Soto, A. M., Developmental effects of endocrine disrupting chemicals in wildlife and humans, *Environ. Health Perspect.*, 101, 378, 1993.

79. Kavlock, R. J., Daston, G. P., DeRosa, C., Fenner-Crisp, P., Gray, L. E., Kaattari, S., Lucier, G., Luster, M., Mac, M. J., Maczka, C., Miller, R., Moore, J., Rolland, R., Scott, G., Sheehan, D.M., Sinks, T., and Tilson, H. A., Research needs for the risk assessment of health and environmental effects of endocrine disruptors: A report of the US EPA sponsored workshop, *Environ. Health Perspect. Suppl.*, 104, 715, 1996.

80. Nagel, S. C., vom Saal, F. S., Thayer, K. A., Dhar, M. G., Boechler, M., and Welshons, W. V., Relative binding affinity-serum modified access (RBA-SMA) assay predicts the relative *in vivo* bioactivity of the xenoestrogens bisphenol A and octylphenol, *Environ. Health Perspect.*, 105, 70, 1997.

81. vom Saal, F. S., Cooke, P. S., Palanza, P., Thayer, K. A., Nagel, S., Parmigiani, S., and Welshons, W. V., A physiologically based approach to the study of bisphenol A and other estrogenic chemicals on the size of reproductive organs, daily sperm production, and behavior, *Toxicol. Ind. Health*, 14, 239, 1997.

82. Howdeshell, K. L., vom Saal, F. S., Thayer, K. A., Benson, S., Baerwald, C., and Welshons, W., Prenatal exposure to an environmentally relevant dose of bisphenol A accelerates puberty in female mice, Program of the Estrogens in the Environment IV, Bethesda, MD, 1997.

83. Colerangle, J. B. and Roy, D., Profound effects of the weak environmental estrogen-like chemical bisphenol A on the growth of the mammary gland of noble rats, *J. Steroid Biochem. Molec. Biol.*, 60, 153, 1997.

84. Steinmetz, R., Brown, N. G., Allen, D. L., Bigsby, R. M., and Ben-Jonathan, N., The environmental estrogen bisphenol A stimulates prolactin release *in vitro* and *in vivo*, 138, 1780, 1997.

85. Stumpf, W. E., Narbaitz, R., and Sar, M., Estrogen receptors in the fetal mouse, *J. Steroid Biochem.*, 12, 55, 1980.

86. Djoesland, O., Androgen metabolism by rat epididymis: effects of castration and antiandrogens, *Steroids*, 27, 47, 1976.

87. Tindall, V. J., French, F. S., and Nayfeh, S. N., Estradiol-17B inhibition of androgen uptake and binding in epididymis of adult male rats *in vivo*: a comparison with cyproterone acetate, *Steroids*, 37, 257, 1981.

88. Kuiper, G. G. J. M., Enmark, E., Pelto-Huikko, M., Nilsson, S., and Gustafsson, J.-A., Cloning of a novel estrogen receptor expressed in rat prostate and ovary, *Proc. Natl. Acad. Sci. U.S.A.*, 93, 5925, 1996.

89. Kuiper, G. G. J. M., Carlsson, B., Grandien, K., Enmark, E., Häggblad, J., Nilsson, S., and Gustafsson, J.-A., Comparison of the ligand binding specificity and transcript tissue distribution of estrogen receptors alpha and beta, *Endocrinology*, 138, 863, 1997.

90. Paulozzi, L. J., Erickson, J. D., and Jackson, R. J., Hypospadias trends in two US surveillance systems, *Pediatrics*, 100, 831, 1997.

91. Carlsen, E., Giwereman, A., Keding, N., and Skakkebaek, N., Declining semen quality and increasing incidence of testicular cancer: is there a common cause? *Environ. Health Perspect.*, 103 (Suppl 7), 137, 1995.

92. Swan, S. H., Elkin, E. P., and Fenster, L., Have sperm densities declined? A reanalysis of global trend data, *Environ. Health Perspect.*, 105, 1228, 1997.

12

Metal Ions and Prostate Cancer

Shuk-Mei Ho

CONTENTS

12.1 Abstract

Metal ions are significant contaminants of the environment. Yet, their impacts
on normal and malignant prostatic functions are poorly understood. Studies
implicating metal ions as environmental risk factors for the prostate are
limited and have been focused mainly in the area of prostate cancer. Information on heavy-metal-ion influences on the other two prostatic diseases,
benign prostatic hyperplasia and prostatitis, is virtually nonexistent. Data
from a relatively limited number of studies have identified zinc as a crucial
intracellular trace element of the prostate. Zinc ion is present in high concentrations in normal and benign hyperplastic prostates and may play a role
in regulating androgenic action and intermediate metabolism. Prostatic
secretion of the metal ion into seminal plasma may affect sperm viability.
Marked reduction in tissue zinc content is noted during aging and neoplastic
transformation of the gland. In parallel, serum and urinary zinc concentrations in prostate cancer patients are consistently reduced when compared to
those found in healthy controls. Epidemiological studies, which have aimed
at establishing a correlation between dietary intake of zinc and prostate
cancer risk, have yielded inconclusive data. Human exposure to cadmium

is normally via food, air and water contamination. However, occupational exposure and cigarette smoking may contribute significantly to the overall bodily burden. In animal and cell culture studies, cadmium is a proven carcinogen of the prostate, although its mechanism of action is entirely unclear. In human studies, only weak association has been found to exist between cadmium exposure and prostate cancer risk. One study has, however, indicated a stronger correlation between cadmium exposure and evolution of an aggressive form of prostatic adenocarcinomas. Finally, results from a handful of investigations suggest that both copper and arsenic may have potential carcinogenic action in the prostate.

12.2 Introduction

The prostate is perhaps the most disease-prone organ of the aging human male. Prostatic adenocarcinoma, benign prostatic hyperplasia (BPH), and prostatitis are common disorders found in the aged human gland.[1-3] Additionally, adenosis or atypical adenomatous hyperplasia (AAH) and prostatic intraepithelial neoplasia (PIN) are often identified incidentally in autopsy, biopsy, and transurethral resection samples of the prostate.[4,5] The etiologies of these prostatic diseases or pathological conditions are poorly understood. Aging appears to be the single common determinant for these diseases/pathologies. Epidemiologic and basic research studies have, however, identified separate endogenous and exogenous risk factors for each of these conditions.[1-5] Studies implicating environmental pollutants as causative factors of prostatic diseases are scarce, and they are limited almost exclusively to prostate cancer. Among environmental factors, metal ions and environmental estrogens are likely of importance.[1] The impacts of environmental estrogens on prostatic development and functions have been reviewed in this volume by Dr. Frederick vom Saal in Chapter 11. Hence, discussions in this chapter will focus only on heavy metal ions as disruptors and disease-causing agents of the prostate.

12.3 Zinc

It has long been known that the prostate has the highest concentration of zinc.[6,7] The zinc content is high in the epithelial cells and low in the stromal components.[8,9] Subcellular distribution favors the nuclear fraction, but substantial levels are also found in the cytosol[10] and mitochondria.[11] In the rat prostate, the lateral lobe contains several-fold higher zinc contents than the dorsal and ventral lobes.[11] Both testosterone and prolactin have been shown to increase zinc contents in the lateral lobe of the rat prostate gland. The precise physiological roles of zinc in the gland are unknown. *In vitro* studies have demonstrated that zinc enhances binding of androgen-androgen receptor complexes to cell nuclei[12] and increases total androgen uptake by prostatic tissues.[10] It has also been suggested that zinc inhibits mitochondrial m-aconitase activity and citrate oxidation.[11] Neutralized zinc, injected directly into the rat prostate, reduces prostatic weight and 5α-reductase activity.[13] Large quantity of zinc is apparently secreted into prostatic fluid and reaches the seminal plasma, where it plays a role in extending the functional life span of the ejaculated sperm.[7]

The American diet is often deficient in zinc,[6] hence a question arises as to whether dietary intake of zinc influences disease development in the prostate. Epidemiological data revealed conflicting data. In a Utah study, in which 358 cases were compared to 679 controls, weekly intake of zinc was found to have little association with prostate cancer.[14] In contrast, when a Hawaii population with 452 cases of prostate cancer and 899 age-matched controls was studied, weekly zinc intake, adjusted for age and ethnicity, was found to be greater for prostate cancer cases than for healthy controls.[15] The latter study thus implicates dietary zinc as a risk factor for prostate cancer.

When zinc contents in expressed prostatic fluids from healthy men and patients suffering from chronic prostatitis, adenoma, or adenocarcinoma were analyzed, a marked reduction (>90%) in zinc level was observed only in fluid samples from cancer patients.[16] These findings were in accord with those reported in an earlier study on zinc contents in post-prostatic-massage urine[17] and in serum samples. Marked reductions in plasma zinc levels were noted in patients with prostate cancer when compared to healthy subjects or BPH patients.[18-23] Further declines in serum zinc levels were observed after cancer patients had undergone androgen ablation therapies.[20,23] In one study,[22] aging was shown to associate with significant declines in tissue zinc contents. Collectively, these data clearly indicate that zinc is present in high concentrations in normal and hyperplastic human prostates, but its levels are considerably reduced with advancement of age or neoplastic transformation. Future mechanistic investigations are needed, however, to discern (1) whether the carcinogenic process, per se, perturbs zinc metabolism/homeostasis in the prostate, and (2) whether a reduction in zinc content, either in circulating or at the tissue level, predisposes the gland to neoplastic transformation. Importantly, environmental influences, such as dietary habits or cadmium exposure (see next section), that affect prostatic zinc content, may have major consequences in disease development of the gland.

12.4 Cadmium

Cadmium (Cd) is a significant environmental contaminant as a result of zinc mining and smelting, sewage-sludge disposal, various industrial uses, such as making tires and batteries, and combustion of municipal waste and fossil fuels.[24,25] Worldwide production is over 18,000 tons/year[26] leading to contamination of the air. About 4,000 tons of cadmium are used yearly in the U.S., roughly 50% for the plating of metals and another 50% for pigments, batteries, stabilizers in plastics, metallurgy, nuclear reactor rods, the semiconductor industry, and as catalysts.[27] Accordingly, Cd contamination in food, soil, air, and water can be high in certain industrial and cosmopolitan areas.[28-30] Apart from occupational exposure, the general population is probably exposed to low doses of Cd through dietary consumption of contaminated fish, drinking water, inhaling polluted air, and cigarette smoking.[29-31] This metal ion is frequently found in the National Priorities List sites and The National Toxicology Program (NTP) has classified it as a potential human carcinogen.[30] In its inhaled forms, Cd induces lung cancer in human and rodents, and systemic exposure to this metal ion leads to tumor development in rodent prostate, testis, and site of administration.[30-32]

Cd exposure has been linked to human prostatic cancer in some but not all epidemiological studies.[31,32] Among 522 Swedish workers exposed to cadmium for at least 1 year in a nickel-cadmium battery plant, the mortality rate for prostate cancer was increased in a dose- and latency-dependent manner.[33] Similarly, in a Utah population-based case-control study, occupational exposures to Cd were found to result in a small increase in prostate cancer risk.[34] A high incidence of the cancer was observed in certain areas of Spain, where Cd was naturally found in abnormally high concentrations in the stream sediments.[35] In a case-referent study of 345 prostate cancer cases, a significantly higher risk was found in cases who had the most frequent occupational exposure to Cd.[36] Contrary to the aforementioned studies, other reports unveiled no association between Cd exposure and the disease. In a population-based case-control study in Utah, in which 358 cases of prostate cancer were compared with 679 controls, no association was found between prostate cancer and dietary intake of cadmium.[14] In a cohort mortality study of Cd-exposed workers, no increased risk form prostate cancer was noted in a 5-year follow-up study.[37] Using the method of regression models in life tables to compare the estimated Cd exposures of those dying from prostate cancer with those of matching survivors, a study on a cohort of 3,025 nickel-cadmium battery workers revealed no evidence of association between occupational Cd exposure and prostate cancer.[38] In general studies that revealed a positive correlation between Cd exposure and prostate cancer, only weak associations have been found.[34-37] A stonger association was, however, noted for the more aggressive cancers of the prostates (OR = 1.7).[34] Overall, analyses of tissue Cd contents revealed higher Cd contents in prostate cancer specimens when compared to those present in normal or BPH tissues.[21,39,40] Interestingly, the highest concentrations of the metal ion were found in poorly differentiated carcinomas,[39] hence perhaps suggesting that a dose-response relationship exists between Cd and prostate cancer progression.

In laboratory rats, injection of low doses of Cd (0.03 mmol/kg b.w.) induced apoptosis in the prostate within 48-h post-treatment.[41] Over a longer time frame, single exposure to a low dose of Cd induced atypical hyperplasia, dysplasia, adenomas, and adenocarcinomas in the ventral prostate (VP, 34% incidence), but not for the other lobes of the rat gland.[42] Exposure of rats to higher Cd doses caused testicular regression, which in turn led to atrophy of the prostate.[42,43] When Cd was injected directly into the VPs of rats, high incidence of severe dysplasia and invasive carcinomas occurred within a relatively short period of time (270 d).[44] Cd also enhanced the potency of other chemical carcinogens, such as that of DMBA in carcinoma induction in the VP.[45] *In vitro*, Cd causes malignant transformation of rat VP epithelial cells.[46] The unique susceptibility of the VP to Cd-induced carcinogeneity may be due to the lack of substantial expression of metallothionein (MT), a Cd-Cu-Zn-binding protein, with putative antioxidant activity, in the rat VP.[47,48]

Cd seems to affect a multitude of cellular functions,[49] yet no single mechanism has been identified as the principal cause of Cd carcinogeneity in the prostate.[50] Cd tends to distribute rather evenly between the epithelial and stromal components.[8,39] Its contents have been shown to inversely associated with testosterone levels in epithelial preparations from BPH specimens, and hence may indirectly influence prostatic functions through modulation of androgenic action.[8] Exposure of cultured human prostatic epithelium to the metal ion induces cell proliferation.[51] Interestingly, the growth stimulatory action of Cd on human epithelial cells could be blocked by the antioxidant trace element, selenium, thus suggesting that the mitogenic action of the metal ion may be mediated via induction of a pro-oxidation state in the cells.[51] In many nonprostatic tissues, Cd is known to induce oxidative stress.[52] Increased intracellular oxidant burden is well recognized as a condition for DNA damage and tumor initiation. If a similar cellular phenomenon occurs in prostate cells, it would explain why the metal ion is carcinogenic to the prostate.

Interestingly, in animal studies, zinc has the ability to modify the carcinogenic potential of cadmium.[53] Administration of of zinc apparently potentiated or inhibited, dependent on dose and route of administration, the carcinogenic effects of cadmium in the rat ventral prostate. In the human prostate, there seems to have a distinct antagonistic effect between Zn and Cd.[21,39,40,54] Marked reduction in tissue zinc contents and elevation in Cd contents were consistently observed in prostatic cancer specimens. These findings suggested that a high zinc content may confer protection against Cd-carcinogeneity/toxicity to prostatic cells. Conversely, zinc deficiency, at bodily or cellular level, may exacerbate the cytotoxic effects of Cd in the prostate.

12.5 Copper, Nickel, and Arsenic

Copper and nickel are commonly found to coexist with Cd as environmental pollutants.[30] It is therefore conceivable that the reported effects of Cd on the prostate may, in part, be due to the adverse action of copper or nickel contaminants. However, epidemiological data in support of this hypothesis are nonexistent, and not a single study has focused on the toxicity/carcinogeneity of these two compounds in the human prostate. In an animal study, nickle chloride added to the drinking water in 5 and 50 ppm were shown to have no effects on the morphology and ultrastructure of the rat prostate.[49] Among all the other metal ions, only arsenic has been found to associate with prostate cancer in one epidemiological study.[55]

12.6 Summary

From this literature review it has become apparent that information on the effects of metal ions on prostatic functions is sketchy. Although Cd has been identified as a potential environmental carcinogen for the human prostate, its mode of action remains largely unknown. Zinc ion, on the other hand, appears to be needed to maintain normal prostatic functions. Since metal ions bind to common cellular proteins, it is conceivable that zinc homeostasis may influence accumulation rates of various metal ions in the prostate. Future studies that focus on synergism/antagonism of zinc and other metal ions will help unveil the true significance of environmental metal ions in prostatic disease development.

Acknowledgment

This work was supported in part by the NIH Grant CA-62269.

References

1. Ho, S.-M., Lee, K.-F., and Lane, K., Neoplastic transformation of the prostate, in *Prostate Basic and Clinical Aspects*, Naz R. K., Ed., CRC Press, Boca Raton, FL, 1997, 73.
2. Petrovich, Z., Ameye, F., Baert, L., Bichler, K. H., Boyd, S. D., Brady, L. W., Bruskewitz, R. C., Dixon, C., Perrin, P., and Watxon, G. M., New trends in the treatment of benign prostatic hyperplasia and carcinoma of the prostate, *Am. J. Clin. Oncol.*, 16, 187, 1993.
3. Blumenfeld, W., Tucci, S., and Narayan, P., Incidental lymphocytic prostatitis. Selective involvement with nonmalignant glands, *Am. J. Surg. Pathol.*, 16, 975, 1992.

4. Epstein, J. I., Adenosis (atypical adenomatous hyperplaia): histopathology and relationship to carcinoma, *Pathol. Res. Pract.*, 191, 888, 1995.

5. Bostwick, D. G., Oian, J., and Frankel, K., The incidence of high grade prostatic intraepithelial neoplasia in needle biopsis, *J. Urol.*, 154, 1791, 1995.

6. Vallee, B. L., Biochemistry, physiology and pathology of zinc, *Physiol. Rev.*, 39, 443, 1992.

7. Bedwal, R. S. and Bahuguna, A., Zinc, copper and selenium in reproduction, *Experientia*, 50, 626, 1994.

8. Lahtonen, R., Zinc and cadmium concentrations in whole tissue and in separated epithelium and stroma from human benign prostatic hypertropic glands, *Prostate*, 6, 177, 1985.

9. Feustel, A., Wennrich, R., and Dittrich, H., Zinc, cadmium and selenium concentrations in separated epithelium and stroma from prostatic tissues of different histology, *Urol. Res.*, 15, 161,1987.

10. Leake, A., Chrisholm, G. D., Busuttil, A., and Habib, F. K., Subcellular distribution of zinc in the benign and malignant human prostate: evidence for a direct zinc androgen interaction, *Acta Endocrinol.*, 105, 281, 1984.

11. Liu, Y., Franklin, R. B., and Costello, L. C., Prolactin and testosterone regulation of mitochondrial zinc in prostate epithelial cells, *Prostate*, 30, 26, 1997.

12. Colvard, D. S. and Wilson, E. M., Zinc potentiation of androgen receptor binding to nuclei *in vitro*, *Biochemistry*, 23, 3471, 1984.

13. Fahim, M. S., Wang, M., Sutcu, M. F., and Fahim, Z., Zinc arginine, a 5 alpha-reductase inhibitor, reduces rat ventral prostate weight and DNA without affecting testicular function, *Andrologia*, 25, 367, 1993.

14. West, D. W., Slattery, M. L., Robison, L. M., French, T. K., and Mahoney, A. W., Adult dietary intake and prostate cancer risk in Utah: a case-control study with special emphasis on aggressive tumors, *Canc. Causes Control*, 2, 85, 1991.

15. Kolonel, L. N., Yoshizawa, C. N., and Hankin, J. H., Diet and prostatic cancer: a case-control study in Hawaii, *Am. J. Epidemiol.*, 127, 999, 1988.

16. Zaichick, V. Y., Sviridova, T. V., and Zaichick, S. V., Zinc concentration in human prostatic fluid: normal, chronic prostatitis, adenoma and cancer, *Int. Urol. Nephrol.*, 28, 687, 1996.

17. McCallum, K. A., Kavanagh, J. P., Farragher, E. B., and Blacklock, N. J., Ratio of post-prostatic massage urinary zinc concentration to initial urinary zinc concentration. An improved method of assessing prostatic function, *Br. J. Urol.*, 62, 565, 1988.

18. Whelan, P., Walker, B. E., Kelleher, J., 1983 Zinc, vitamin A and prostatic cancer, *Br. J .Urol.*, 55, 525, 1983.

19. Chirulescu, Z., Chiriloiu, C., Suciu, A., and Pirvulescu, R., Variations of zinc, calcium and magnesium in normal subjects and in patients with neoplasias, *Med. Int..*, 25, 257, 1987.

20. Feustel, A., Wennrich, R., and Schmidt, B., Serum-Zn-levels in prostatic cancer, *Urol. Res.*, 17, 41, 1989.

21. Ogunlewe, J. O. and Osegbe, D. N., Zinc and cadmium concentrations in indigenous blacks with normal, hypertrophic, and malignant prostate, *Cancer*, 63, 1388, 1989.

22. Tvedt, K. E., Halgunset, J., Kopstad, G., and Haugen, O. A., Intracellular distribution of calcium and zinc in normal, hyperplastic, and neoplastic human prostate: X-ray microanalysis of freeze-dried cryosections, *Prostate*,15, 41, 1989.

23. Lekili, M., Ergen, A., and Celebi, I., Zinc plasma levels in prostatic carcinoma and BPH, *Int. Urol. Nephrol.*, 23, 151, 1991.

24. Hoover, R., Epidemiology — tobacco and geographic pathology, in *Lung Biology in Health and Disease, Pathogenesis and Therapy of Lung Cancer*, Harris, C. C., Ed., Marcel-Dekker, New York, 1978, 3.

25. Lloyd, O. L, Respiratory-cancer clustering associated with localized industrial air pollution, *Lancet*, 1, 318, 1978.

26. Commission of the European Communities, *CEC Criteria (Dose/Effect Relationships) for Cadmium*, Pergamon Press, Oxford, 1978.

27. National Institute of Occupational Safety and Health, Current Intelligence Bulletin 42: Cadmium, (DHHS (NIOSH) publication no 84-116), Cincinnati, OH, 1984.

28. Friberg, L., Piscator, M., Nordberg, G. F., and Kjellstrom, T., *Cadmium in the Environment*, 2nd ed., CRC Press, Cleveland, 1974.

29. Waalkes, M. P., Coogan, T. P., and Barter R. A. Toxicological principles of metal carcinogenesis with special emphasis on cadmium, *Crit. Rev. Toxicol.*, 22, 175, 1992.

30. Faroon, O. M., Williams, M., and O'Connor, R., A review of the carcinogenicity of chemicals most frequently found at National Priorities List sites, *Toxicol. Ind. Health*, 10, 203, 1994.

31. Piscator, M., Role of cadmium in carcinogenesis with special reference to cancer of the prostate, *Environ. Health Perspect.*, 40, 107, 1981.

32. Saldivar, L., Luna, M., Reyes, E., Soto, R., and Fortoul, T. I., Cadmium determination in Mexican-produced tobacco, *Environ. Res.*, 55, 91, 1991.

33. Elinder, C. G., Kjellstrom, T., Hogstedt, C., Andersson, K., and Spang, G., Cancer mortality of cadmium workers, *Br. J. Ind. Med.*, 42, 651, 1985.

34. Elghany, N. A., Schumacher, M. C., Slattery, M. L., West, D. W., and Lee, J. S., Occupation, cadmium exposure, and prostate cancer, *Epidemiology*, 1, 107, 1990.

35. Garcia Sanchez, A., Antona, J. F., and Urrutia, M., Geochemical prospection of cadmium in a high incidence area of prostate cancer, Sierra de Gata, Salamanca, Spain, *Sci. Total Environ.*, 116, 243, 1992.

36. van der Gulden, J. W., Kolk, J. J., and Verbeek, A. L., Work environment and prostate cancer risk, *Prostate*, 27, 250, 1995.

37. Kazantzis, G., Lam, T. H., and Sullivan, K. R., Mortality of cadmium-exposed workers. A five-year update, *Scand. J. Work Environ. Health*, 14, 220, 1988.

38. Sorahan, T. and Waterhouse, J. A., Mortality study of nickel-cadmium battery workers by the method of regression models in life tables, *Br. J. Ind. Med.*, 40, 293, 1983.

39. Feustel, A. and Wennrich, R., Determination of the distribution of zinc and cadmium in cellular fractions of BPH, normal prostate and prostatic cancers of different histologies by atomic and laser absorption spectrometry in tissue slices, *Urol. Res.*, 12, 253, 1984.

40. Habib, F. K., Hammond, G. L., Lee, I .R., Dawson, J. B., Mason, M. K., Smith, P. H., and Stitch, S. R., Metal-androgen interrelationships in carcinoma and hyperplasia of the human prostate, *J. Endocrinol.*, 71, 133, 1976.

41. Yan, H., Carter, C. E., Xu, C., Singh, P. K, Jones, M. M., Johnson, J. E., and Dietrich, M. S., Cadmium-induced apoptosis in the urogenital organs of the male rat and its suppresion by chelation, *J. Toxicol. Environ. Health*, 52, 149, 1997.

42. Waalkes, M. P., Rehm, S., Riggs, C. W., Bare, R. M., Devor, D. E, Poirier, L. A., Wenk, M. L., Henneman, J. R., and Balaschak, M. S., Cadmium carcinogenesis in male Wistar [Crl: (WI)BR] rats: dose response analysis on tumor induction in the prostate and testes and at the injection site, *Canc. Res.*, 48, 4656, 1988.

43. Waalkes, M. P., Rehm, S., and Devor, D. E., The effects of continuous testosterone exposure on spontaneous and cadmium-induced tumors in the male Fischer (F344/NCr) rat: loss of testicular response, *Toxicol.Appl. Pharmacol.*, 142, 40, 1997.

44. Hoffmann, L., Putzke, H. P., Kampehl, H. J., Russbult, R., Gase, P., Simonn, C., Erdmann, T., and Huckstorf, C., Carcinogenic effects of cadmium on the prostate of the rat, *J. Canc. Res. Clin. Oncol.*, 109, 193, 1985.

45. Shira, T., Iwasaki, S., Masui, T., Mori, T., Kato, T., and Ito, N., Enhancing effect of cadmium on rat ventral prostate carcinogenesis induced by 3,2'-dimethyl-4-aminobiphenyl, *Jpn. J. Canc. Res.*, 84, 1023, 1993.

46. Terracio, L. and Nachtigal, N., Oncogenicity of rat prostate cells transformed *in vitro* with cadmium chloride, *Arch. Toxicol.*, 6, 450, 1988.

47. Coogan, T. P., Shiraishi, N., and Waalkes, M. P., Minimal basal activity and lack of metal-induced activation of the metallothionein gene correlates with lobe-specific sensitivity to the carcinogenic effects of cadmium in the rat prostate, *Toxicol. Appl. Pharmacol.*, 132, 164, 1995.

48. Ghatak, S., Oliveria, P., Kaplan, P., and Ho, S. M., Expression and regulation of metallothionein mRNA levels in the prostates of Noble rats: lack of expression in the ventral prostate and regulation by sex hormones in the dorsolateral prostate, *Prostate*, 29, 91, 1996.

49. Battersby, S., Chandler, J. A., and Morton, M. S., The effect of orally administered cadmium on the ultrastructure of the rat prostate, *Urol. Res.*, 10, 123, 1982.

50. Boffetta, P., Methodological aspects of the epidemiological association between cadmium and cancer in humans, *IARC Sci. Publ.*, 118, 425, 1992.

51. Webber, M. M., Selenium prevents the growth stimulatory effects of cadmium on human prostatic epithelium, *Biochem. Biophys. Res. Commun.*, 127, 871, 1985.

52. Beyersmann, D. and Hechtenberg, S, Cadmium, gene regulation, and cellular signalling in mammalian cells, *Toxicol. Appl. Pharmacol.*, 144, 247, 1997.

53. Waalkes, M. P., Rehm, S., Riggs, C. W, Bare, R. M., Devor, D. E., Poirier, L. A., Wenk, M. L., and Henneman, J. R., Cadmium carcinogenesis in male Wistar [Crl:(WI)BR] rats: dose-response analysis of effects of zinc on tumor induction in the prostate, in the testes, and at the injection site, *Canc. Res.*, 49, 4282, 1989.

54. Feustel., A., Wennrich, R., Steiniger, D., and Klauss, P., Zinc and cadmium concentration in prostatic carcinoma of different histological grading in comparison to normal prostate tissue and adenofibromyomatosis (BPH), *Urol. Res.*, 10, 301, 1982.

55. Barthel, E., [Cancer risk in pesticide exposed agricultural workers (author's trans.)], *Arch. Geschwulstforsch*, 51, 579, 1981.

Index

A

ACI rat, 142, 147
Acridine orange staining, 240
Adenosis, 330
Adipose tissue, PCB levels in women with
    breast cancer, 188
Adrenal gland neoplasias, 149
Adrenocortical tumors, 143
Aging
    impotence and, 280, 284–285, 287
    prostate disease and, 330
    tissue zinc content and, 331
AhR nuclear translocator, See Arnt protein
Akineton, 292
Albumin, estrogen-induced cell proliferation
    and, 135–136
Alcohol
    fetal vs. postnatal testicular function effects,
        256
    male sexual dysfunction and, 293
    phytoestrogens, 102
Aldactone, 290
Aldehyde-3-dehydrogenase, 192
Aldomet, 290
Alfalfa, 92
Alfalfa sprouts, 94
Alkylating agents, ovotoxicity, 70–71
6-Alkyl-1,3,8-triCDF, 203–205
Alligators, feminization of males, 4, 227, 281
Allyl alcohol (AA), 74
Alpha$_2$-agonists, 290
American dwarf palm, 264–265
Amicar, 292
Amino acids, soy cardioprotective effects, 112
Aminoglutethimide, 233
Amphetamines, 293
Amphibians, 6–7, 227
Anabolic steroids, 232
Androgen insensitivity syndrome, 257
Androgen receptor, 235, 259
    antagonists, 5, See Androgen receptor
        antagonists
    DNA binding, 259–261

prostate development, 311
sex differentiation and postnatal
    development, 249–250
testosterone binding, 259
testosterone short-loop negative feedback
    effect, 254
vinclozolin antiandrogenic activity, 235, 266
Androgen receptor antagonists, 5, 248,
    259–265, 297–298, See also
        Antiandrogens; Kepone
    DDT metabolites, 263–264
    exogenous androgens, 261–262
    permixon (palm tree product), 264–265
    progestins, 262–263
    screening and hazard assessment, 266–267
    vinclozine (fungicide), 263
    xenoestrogens, 262
Androgen response element, 259
Androgen supplementation, 287, 296
Androgens, See specific substances
Androstenedione, 249
Animal feed, 101–102
Anogenital distance, 103
    antiandrogenic effects, 263
    aryl hydrocarbon receptor agonists and, 298
    DDT effects, 289
Antabuse, 292
Antiandrogens, 5, See also Male infertility;
    specific substances
    5-α-reductase inhibitors, 248, 257–259
    androgen receptor antagonists, 248,
        259–265, 297–298, See also Kepone
    DDT metabolites, 263–264
    exogenous androgens, 261–262
    permixon (palm tree product), 264–265
    progestins, 262–263
    vinclozine (fungicide), 263
    xenoestrogens, 262
    chemotherapeutic agents, 258, 261
    effects on Leydig cell
        testosterone-producing function
        androgens, 254–255
        cell viability, 256
        estrogens, 255–256